SATIETOPATHY

It's Not Your Fault
That You're Overweight

DEREK MUSE MD, FOMA

This book is dedicated to my wife and best friend Emily, who's countless hours of listening, encouraging, and helping with editing have made this book so much more than it ever would have been.

CONTENTS

CHAPTER 1
WE'VE GOT A BIG PROBLEM

JUST A GLANCE in any direction at shopping malls, airports, and theaters will tell you that we are in big trouble. People of all ages, races, and socioeconomic classes weigh a lot more than just a few decades ago. Recent studies have confirmed what we all have observed, that more than two-thirds of the United States population is now overweight, and more than one-third is obese (Flegal, 2016). This rapid expansion of the obesity problem has occurred despite significant advances in our understanding of nutrition and despite a myriad of diet experts telling us what we should do to be thin. Most people who are overweight have tried to follow the advice of these experts and have lost weight, only to gain it back, and more. The weight-loss recommendations made by these experts have failed our country so profoundly over the last three to four decades that we must resoundingly state that what they have and are advising the overweight to do is just not helpful in preventing the progression of the obesity epidemic in our country. We need to intensify our efforts to discover how to prevent long-term weight gain in the first place, and how to help those who have gained excess weight to lose it and keep it off.

I would like to take a moment to make it clear that the word *obesity* is used in this book as a medical term to describe individuals who have a body mass index (BMI) that is greater than or equal to 30. Although the medical term *overweight* officially refers to individuals who have a BMI that is greater than or equal to 27 and is less than 30, I will use the term *overweight* to describe individuals who are obese as well. I am doing this because society has assigned a negative connotation to the medical terms *obese* and *obesity*. I would like for my book to be as inoffensive as possible. On the other hand, I will at times need to use the words *obese* and *obesity* when they are needed to describe disease's states or when they are needed to report the results of medical studies. I apologize in advance for any discomfort that this might cause for any reader.

Increasing obesity in the US is a major health concern. While it is true that otherwise healthy obese people can sometimes live to an old age, it is also true that few obese people remain completely healthy throughout their lives. Obesity both causes and makes worse a host of medical problems, leading to a loss of quality of life and an increase in medical expenses, suffering, and premature death.

One of the most common health problems associated with obesity is type 2 diabetes. The incidence of type 2 diabetes has almost doubled in the US in the last two decades (Selvin, 2014) and is expected to double again in the next one to two decades. The cost to the country for the treatment of these new diabetics is high enough now but will be staggeringly higher in 10 to 20 years when these diabetics will begin to have premature kidney failure, loss of vision, and lower-extremity amputations, as well as disability and death from strokes and heart attacks. The cost associated with treating obesity-related type 2 diabetes, and its consequences, exceeds the expense of treating smoking-related disease (Moriarty, 2012). Type 2 diabetics have a similar risk for stroke and heart attack as do smokers but must be treated with expensive medications to keep their diabetes in control for many years in an effort to prevent these events. Smokers don't cost the health care system much until their first heart attack or stroke or until they develop cancer or emphysema.

In addition to type 2 diabetes, other serious medical problems that are caused by obesity, or are worsened by obesity, are stroke, heart attack, heart failure, high blood pressure, deep-vein blood clots, pulmonary embolism, asthma, emphysema, pulmonary hypertension, sleep apnea, high bad cholesterol, low good cholesterol, breast cancer, uterine cancer, prostate cancer, colon cancer, and depression. Less serious obesity-related medical problems are arthritis of the hips and knees, urinary stress incontinence, fatigue, varicose veins, and chronic low back pain. Minor medical problems associated with obesity include neuromas of the feet, rashes in skin folds, leg swelling, breast growth in men, unwanted hair growth women, male-pattern hair loss in females, male impotence, decreased fertility in both men and women, and female menstrual irregularities.

In addition, obese patients experience a number of adverse consequences related to quality of life. Obese patients are less likely to marry (Gortmaker, 1993), to get a college education (Cohen, 2013), and to be hired for a job (Flint, 2016). They are discriminated against socially at many levels, including being assumed to have poor self-control and to be lazy (Puhl, 2010). They are often excluded from social circles and social events, beginning even in grade school. The obese struggle to exercise, to play sports with friends, and to participate in physical activities with their children.

Alleviating the physical and social suffering of individuals with obesity and controlling the staggering costs caused by obesity are a national priority. Everyone is affected by obesity, either directly or indirectly, because at least a few of every thin individual's family members, friends, co-workers, and neighbors suffer from the negative effects of obesity.

The primary question that all of us would like to have answered is why are so many people obese? Some insist that obesity is completely self-inflicted, while others blame the modern food environment. Others attempt to pin the cause on food additives, hormones fed to animals, and chemicals released from plastics. No clear answer has emerged to explain the explosion in the number of obese people in the world.

There is no shortage of proposed solutions for the obesity epidemic. A host of well-meaning individuals, societies, medical professionals, supplement manufacturers, and exercise facilities have come up with numerous solutions to help the obese lose weight. However, because they all lack an adequate understanding of why overweight people struggle so much with their weight, their advice is ineffective, confusing, and sometimes even dangerous. Some have even resorted to telling downright lies about what works for weight loss to cash in on the money that obese individuals are willing to spend to try to lose weight. For example, the most common advice given to the overweight individual is to, "Just push away from the table." The people who say this are rarely themselves weight challenged. They figure that since they are thin and that they seem to always know when to quit eating, that the solution to obesity is for obese people to just listen to their bodies telling them when they're full. However, anyone who struggles with their weight knows this advice doesn't help.

Through years of observation and interviews with my patients, and after conducting a confirmatory study at my office clinic, I believe I have been able to identify a significant contributor to the worldwide burgeoning problem of obesity. Certainly, the concepts I will present in this book are a work in progress. I know that my single small study and my theories will need further study and confirmation, followed by additional refining, as new data becomes available. However, I feel an urgent need to present my research and my theories now, in hopes that it might help to stem the worldwide tsunami of obesity and to help mitigate the suffering of my fellow men and women.

In attempting to explain why the obese individuals of this world have so much trouble losing weight and keeping it off, it is necessary to understand the normal human hunger and satiety response. The human body is just a machine that our intelligence lives in. It is truly an amazing machine, but it is a machine just the same. As a machine, it can work perfectly, or it can suffer from any number of genetically predisposed or acquired diseases. In its ideal state, the human machine is designed with biochemical circuitry in the brain that subconsciously ensures that the body neither overconsumes, nor under consumes, calories. However, this circuitry is not working properly to some degree for about 85% of the world's population, leading them to gain weight over time when food is plentiful, inexpensive, and engineered to be irresistible. Some gain weight faster than others.

On the other hand, 15% of the world's population consumes just the right number of calories each day, day in and day out, leading them to maintain their weight at a healthy level for their whole lives. We all know people like this. They are the ones that are staying slim despite being surrounded by an overabundance of very palatable food, despite having sedentary desk jobs, and even despite not exercising.

This leads me to an important point. The root of the problem with obesity is not the inability to lose weight, but the inability to maintain weight. Most overweight individuals have lost weight at least once before, only to gain it back almost every time. Less than 10% of obese individuals who have lost weight have successfully kept the weight off for more than a few years. The inability to maintain weight comes from one or more defects in the biochemical circuitry in the brain that is supposed to mostly subconsciously tell us to stop eating when we have eaten enough to meet our calorie needs. The presence of these defects in the biochemical circuitry of the brain makes the inability to maintain weight a disease, not a lack of character or a lack of self-control. In doctor terminology, lacking these biochemical signals is a pathological condition of an inability to appropriately feel satiety. I have therefore chosen to name this disease Muse's Satietopathy and will refer to this disease by this name for the remainder of this book.

CHAPTER 2
MUSE'S SATIETOPATHY

CONSIDER A GROUP of 10 to 15 mostly sedentary individuals who are seated at a large table at a restaurant for dinner. The diners are of all different levels of being overweight. The members of the dining party are hungry from not having eaten anything for the past four to five hours. When the food is served, they all start eating with gusto. After consuming a third, or maybe half, of the meal that they have ordered, roughly two-thirds of the group will put down their forks. Those who put down their forks don't exclaim that they are feeling stuffed, bloated, or sick; they just stop eating, even if they are in the middle of an engrossing conversation. The remaining diners continue eating without stopping until the food on their plates is gone. They then look around hungrily for more to eat.

After 10 to 15 minutes, about three-fourths of the group that put their forks down before consuming all the food on their plates will pick their forks up and start eating again. Some will take just a few additional bites and then put their forks down yet again. The rest will keep eating, possibly until the plates are empty.

After all the diners have stopped eating, the server then approaches and asks who wants dessert. Those who put their forks down and didn't pick them up again will say they are too full for dessert. The rest will most often order dessert. Once the desserts arrive, are sampled, and are found to be delicious, those who ordered dessert will try to talk the others that didn't order dessert into trying a bite of their dessert. If they are successful, those who didn't order dessert will take a bite or two of the dessert, and then they might say, "If I eat any more, I'm going to be sick." After the meal is over, the diners that didn't finish their plates of food and that ate only a few bites of dessert will stand up to leave, may hold their upper stomachs and say, "I can't believe I ate that much. Now, I'm sick." We have all seen this scenario play out in real life, time and time again. We all have observed that diners who don't eat all their meals and that have no more than a few bites of dessert are invariably thinner than other diners.

How do the thinner diners in the scenario above, as well as all thin sedentary individuals, know when to stop eating? They experience three distinctly different orchestrated signals that tell them to stop at exactly the moment when they have consumed an adequate number of calories to meet their body's needs. The three signals are powerful and when all three are present, they are nearly impossible to ignore. These signals are inherited genetically, although they are not always fully expressed in every person who inherits them. The signals mostly cannot be lost if you have them and cannot be gained if you don't have them.

To set the stage for the satiety signals, I'd like you to consider a fictitious sedentary person who eats 2,000 calories per day, burns 2,000 calories per day, and has a stomach that holds up to 2,000 calories of an average variety of food. Of course, the same stomach could hold more or less calories, depending on the calorie density of the foods eaten. If this fictitious person were to eat 2,000 calories of food until the stomach was full, the stretch receptors in the stomach wall would fire off, telling the brain to inform the person's conscious mind that they are now feeling pain, cramping, and bloating. These sensations would then convince the person to stop eating before the food filled up their esophagus and started flowing into their lungs. If this fictitious person did eat 2,000 calories of food in one sitting, then they would have to not eat for the next 24 hours in order to not gain weight, since they are only burning 2,000 calories per day. However, since many humans eat three meals a day, this fictitious person should only consume about 650 calories per meal so that their three meals per day will equal their calorie need of 2,000 calories per day. What does the stomach of this fictitious person look like when it has 650 calories of average food in it? It looks like a hot air balloon without enough air in it. The stretch receptors of the stomach are not firing off, telling the brain that the person is full. Instead, there are nerve and hormonal signals coming from the stomach, intestine, pancreas, and fat cells that travel to the brain and tell the brain to feel a sensation of fullness.

With that example in mind, the three signals that cause a person to stop eating at a meal, or satiety signals, are:

1. Fullness – This is not a painful fullness, a bloated feeling, or cramping, but just a knowledge that a person needs to stop eating. It lasts 10 to 15 minutes. It occurs at a different point in each meal for each individual, depending on the caloric content of the food in the meal, the calories consumed in the last 24 hours, and the calories burned in the last 24 hours. Except in high performance athletes and construction workers, who must eat large amounts of food to meet their calorie needs, this signal comes from the brain and not from the stomach. About 60% of the individuals in the study I conducted at my office had this signal. The study population for my study was mostly white and North American. I don't have information on the percentage of people who have this signal among other races in North America, or among the populations of the other countries around the world. In my experience, the presence of this signal is black and white; either you have it or you don't. Those who don't have this signal have no understanding of what this signal feels like and they often mistake the pain, bloating, and fullness that they get from overeating as their "full" signal. One patient who didn't have this signal asked me if maybe this signal felt like having to sigh near the end of a meal. However, the need to sigh for this person meant that they had eaten too much and that their full stomach was compressing their lungs.

   Knowing the effects and duration of the hormone cholecystokinin that is produced by the small intestinal wall, I'll make an educated guess that rising cholecystokinin levels stimulated by food entering the small intestine are the primary inducer of this signal in the brain (Hajishafiee, 2019) (Lieverse, 1995). As I will discuss later, there are at least eight known hormones produced by the intestine, pancreas, and fat cells that rise with eating to cause satiety (Austin, 2009).

Is the full signal enough by itself? No. It fades after 10 to 15 minutes and the individual can pick up their fork and start eating again. There must be a second signal.

2. Loss of Savor – This is a loss of the pleasure and enjoyment of eating. Once triggered, it lasts for about four hours. It is what keeps an individual at a meal from picking up their fork and starting to eat again. It is also what keeps an individual from eating more of the previous meal, or snacking on other food, two to three hours after a substantial meal. Only 15% of the individuals in the study I performed at my office had this signal.

    My hypothesis is that the loss-of-savor signal comes primarily from leptin being released by the fat cells of the body in response to eating (McDuffie, 2004). This theory needs to be studied further for confirmation. In addition, there could be other satiety hormones that could be adding to this signal.

    Are the fullness signal and the loss-of-savor signal enough to stop a person from overeating? A person could still be convinced to try an extra bite of food, which would then cause weight gain over time. There must be a third signal.

3. Nausea – It is a warning to stop overeating. It is not painful, cramping, or bloating. It feels like you've been punched in the gut or like you have the stomach flu. For individuals who experience this signal, it triggers with eating just one or two bites of food beyond when the full signal and/or loss-of-savor signal first triggered the individual to stop eating. When triggered, the nausea can last two to twenty-four hours, depending on the degree of overconsumption. About 50% of

the individuals in the study I performed at my office had this signal. This signal is also variable from person to person. Some people only have this signal a few times a year, such as at Thanksgiving and Christmas. A person is considered not to have this signal unless this signal occurs every time they overeat.

I have theorized that this signal is primarily coming from the effects of the satiety hormones PYY (Degen, 2005) and GLP-1 (Shah, 2014) that are produced by the small intestinal wall. Further research is needed to prove this theory.

The goal of the study that I performed at my office was to prove that, depending on which of these three satiety signals a person had or didn't have, they could be classified into one of five distinctly different satiety types that I called the Muse Satiety Types. The study then predicted their long-term risk for weight gain based on their Muse Satiety Type, as is indicated in Figure 1. In the figure, the √ mark indicates the presence of the satiety signal and an X mark indicates the absence of the satiety signal.

Muse Satiety Types					
	1	**2**	**3**	**4**	**5**
Fullness	√ or X	√	√	X	X
Loss of Savor	√	X	X	X	X
Nausea	√ or X	√	X	√ (late)	X
20-Year Weight Gain Risk (lbs.)	0-25	15-50	30-125	50-150	75-600
Lifetime Cumulative Weight Loss (lbs.)[1]	0	10-30	30-100	50-800	200-2000
Population Frequency	15%	25%	20%	25%	15%

Figure 1 - Muse Satiety Types

[1] *The term lifetime cumulative weight loss is defined in my practice as the sum of all the weight a person has lost during all the times in their life that they have lost weight. It doesn't count any of the weight that was regained. Any type of weight loss counts, although the weight lost in the first year after a pregnancy doesn't count.*

Before discussing the information in Figure 1, it is important to stress that the examples of members of the different Muse Satiety Types that I am going to be describing in the rest of this chapter are based on those individual's eating patterns while sedentary. This is because an individual who burns 4,000 or more calories per day due to their job, heavy involvement in sports, or hyperactivity, has to eat all day long to keep up with their calorie needs, no matter what Muse Satiety Type they are. Determining which Muse Satiety Type that very active individuals belong to is more difficult, but it can be done by assessing how they eat after three days of inactivity.

Muse Satiety Type 1

To best understand the struggles of members of Muse Satiety Types 2 to 5, it is necessary to understand those who are members of Muse Satiety Type 1. Members of Muse Satiety Type 1 all experience the loss-of-savor signal, causing them to consistently lose the pleasure and enjoyment of eating at the appropriate time during each meal.

For the time being, let's ignore the X's in the column in Figure 1 for Muse Satiety Type 1s and assume that they also all feel the satiety signals of fullness and nausea.

Referring back to the example of the diners at the restaurant, if a Muse Satiety Type 1 hasn't eaten for four or more hours and they are then served one of their favorite meals at a restaurant, they will start eating with gusto, just like the members of the other Muse Satiety Types. If you had asked them how much of their plate of food they were going to eat before they started, they would have likely said, "Most of it," since before starting to eat, they were feeling just as hungry as everyone else. As they approach the number of calories needed to equal just what they have burned in calories for the previous day, they begin to feel full and lose savor for the food they are eating. The feelings of fullness and loss of savor increase rapidly with just a few more bites of food. They then put down their forks and stop eating. The fullness and loss of savor signals that they feel are undeniable. When they feel them, they don't complain of pain or fullness, then just stop, even in the middle of a fascinating conversation.

The feelings of fullness and loss of savor occur at different levels of calorie intake at every meal, depending on the calories burned and the calories consumed in the previous 24 hours. Members of Muse Satiety Type 1 often remark that their stomach has shrunk down to a certain small size and that that is how they know when to stop eating. However, it has been shown that individuals who exercise on some days but not on others report that they eat the same amount of food every day since, to them, they eat until they feel full, filling up their small stomachs. In reality, with researchers watching their calorie intake, these individuals are eating more the day after they exercise and less the day after they don't exercise (Pomerleau, 2004). The full feeling that these individuals experience is not coming from the wall of their stomach being stretched, but is coming from their brain, or more specifically, the hypothalamus in their brain. Biochemical circuitry in the hypothalamus is keeping track perfectly of the calories consumed and burned by these individuals and tells them they are full exactly at the proper bite. Otherwise, they wouldn't be able to maintain a consistent weight long term. If their satiety system were to let them eat even one extra bite of food per meal, that would result in a weight gain of up to six to 10 pounds per year. It is amazing how accurate the human satiety system is when it is working correctly.

If needed, the human stomach is designed to be able to hold a large amount of food from a meal, such as when a person is burning a large number of calories per day from exercising. Depending on the person's height, the human stomach can hold up to two liters of food and possibly even up to four liters of food (Geliebter, 1992) (Cheng J. , 2000). Two liters of ice cream can be about 2,000 calories, while two liters of macadamia nuts would be about 4,000 calories. Wow! To illustrate this further, the Olympic swimmer Michael Phelps reported he consumed more than 8,000 calories per day when he was training for the Olympics (Zelman, 2008). Therefore, in the hours in between training, he was probably consuming three 2,000-plus calorie meals, as well as about 2,000 calories of snacking throughout the day, just to keep up with the calories he was burning. It is important to note that the stomach sizes of thin and obese individuals of the same height are about the same (Roque, 2006).

Since the loss of savor signal lasts for four hours, it protects Muse Satiety Type 1s from snacking over the next four to five hours until the next meal. When presented with a favorite snack two hours after a substantial meal, a Muse Satiety Type 1 will accept the snack and maybe take one bite, but then not finish the rest, even though the remainder of the snack might sit right in front of them on their kitchen counter, or on their work desk, for the next two to three hours.

More than once in the past, while my wife and I have been playing cards with friends after dinner, I have tried to eat a piece of candy only when my wife ate a piece of her candy. She's a member of Muse Satiety Type 1 and I am not. She would eat her first piece of candy and then so would I. Then, over an hour would go by before she ate another piece, if she ever even ate another one. My next piece of candy would sit there right in front of me, screaming to be eaten. When I would ask her to please eat her next piece of candy so that I could eat another of mine, she would say that she didn't feel like it, and then would keep playing. It was like the candy wasn't even there.

Muse Satiety Type 1s feel nausea if they try to eat past the loss of savor signal. Consider again the example of the Muse Satiety Type 1s at the restaurant. The server returned to the table when all the diners at the table had stopped eating and asked if anyone wanted dessert. While most at the table that weren't Muse Satiety Type 1s ordered dessert, the Muse Satiety Type 1s declined dessert, stating that they were too full for dessert. Fifteen minutes later, the server returned with visually appealing desserts and with extra utensils for everyone to share a bite or two. Even though the Muse Satiety Type 1s had lost their savor, their tongues still wanted a taste of the scrumptious desserts. After a bite or two of the delicious desserts, the Muse Satiety Type 1s started to feel nausea with overeating and said aloud, "If I eat another bite, I'm going to get sick." If they then ate the extra bite, they would have begun to feel nausea as a warning from their hypothalamus that they were overeating. Virtually always, the Muse Satiety Type 1s that feel nausea with overeating will then immediately stop eating, because nausea is a highly effective motivator for all humans to stop eating.

However, some powerful motivators will cause Muse Satiety Type 1s that experience nausea with overeating to eat a bite or two past when they start to feel nausea. Examples are pressure from others to not waste food from an expensive meal, or pressure from a family member or friend to try the food they made, or they will be offended. In those rare cases, each bite taken past the point of feeling nausea will cause the nausea to become more intense and to last longer, even up to 24 hours. Given enough nausea, the Muse Satiety Type 1 finally will have to quit eating.

I am not a Muse Satiety Type 1 and I have never experienced nausea from overeating a single time, no matter how much I have eaten and no matter how rich the food has been. In restaurant situations like the example above, I have been mystified in the past by Muse Satiety Type 1's declaration of nausea after just a few bites of desert, especially since by the time that they are talking about nausea, I have usually already finished my dessert and have started on someone else's dessert, if they will give it to me. Naively, I used to think that the Muse Satiety Type 1s must have a disease. But now I know that I am the one who has a disease, since I never feel the nausea signal when I overeat.

Muse Satiety Type 1s can avoid the feeling of nausea with overeating if they don't eat past their loss of savor signal. The memory of triggering the nausea by overeating in the past burns bright in a Muse Satiety Type 1's mind, long after the meal at which the nausea was triggered, making them hesitant to even try to overeat for days and weeks afterward. My wife, who is a Muse Satiety Type 1, will consider not returning to certain restaurants where she has eaten enough to trigger her nausea signal in the past, even though she liked the food at the restaurant enough to overeat it.

Many of my Muse Satiety Type 1 patients have reported to me that their nausea signal will even trigger after the first few bites of breakfast. Because of the nausea, some of my Muse Satiety Type 1s have had to permanently stop eating breakfast. They feel perfectly fine when they eat only lunch and dinner each day. However, they come to me worried that it is unhealthy for them to be skipping breakfast. The advice that I give these thin Muse Satiety Type 1 patients, after first making sure that they are otherwise healthy, is that it's okay for them to wait until lunch for their first meal of the day. They really don't have much choice in the matter, since no one can eat when nauseated.

Due to their having the satiety signal of loss of savor, along with the signals of fullness and nausea with overeating, Muse Satiety Type 1s have little risk for weight gain long term. The average 20-year weight gain for Muse Satiety Type 1s is zero to 25 pounds. Since that is very little weight to gain, most have never needed to diet. I'm not saying that the 10 or 20 pounds that Muse Satiety Type 1s gain over 20 years is okay with them. For a woman, even a five-pound weight gain makes it hard to wear certain outfits and a ten-pound weight gain moves a woman up a dress size, or even two. In addition, a 10 to 15-pound weight gain every 20 years can result in 30 to 45 pounds of total weight gain during a person's lifetime, which can aggravate a host of medical conditions later in life, as has been discussed previously. If a Muse Satiety Type 1 does gain 10 pounds over a 20-year period, then it is just as hard for them to lose that 10 pounds as it is for any another person of the same size and sex, no matter their Muse Satiety Type. It's just that it will be much easier for Muse Satiety Type 1s to keep the weight off once they have lost it.

According to my office study, about 15% of the population is a Muse Satiety Type 1. The average lifetime cumulative weight loss for Muse Satiety Type 1s in my experience has been zero pounds.

Muse Satiety Type 2

Members of Muse Satiety Type 2, which in my research accounted for about 25% of the individuals in the study, are missing the signal for loss of savor. Muse Satiety Types 2s still feel the fullness signal and still experience nausea with overeating.

If a Muse Satiety Type 2 were to eat a meal side by side at a restaurant with a Muse Satiety Type 1 of the same age, sex, body size, and level of activity, they would both feel full at the same point and would stop eating. As previously explained, the feeling of fullness is the point where their brains have determined that they have consumed exactly the number of calories needed to equal the number of calories burned in the previous day or days. For these two individuals, any additional calories consumed beyond the point of fullness will always be excess energy consumed and will always have to be stored as fat.

After 10 to 15 minutes, the feeling fullness will fade for the Muse Satiety Type 2. Since the Muse Satiety Type 2 hasn't lost their savor, the food will look just as appealing as it did when they started eating. The Muse Satiety Type 2 will pick up their fork and start eating again. Gratefully, they are only able to overeat a few bites before they trigger the nausea signal. They then must stop eating and put their fork down. They won't be able to finish their food. Different from the Muse Satiety Type 2, the Muse Satiety Type 1 will have lost their savor for their food and will not have picked up their fork again.

The members of Muse Satiety Type 1 and Muse Satiety Type 2 will take their restaurant food home at that point, thinking that they will eat it later when they are hungry again. However, the Muse Satiety Type 1 has lost their savor for the next four hours and won't even think of the leftovers sitting in the fridge during that four hours. If the Muse Satiety Type 1's leftovers get eaten, it is not by the Muse Satiety Type 1, but by the other Muse Satiety Types in the house. On the other hand, since the Muse Satiety Type 2's savor is not gone, they will pull out the leftovers after a few hours and they will eat a few more bites on and off until the next meal, being careful not to trigger the nausea signal.

Muse Satiety Type 2s are pure snackers. Because of their excess snacking, they can gain 15 to 50 pounds over a 20-year period. I am providing a range because some individuals who start to gain weight will try to keep from gaining weight by snacking less than others, exercising more than others, and dieting more often than others. Each of these efforts protects somewhat against weight gain over time. Since most of the Muse Satiety Type 2s will have tried dieting at least a few times in their life, they report an average lifetime cumulative weight loss of about 10-30 pounds when asked.

I don't see very many Muse Satiety Type 2s in my weight-loss clinic, since people who are 10 to 30 pounds overweight don't usually go to a medical provider for help, choosing instead to work on their weight by themselves. However, some Muse Satiety Type 2s can gain more than just 15-50 pounds, if they:

- Grew up in a home where there was unrestricted snacking.
- Had multiple pregnancies close together.
- Took certain medications that enhance snacking.

The Muse Satiety Type 2s that I have seen who have gained 50 or more pounds have been particularly frustrated. They have usually done their best to stop snacking by the time that they see me and therefore have remained about the same weight for years. They tell me that they eat just like the Muse Satiety Type 1s that they know, but that the Muse Satiety Type 1s that they know are skinny and they aren't. The solution for these Muse Satiety Type 2s is simple. They need to get the weight off and then, as long as they don't resume snacking, it will be easier for them to keep the weight off that they have lost, at least as compared to the members of Muse Satiety Types 3 to 5. In my observation, only a few of the Muse Satiety Type 2s that I have seen in my office have had to return in a few years because they have regained all the weight that they lost.

Muse Satiety Type 3

Like members of Muse Satiety Types 1 and 2, sedentary members of Muse Satiety Type 3 will stop eating at a restaurant when they reach their full signal. However, as soon as the full signal passes, the Muse Satiety Type 3s pick up their forks and start eating again because they haven't lost their savor. Since they don't experience nausea, they can even finish their plate of food. They will have to store every bite eaten past their full signal as fat. The body has already told them, albeit ineffectively, that they have satisfied their energy needs for that meal. But, due to the lack of signals of loss of savor and nausea as a warning not to overeat, Muse Satiety Type 3s overconsume at almost every meal if they stay near the meal for longer than 10 minutes. If Muse Satiety Type 3s don't finish their food at the meal, they will save it but will then pull it out in a couple of hours to eat some more.

Due to chronic overconsumption of calories at each meal and excess snacking, Muse Satiety Type 3s can gain 50 to 125 pounds over a 20-year period. Again, there is a range of weight that can be gained, and it is due to some trying harder to avoid weight gain than others. Some Muse Satiety Type 3s will notice that they are getting heavier and will reduce their calorie intake, leading to less weight gain over time. Some will exercise more than others, which will help them to maintain weight. Some will diet more often and therefore will gain a smaller amount of weight over time. Gaining 50 to 125 pounds of excess weight causes significant health problems for Muse Satiety Type 3s. Muse Satiety Type 3s accounted for about 20% of the population of the study that I performed at my office.

Muse Satiety Type 3s, as well as Muse Satiety Type 2s, are most often thin until they reach their mid-twenties. When Muse Satiety Type 2s and Muse Satiety Type 3s were children and were eating a meal with their family, as soon as they felt the full signal they likely asked to be excused from the table and went elsewhere to play. Ten to 15 minutes later, when the full signal had passed and they were hungry again, they were often too busy to stop playing to go back to the kitchen to look for more to eat. If they had returned to the kitchen for more food, they most often would have found that the previous meal was put away. Many households have pretty strict rules about younger children not getting food out and serving themselves in between meals. The Muse Satiety Type 2s and Muse Satiety Type 3s that had come to the kitchen looking for a snack would have most often left the kitchen hungry. In the few households where there was highly palatable food consistently on the kitchen counter in between meals, the children who were Muse Satiety Type 2s and 3s would have snacked on and off in between meals and would have gained a significant amount of weight during their childhood.

In their teens, Muse Satiety Type 2s and 3s are most often so busy with sports and playing with friends that they aren't around food enough to snack excessively, and so they mostly remain thin. In their late teens and early twenties, many Muse Satiety Type 2s and 3s sit in class, study in the library, and work at jobs where it is socially unacceptable or even forbidden to eat. Additionally, they often don't have a lot of extra money with which to purchase snack food. They usually remain very active when they aren't in class or studying. The ones that do work usually have jobs that require them to be on their feet and moving the whole time they are at work. Because of these and other factors, their weight remains relatively constant. It isn't until the Muse Satiety Types 2 or 3 get their own places with pantries full of their own food that they can eat 24 hours a day, start work at a business that has a kitchen that is always stocked with food, or can finally afford a stash of food at their desk, that they start to gain weight. Some Muse Satiety Type 3s have asked me if a person can be a Muse Satiety Type 1 when they are young and then become a Muse Satiety Type 3 later in life. After careful discussion of their eating habits as children, I have helped them to understand that they have always been a Muse Satiety Type 3.

Muse Satiety Type 4

Of the individuals studied in my office, 25% were Muse Satiety Type 4s. Muse Satiety Type 4s are missing their fullness signal, meaning that they can eat past their calorie needs for the day and feel no sensation whatsoever that they have done so.

As previously mentioned, the human stomach is a variable-sized storage container, able to expand to take in whatever calories are needed to replace what has been burned in the previous day, at least up to its maximum capacity. Within a few bites before reaching the stomach's maximum capacity, the stretch receptors in the stomach wall fire off, telling the brain that the individual must stop eating, or else the food is going to go up their esophagus and into their lungs. Members of Muse Satiety Types 1 through 3 that are sedentary feel full long before their stomachs reach their maximum capacity, due to rising satiety hormones from the small intestine, pancreas, and fat cells. However, Muse Satiety Type 4s can eat past the point where they should have felt a fullness signal. Since they also don't lose their savor, they just keep on eating at meals, through their first plate of food and possibly on to their second. They are saved by the third satiety of signal of nausea, although it appears later than it should and is milder than for Muse Satiety Type 1s and 2s. Muse Satiety Type 4s tell me their nausea feels more like the nausea from a stomach flu and not like the feeling of a gut punch that members of Muse Satiety Types 1 and 2 have told me about. The nausea can come on gradually, or it can come on suddenly. Muse Satiety Type 4s might take their leftover food home from a restaurant, but since they triggered the nausea by overeating, they won't have any desire to pull the leftovers out for a snack a few hours later.

Due to their significant overeating, Muse Satiety Type 4s can gain 75 to 150 pounds over a 20-year period. Again, the degree of weight gain over time varies with how hard they have tried to avoid overeating, how much they exercise, and how often they have serially dieted. Most of the Muse Satiety Type 4s will have tried multiple diets and will have a lifetime cumulative weight loss of 50 to 800 pounds. In my practice, I have only met a few Muse Satiety Type 4s that have repeatedly gained and lost more than 300 pounds cumulatively.

Muse Satiety Type 5

Members of Muse Satiety Type 5 don't have any of the three satiety signals. They don't feel full, so they eat past their calorie needs at each meal without any clue that they are doing so. They don't lose their savor, so that the last bite of a meal is just as exciting and pleasureful as the first. They never experience nausea, no matter how much food they eat and no matter how rich in sugars and fat the food is. They only thing that stops them from eating is that they finally reach the maximum capacity of their stomachs, at which point they finally know that they have to stop due to worsening pain, cramping, and bloating. But they still don't lose their savor. They leave the table feeling stuffed, even feeling the food sloshing up into their esophagi, but at the same time feeling confused by the fact that they still feel hungry. Eating is pure pleasure for Muse Satiety Type 5s, with very little negative consequences, except that after a while they get so big that they can't see their waist to button up their jeans or their feet to tie their shoelaces. Muse Satiety Type 5s comprised approximately 15% of the population in the study done at my office.

Muse Satiety Type 5s are the only true binge eaters. If you can get them to reveal themselves, most of them can tell you of times in the past where they ate whole cakes, whole boxes of cereal, whole plates of cookies, whole jars of nuts, whole loaves of bread, whole family size bags of candy, etc., all within a matter of hours. Even the Muse Satiety Type 5s that don't binge on tasty carbs between meals will still binge by taking seconds and thirds at meals. Members of the other Muse Satiety Types have at least one signal that prevents them from binge eating. Members of the other Satiety Types can't even imagine eating as much as Muse Satiety Type 5s can eat, because it would make them lose interested in eating, feel full, or feel sick.

Because of their lack of signals, Muse Satiety Type 5s can gain a tremendous amount of weight over a 20-year period. It is not uncommon for a Muse Satiety Type 5 to gain 20 to 50 pounds in a year. Some lose most of the weight they gain each year, but others don't try to diet at all. Those who don't try can gain up to 600 pounds of excess body fat over time, leaving them unable to work, suffering from numerous medical problems, and even suffering death. For the Muse Satiety Type 5s that fight the weight gain each year by repeated dieting, the lifetime cumulative weight loss can be staggering. I have listed in Figure 1 the lifetime cumulative weight loss of 300 pounds or more for Muse Satiety Type 5s, but I have routinely heard numbers up to 2,000 pounds from some of my Muse Satiety Type 5 patients. Any individual who states that their lifetime cumulative weight loss is greater than 300 pounds is most certainly a Muse Satiety Type 5. It does take a little coaxing at times to get a Muse Satiety Type 5 to admit, even to themselves, how much weight they have gained, lost, and then gained again in their lifetimes. The most anyone has ever told me was a patient who started dieting at age 10 and had lost and regained 40 pounds a year for 50 years, or 2,000 pounds.

This is as good a time as any for me to let the cat out of the bag. I am a Muse Satiety Type 5. My lifetime cumulative weight loss is approaching 1,500 pounds. I am a binge eater in a tenuous state of recovery. Being a Muse Satiety Type 5 is what has driven me to try to understand my illness and subsequently everyone else's. I knew from the beginning that I felt something different than others when it came to feeling full at the end of a meal, but I had no clue what it was. I remember well a time when I was 17-years old and had just finished eating all of my dinner, all of the food on my five brothers' and sisters' plates, all of the extra food in the pans on the stove, and 12 slices of homemade whole-wheat bread spread with peanut butter and honey with multiple glasses of milk. I felt painfully bloated but was still hungry. I walked away from the kitchen with food sloshing high in my chest wondering why I could eat so much and still be hungry. My parents and brothers and sisters were long gone from the kitchen, since none of them were Muse Satiety Type 5s.

Over the years, the explanations that I have heard about low metabolism, food addiction, and being trained to eat all my food as a child just haven't made sense. When I married my sweetheart, Emily, who is a Muse Satiety Type 1, I quickly came to realize that there was a world of difference in the way we felt full at mealtimes, and I could hardly believe that she just wouldn't snack between meals. I started the journey of trying to figure this whole satiety disease thing in about 2007. At that time, I had the limited knowledge of people like my wife at one extreme, people like me at the other extreme, and other people somewhere in between. Since I have never felt any of the satiety signals, it took talking to hundreds of people and then having them tell me how they experienced satiety for me to realize that there were at least two distinct satiety groups between my wife and me. It wasn't until I completed the research study in my office in 2011 that I discovered another type, Muse Satiety Type 4, that developed nausea late when they overate.

Now that I have finally ferreted out the fact that there are five distinct Muse Satiety Types, no one stops me in my presentations and tells me that what I am saying doesn't apply to them. Teaching my patients what Muse

Satiety Type they are and what strategies will work for their Muse Satiety Type for long-term weight maintenance has been a powerful tool in my practice. My patients are staying thinner, or at least thinner longer, after completing their diets. It's exciting. It's wonderful. Knowledge is power and it's motivating. Knowing your Muse Satiety Type doesn't make weight loss any easier, since it's just plain hard work for everyone. Knowing your Muse Satiety Type makes weight maintenance easier and more likely to be successful, but it is still hard, even harder than weight loss. Central to weight maintenance is the knowledge and acceptance of Muse's Satietopathy as a disease that can be controlled and not as a lack of character or a lack of self-control. Accepting this knowledge gives my patients the power to succeed. That is why I am writing this book, to share this important and life-changing knowledge with everyone.

Muse's Satietopathy

As discussed above, the lack of one or more of the Muse Satiety Signals often results in an inability to maintain weight. The inability to maintain weight is a disease which I have chosen to call Muse's Satietopathy. I am defining Muse's Satietopathy as a disease of satiety caused by the genetic absence of one or more satiety signals, leading to a propensity to gain weight over time. Using the predicted weight gain from the five Muse Satiety Types in my study and my clinical experience, I have graphed my estimation of the projected average weight gain from age 20 to age 60 for each Muse Satiety Type in Figure 2.

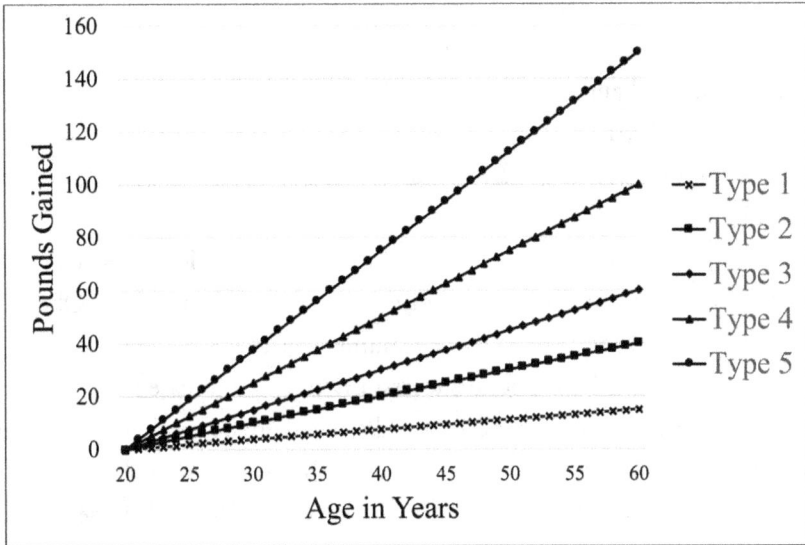

Figure 2 - Estimated Weight Gain Over Time for Each Muse Satiety Type

In Figure 2, it can be seen that Muse Satiety Type 1s gain an average of less than 20 pounds in 40 years, while the other Muse Satiety Types gain much more than that. The Muse Satiety Type 1s can't gain more than the other types, since they aren't able to overeat even if they try because they feel full, lose their savor, and experience nausea. Try as they might, the members of the other Muse Satiety Types keep gaining.

Muse's Satietopathy is the first of three diseases behind obesity. The other two diseases behind obesity will be discussed later in this book. Obesity, or having excess body fat on one's body, is not a disease itself but a symptom of poorly controlled Muse's Satietopathy. There are other common diseases that can be used to further illustrate this point. High blood sugar in a diabetic is not a disease itself but is a symptom of poorly controlled diabetes. Elevated blood pressure is not a disease itself but is a symptom of poorly controlled hypertension. High cholesterol is not a disease itself, but a symptom of poorly controlled hyperlipidemia. In each of these diseases, there is a genetic defect in the body that results in an inability of most individuals to control their disease by diet and exercise alone. Medication is almost always required to keep blood pressure, blood sugar, and blood cholesterol in a normal range. The same principal applies to Muse's Satietopathy. Mark my words: in the next 10 to 20 years, it will be commonplace to treat individuals who show signs of Muse's-Satietopathy-related weight gain with a goal to return their weight to normal and keep it there.

In July 2012, I was thrilled to learn that the American Association of Clinical Endocrinologists had declared that there was enough significant clinical evidence to declare obesity as a disease (Mechanick, 2012). I was even more pleased when, in July of 2013, the American Medical Association (AMA) also declared obesity as a disease (AMA Resolution On Obesity, 2013). The more that the medical community can accept obesity as a disease, the more that we will be able to successfully treat the disease of obesity. As helpful as the declaration of obesity as a disease might be, it still doesn't focus on the real disease underlying obesity, namely Muse's Satietopathy. Focusing on obesity as only a disease results in the false belief by both patients and medical providers that a person is cured once they have lost weight. Focusing instead on Muse's Satietopathy as the cause of obesity promotes the idea that Muse's Satietopathy requires long-term medical treatment to maintain weight, just like patients with diabetes, hypertension, and hyperlipidemia require long-term medical treatment to stay in control.

In decades past, it was believed by medical providers that diabetes, hypertension, and hyperlipidemia could be treated by diet and exercise alone. Sure enough, some individuals could control those diseases by diet and exercise alone, but most could not. In the case of hyperlipidemia, diet only lowers bad cholesterol by about 15%, which is not enough for most patients who are higher risk for heart disease (Scirica, 2005). The problem is that if everyone eschews medication and chooses instead to try diet and exercise to control these diseases, then the majority will fail to adequately control their disease, and many will suffer serious consequences of their uncontrolled disease. In modern times, it is widely understood that medical treatment for these diseases should be started at the time of first diagnosis, with diet and exercise being used as additional treatments on top of medication.

The same principal applies to the disease of Muse's Satietopathy. In a meta-analysis of 29 long-term weight-loss studies, 80% of the weight that was initially lost was regained within five years (Maintenance of lost weight and long-term management of obesity, 2018). Therefore, just like with the other diseases mentioned above, at the first sign of failure to maintain weight after a diet, a reassessment of treatment needs to occur immediately to improve its efficacy. In addition, the treatment that is effective in maintaining weight should never be stopped.

It may go without saying, but Muse Satiety Type 1s don't have the disease of Muse's Satietopathy. Muse Satiety Type 2s through Muse Satiety Type 5s have the disease of Muse's Satietopathy in varying degrees.

It is interesting to point out that animals can have the same problem that humans do with stopping eating even after they have met their calorie needs. Our household dog, a dachshund named Tegan, must be fed a measured meal twice a day and no more than that. If we leave extra food out for her, she eats all of it until she is bloated. She will eat whatever she can find in between meals. If well-meaning members of my family can't resist her whining for food all day long and feed her extra food, she gains weight. On the other hand, some other dog owners tell me that they can put food in their dog's bowl and their dog will only eat what it needs and then walk away. A veterinarian that I spoke with, who sees mostly people's pets, says this polarization of eating behavior can be seen in most mammals and in birds, although this has not been studied and quantified.

Humans have an inborn tendency to overserve themselves at mealtimes in my observation, which can create a problem for individuals in Muse Satiety Types 3 to 5. A number of years ago, I was waiting for a meeting at my church with another member. He was delayed, and there wasn't much to do while I waited. As I wandered around the church, I noted, to my surprise, that the women from my church had recently eaten dinner in the church gymnasium and had left their plates uncleared on the tables to attend a lecture in another room. It seemed obvious to me that their speaker must have had to leave quickly, so they had done the unheard of and left every one of their plates at their tables. Certainly, I reasoned, they were planning to return after the speaker finished to clear their plates. I decided to make myself useful and began clearing the plates. About every three place settings had food left on the dinner plate, juice left in the glass, and a partially eaten dessert. The other two-thirds of the place settings had no food left on the plate, no remaining juice in the glass, or no more dessert. The difference was so stark. The fact that humans are programmed to overserve themselves in times of plenty is a real problem for those who are overweight. Those who are overweight will serve themselves the same size plate of food as the members of Satiety Type 1 but will finish the plate of food at every meal, causing them to consume extra calories and gain weight.

Benefits of Knowing Your Muse Satiety Type

Knowing your Muse Satiety Type can help individuals accept that fact that their obesity is not the result of a lack of character or a lack of self-control. As I have spoken these words to my overweight patients, tears have frequently come to their eyes. The guilt and self-blame that overweight individuals heap on themselves is immense. Sure, there is additional shame that comes from the ridicule of others. But that is nothing compared to the self-loathing that so many of the overweight feel, including myself. I never look at my body as a whole in the mirror when I am dressing each morning, at least until I am dressed. I am too ashamed and disgusted by how my overweight my body looks in the mirror to even glance at it. So many of my patients feel exactly the same. We are our own worst critics.

One of the main purposes of writing this book is to get the message out to overweight people everywhere to stop feeling guilty over your difficulties with maintaining your weight. It is not your fault that you were born with one of the Muse's Satietopathies. It is not your fault that you can't seem to control your weight no matter how hard you try. It is no more your fault that you can't control your weight than it is the fault of a diabetic that can't control their blood sugar by diet and exercise alone. All of the Muse Satiety Type 3s, 4s, and 5s struggle. None of them "get it all figured out" and then never have to struggle with their weight again. The few that stay thinner long term are fighting tooth and nail to stay there. They are barely hanging on to their weight loss, but you can't tell by looking at them. And they are not going to tell you how hard they are working to maintain their weight.

One of the Muse Satiety Type 5s in my office, a young woman in her 20s, came to see me in the recent past. She had lost 70 pounds on one of my diet programs three years previously and three years later was still only

10 pounds over her ideal weight. She looked and felt great. She told me that day in the office that when other women would tell her about their struggles with their weight, they often would say to her, "Oh, but you wouldn't understand. You have never struggled with your weight." Little did these other women know how much she has struggled. Knowing she was a Muse Satiety Type 5 and that no Muse Satiety Type 5 can maintain weight without tremendous effort, I asked her the sentinel question: how much weight had she repetitively lost in the last year to remain at her current weight? Thirty pounds was her answer. Thirty pounds! I told her how proud I was at how hard she was working. Being a Muse Satiety Type 5 myself, I understand just how hard it was for my patient.

Knowing your Muse Satiety Type can help you to understand the power of listening to the signals that you do have. For the Muse Satiety Type 1s, who are still at risk of gaining 10 or 15 pounds over a 20-year period in this modern era of highly palatable, plentiful, and inexpensive food, it is to never eat those one to two bites that you can fit in between the full signal and before the onset of the nausea. For the Muse Satiety Type 2s, it is to stop snacking. For the Muse Satiety Type 3s, it is to throw away your food as soon as you feel the full signal, because if you save it, you will start eating it again later, even though you tell yourself that you won't. These solutions for Muse Satiety Types 1, 2, and 3 are just the beginning. I will devote a whole chapter later in the book to discuss weight maintenance. Unfortunately for Muse Satiety Type 4s and Type 5s, they don't have signals that are adequate to stop them from overeating at each meal. To members of Muse Satiety Types 4 and 5, realizing the first three Muse Satiety Types get a full signal right at the point that they meet their calorie needs at each meal seems almost too good to be true, magical even, since they have never experienced that signal once in their lives. Any signal that they might get comes way too late to prevent overconsumption.

I want to stress that what I have been discussing so far addresses the difficulty that most of the human population has with maintaining weight long term based on their Muse Satiety Type. A person's Muse Satiety Type, on the other hand, doesn't have a lot to do with success at weight loss, since weight loss is just as hard for members of all five Muse Satiety Types. If a

Muse Satiety Type 1 has 20 pounds of fat to lose, then it is just as hard for them to lose the 20 pounds of fat as it is for a Muse Satiety Type 5. However, it is true that the Muse Satiety Type 1 will have a much easier time keeping the weight off long term once they have lost it.

CHAPTER 3
DETERMINING YOUR MUSE SATIETY TYPE

IT IS NOT always obvious to some individuals which Muse Satiety Type they belong to, even after listening to me lecture on this topic or after having read the previous chapter. This next chapter aims to help individuals to accurately determine what Muse Satiety Type they belong to. The key to determining an individual's Muse Satiety Type is determining which of the three satiety signals of feeling full, losing savor, and experiencing nausea with overeating that the individual has or doesn't have.

Before I proceed, I want to be clear that it is nearly impossible to determine an individual's Muse Satiety Type during times that the individual is non-sedentary. For the purposes of this chapter, we'll define sedentary as when an adult individual has not been exercising for at least three days. A non-sedentary individual will be considered a person who burns at least 1,000 calories per day above the calories they would burn if they were sedentary. This level of calorie burn can occur in individuals who exercise strenuously for two or more hours per day, or in individuals who work hard at manual labor for eight or more hours per day. This level of calorie burn can also occur in very hyperactive individuals who can't sit still for more than a few minutes all day long. The assumption for the rest of this chapter will be that the individuals who we are discussing are sedentary. If non-sedentary individuals desire to determine their Muse Satiety Type, then they will have to be sure to only answer the questions below for times in their lives where they have been sedentary for at least three days.

The First Satiety Signal of Feeling Fullness

Let's start with the first signal, the sensation of feeling fullness at the exact point in a meal where the individual has consumed enough to meet their calorie needs. As previously pointed out in Chapter 2, this signal lasts about 10 to 15 minutes and occurs during meals at different levels of calorie consumption each day, since individuals don't burn the same number of calories every day and therefore don't have the same calorie needs every day.

The question that I used in my research study in 2011 to determine whether a person had this signal was:

If you are served a substantial meal at a favorite restaurant and you let yourself go, do you usually:

A. Stop eating when you feel full and then not eat any more of your meal.
B. Stop eating when you feel full, but after the fullness fades, you keep eating.
C. Finish all of your food without stopping and without feeling full.

If your answer is A or B, then you have the fullness satiety signal. If your answer is C, then you don't have the satiety signal of feeling full. If you're still not sure of your answer to this question, then consider this slightly different way of asking the question above:

If I were to take you to your favorite restaurant and were to serve you a large plate of your favorite food, would you typically (1) finish eating the whole plate of food within 15 minutes, or (2) would you have to stop part way through and take a break for a while before you finished eating the plate of food?

If the first scenario is true for you, then you don't have the fullness satiety signal. If the second scenario is true for you, then you do have the satiety signal of fullness.

In my experience, I have found the fullness satiety signal to be black and white. Either you have it or you don't. Some individuals have told me that they feel the signal, but that it is not very strong, so they could eat past it if they chose to do so. The people who tell me this are usually significantly overweight, or at least have lost and gained a lot of weight during their lifetime. If such a person tells me that they have lost and gained more than 150 pounds in their lifetime, then I know that they are really a Muse Satiety Type 4 or 5 and that whatever sensation of fullness they do feel comes too little and too late to prevent overeating.

A few individuals have asked me if the feeling of needing to sigh or burp is their feeling of fullness. Unfortunately, a feeling of the need to sigh or burp is not the fullness signal. The people who have told me this also tell me that they can keep eating after they sigh or burp. The feeling of the need to sigh is the result of an overfilled stomach compressing the lower portion of the lungs. The feeling of the need to burp occurs when the upper stomach senses extra gas and contracts to expel it into the esophagus and then to the mouth. Once the excess air has passed, there is more room to continue eating if the person doesn't feel full.

It can be helpful to recall whether you typically take leftover food home from restaurants or not, when trying to determine if you have the fullness signal. Members of Muse Satiety Type 5 don't have the fullness signal and rarely, if ever, have food left over after restaurant meals. Muse Satiety Type 4s don't have the fullness signal and can eat a whole plate of food before they must stop due to nausea. They usually only take food home from restaurants that serve larger portion sizes. Members of Muse Satiety Type 3 have the fullness signal without the satiety signal, and unless they sit at a restaurant meal for a long time so they can eat more after the full signal fades, they will often take food home. Members of Muse Satiety Types 1 and 2 rarely, if ever, eat all their food at restaurant meals and most often take food home.

The Second Satiety Signal of Loss of Savor

The question that I asked in my research study to determine if people had the second satiety signal of loss of savor is:

> If you are served a favorite snack two hours after a meal at which you ate until you were full, and you let yourself go, do you usually:

A. Eat a little of the snack, but then not finish it before the next meal.
B. Eat the snack a little at a time until it's gone, usually before the next meal.
C. Eat the whole snack without stopping and then look for more.

If your answer is A, then you have the satiety signal of loss of savor. If your answer is B or C, then you don't have the satiety signal of loss of savor.

Some caution needs to be taken in answering this question. First, this question must only be answered by individuals after two to three days of inactivity. As I have expressed before, individuals who are burning 1,000 calories or more per day over what they would burn if they were sedentary must snack frequently to make up for the calories they are burning. Second, this question must be answered only by someone that two hours previously ate their usual diet of food until they were full. People with the satiety signal of loss of savor that are underfed at a meal will snack in the hours after the meal in an effort to make up for the calories they didn't consume at the meal. I have observed this in members of my office staff who have the loss of savor signal that were served a lunch of salad with bitter lettuce, a little chicken, and vinaigrette dressing for lunch. Since the salad didn't appeal to them, they ate very little and didn't trigger their loss of savor signal. I then observed them snacking on cookies and other treats in between meals.

There is quite a range in the amount of snacking that different individuals do in between meals. Both answers B and C qualify a person for not having the signal of loss of savor, but the amount of snacking in between meals can range from nibbling on and off on a 200-300 calorie snack, to eating a whole family-size bag of candy in less than an hour. Many factors play into the quantity of an individual's snacking between meals, including the following:

1. Absence of the third satiety signal of nausea with overeating.

2. Carbohydrate addiction.

3. A snack-filled environment.

4. Time spent with friends, family, and/or associates who snack.

5. Psychological factors of stress, sadness, anxiety, anger, and boredom.

6. Sleepiness, whether due to medication, disease, or sleep deprivation.

One final caveat that needs to be mentioned about the loss of savor signal is that the signal can be blunted partially or completely by the effect of high levels of insulin. Elevated insulin blocks the anti-snacking effect of leptin, a hormone produced by fat cells in response to an individual being overfed. When fat cells already contain an adequate amount of fat for good health, additional calorie consumption and storage in fat cells results in the fat cells releasing the hormone leptin. Leptin then travels through the blood to the brain where it binds to receptors in the hypothalamus, causing the individual to feel loss of savor and no interest in snacking. However, since about 25% of the US population is insulin resistant (Statistics About Diabetes, 2018), just a small amount of excess carbohydrate consumption in people who are insulin resistant can result in higher than normal levels of insulin that then block the binding of leptin to the hypothalamus. This results in a persistent sensation of savor for carbohydrates, even when the fat cells are producing leptin to try to stop the excess consumption from occurring. The excess carbohydrate consumption results in increasing body fat which increases insulin resistance. The more insulin resistant a person becomes, the higher and higher the person's insulin levels rise, and the greater and greater the leptin blocking becomes, leaving the individual ravenously hungry for carbohydrates. The possibility exists that individuals born with the loss of savor signal might partially or completely lose that signal by rising insulin levels caused by increasing insulin resistance.

Many medications, and sometimes pregnancy, have the same effect on snacking as elevated levels of insulin do, although not necessarily by the same mechanism. In cases where a person's loss of savor signal was blunted by medication or pregnancy, the signal usually returns to normal after stopping the medication or when the pregnancy ends. However, if the person has insulin resistance that was made worse by their weight gain, the signal might only return partially or not at all.

The Third Satiety Signal of Nausea in Response to Overeating

The presence of the third satiety signal of feeling nausea in response to overeating can be determined by answering the follow question:
If you eat too much at a meal, do you:

A. Get nauseated or sick to your stomach, <u>most</u> of the time.
B. Get nauseated or sick to your stomach, <u>some</u> of the time.
C. <u>Never</u> get nauseated or sick to your stomach.

If you answered A to this question, then you have an effective nausea signal. Those who answered A are Muse Satiety Type 1s, 2s, or 4s. If you answered B or C to this question, then you don't have the signal of nausea and you are either a Muse Satiety Type 3 or 5. Of the three satiety signals, the signal of nausea in response to overeating is quite variable from person to person. In some individuals, the nausea triggers in response to eating just two bites past the full signal. In others, the signal of nausea triggers only with excessive and prolonged eating, such as at Thanksgiving dinner. To function as a signal with the power to prevent overeating, the nausea must consistently trigger within just a few bites of an effort to eat past the full signal. If the nausea happens only after hundreds of calories of overconsumption and then not every time, then it is weak in its ability to prevent weight gain and is not considered to be present in an individual.

If it is still not clear to you what Muse Satiety Type you belong to, then here are a few additional helpful points. Determine your lifetime cumulative weight-loss value if you are over 20 years old. This can be difficult because many of us have fluctuated up and down 10 or 20 pounds every year or two for most of our adult lives. But, since there has been no net weight loss, we have not considered the downward fluctuations to have been meaningful weight loss. To correctly determine your lifetime cumulative weight-loss value, you have to first decide when in your life that you first began to fluctuate up and down and then subtract that from your current age. I'll use myself as an example. My weight started fluctuating up and down when I lost 30 pounds for wrestling when I was 15 years old. I then gained it all back within months of the end of the wrestling season. Since I am around 60 years old as I write this book, then that means that my weight has fluctuated up and down for about 45 years. Then, you need to determine how much your weight has fluctuated up each year, no matter how you lost it. For me, some years I did big diets and other years I did two or three little diets. All told, I have gained and lost an average of about 25 pounds a year. Multiplying the 25 pounds a year by the 45 years I have struggled, for myself I get 1,125 pounds. I know that sounds crazy for many of you, but as previously mentioned in Chapter 2, I am a Muse Satiety Type 5. Some Muse Satiety Type 5s have told me that they have gained and lost up to 2,000 pounds in their lifetimes.

Most individuals under 30 have not struggled long enough with their weight for their lifetime cumulative weight loss to have clinical meaning. For the purpose of trying to determine what Muse Satiety Type an individual is, those who are between the ages of 20 and 30 will need to estimate their potential 20-year weight gain to get a helpful value. As an example, if a 25-year-old individual has lost and gained 30 pounds a year since the age of 15, then their lifetime cumulative weight loss for the 10 years that they have struggled with their weight would be 300 pounds. To estimate what the individual might gain over a 20-year period, the individual could then multiply their 300 pounds in 10 years by two, resulting in an estimate of a 600-pound cumulative weight loss over 20 years. Of course, the whole goal of this book is to slow down that theoretical weight gain in the next 10 years, so that the real weight gain in the next 10 years had better be a lot less than the predicted 300 pounds. This individual can then use their 20-year weight-gain estimate for their lifetime cumulative weight loss in the paragraph below.

Once you have your lifetime cumulative weight-loss value, it can help you determine your Muse Satiety Type. If you have gained and lost more than

500 pounds in your lifetime, then you are most likely a Muse Satiety Type 5. If you have gained and lost 50 to 500 pounds in your lifetime, then you are most likely a Muse Satiety Type 3 or Type 4, with the difference between these two Muse Satiety Types being whether you frequently get nauseated with overeating. If you have gained and lost less than 50 pounds and don't have nausea with overeating, then you are most likely a Muse Satiety Type 3. If you gained most of your weight from excess snacking as a child, or from medications or pregnancies, but have not gained and lost much since, and you have nausea frequently with overeating, then you are probably a Muse Satiety Type 2.

For people that have been thin their whole life but aren't sure if they are a Muse Satiety Type 1, it is important to understand that there are four subtypes of Muse Satiety Type 1, which are broken down in Figure 3.

Muse Satiety Type 1 Subtypes				
	1a	**1b**	**1c**	**1d**
Fullness	√	√	X	X
Loss of Savor	√	√	√	√
Nausea	√	X	√	X
20-Year Weight Gain Risk (lbs.)	0-10	5-10	10-20	15-25
Lifetime Cumulative Weight Loss	0	0	0	0

Figure 3 - Muse Satiety Type 1 Subtypes

Muse Satiety Type 1s only comprised about 15% of the population I studied, so each of the four sub-types of Muse Satiety Type 1 would represent only about 4% of the population. The 20-year weight-gain risk and the lifetime cumulative weight loss in Figure 3 are estimates, as my study didn't have enough Muse Satiety Type 1s to allow me to determine these numbers more exactly. I also don't know the population frequency of Muse Satiety Types 1a through 1d for the same reason.

People in Muse Satiety Type 1a are the only ones that have all three signals, are the most protected from food overconsumption, and are most likely to maintain weight long term.

Members of Muse Satiety Type 1b feel full at the right time and lose their savor appropriately but do not feel nausea when they try to take a bite of extra food after they have experienced the full signal. They have a slight risk of gaining weight over time.

Individuals in Muse Satiety Type 1c don't feel full when they reach their calorie needs at a meal, but they do feel loss of savor a few moments later and just stop eating. Any extra food they might have overconsumed is subtracted from their next meal and they stay relatively thin over the years.

I have seen two Muse Satiety Type 1d patients in my weight-loss practice. Both were in their 60s, had worked in the restaurant business for their entire adult lives and had each gained about 40 pounds over their ideal weight. Neither had dieted previously. Both lost about 20 pounds over two to three months on a medication-assisted diet in my office and both stopped coming. I have never seen them again.

As best as I can tell, my mother is a Muse Satiety Type 1c and is missing the fullness signal. That is how she passed the absence of the fullness signal to me. She does have the loss of savor signal and the nausea with overeating signal. She has never gained more than 10 pounds over her ideal weight and has never dieted. My father appears to have been a Muse Satiety Type 3 and had the full signal but was missing both the loss of savor signal and the nausea with overeating signal. I unfortunately inherited the lack of all three signals from my parents.

Those of us in Muse Satiety Types 3 through 5 tend to be envious of members of Muse Satiety Type 1a to 1d, since they are mostly staying thin in our obesogenic environment. I have even caught myself saying, after explaining to listeners that Muse Satiety Type 1s will stop eating in the middle of a favorite snack and will never finish it, that Muse Satiety Type 1s are aliens. Everyone laughs at this "skinny joke." Then, I get in trouble later when one of my patients who has heard me make the alien comment tells my Muse-Satiety-Type-1a wife what I said.

If you still can't determine which Muse Satiety Type you belong to, you should see a medical professional that is trained in the use of these questions to determine what your Muse Satiety Type is. That medical professional can help you by reviewing your responses to the questions above to clear up any misunderstandings and possibly to pierce through any denial that some individuals struggle with.

40 | DEREK MUSE

DETERMINING YOUR CHILD'S MUSE SATIETY TYPE

IT IS WITH some hesitation that I write this chapter. Certainly, improving the health of children in the world is of critical importance. Identifying a child's Muse Satiety Type could allow caregivers to more carefully monitor and control the calorie content of the child's diet, helping to reduce the degree of overweightness and obesity that might otherwise occur. At the same time, once a child has been determined to be a member of Muse Satiety Types 2 to 5, and especially Muse Satiety Types 4 and 5 where there is so much weight gain occurring in our children in the present day, then the failure of caregivers to prevent weight gain could be used to incriminate the caregivers both social and legally. In the end, however, what is best for children is of the greatest importance, and that is to identify and start prevention of weight gain early in children who are members of Muse Satiety Types 2 to 5.

Just like in adults, the key to determining a child's Muse Satiety Type is to determine whether or not they have the three satiety signals of feeling full, feeling loss of savor, and feeling nausea in response to eating past the full signal. Determining the presence or absence of the three satiety signals is easier in older children, more difficult in younger children and toddlers, and quite difficult in infants. Sometimes, the exact determination of a child's

Muse Satiety Type is not possible until the child reaches their mid-teens. Most children in their mid-teens and older can have their Muse Satiety Type determined by using the questions and information presented in the previous chapter.

Before I proceed, just like with the adults, I want to make sure to be clear that it is more difficult to determine a child's Muse Satiety Type during times that the child is non-sedentary or is experiencing a growth spurt. For the purposes of this chapter, we'll define non-sedentary as when an older child is involved in indoor and outdoor sports for more than five hours per week. The discussion in the rest of this chapter assumes that the children who we are discussing are otherwise sedentary, even though most sedentary children are still more active than sedentary adults. If the parents of non-sedentary children desire to determine their child's Muse Satiety Type, then they will have to be sure to only answer the questions below for times in their child's life where they have been sedentary for at least three days. It is well-known that infants and prepubertal children experience short periods of growth interspaced with longer periods of little or no growth (Lampl, 1992) (Thalange, 1996). Calorie intake increases during growth spurts. Parents of children who are experiencing a growth spurt will have to answer the questions below for times in their child's life when they have not been growing rapidly.

The First Satiety Signal of Feeling Full

Let's start with the first signal, the sensation of feeling full at the exact point in a meal where the child has consumed enough to have met their calorie needs. As was pointed out in the previous chapter, this signal lasts about 10 to 15 minutes and occurs during meals at different levels of calorie consumption each day, since children don't burn the same number of calories every day and therefore don't have the same calorie needs every day.

The question that I use to determine whether a child has the fullness signal is:

If you were to serve your child a substantial meal of their favorite foods, would your child usually:

A. Stop eating somewhere in the middle of the meal and then not eat any more of their meal, even on occasions where they are at the table for more than 15 minutes.

B. Stop eating somewhere in the middle of the meal, but then, on occasions where they are still at the table for more than 15 minutes, they start eating again.

C. Finish all of the food on their plate most of the time without stopping.

If the answer is A or B, then your child has the satiety signal of feeling full. If the answer is C, then your child doesn't have the satiety signal of feeling full. In my experience, I have found the satiety signal of feeling full for about 10 to 15 minutes to be mostly black and white for children, just like it is for adults. Either your child has this signal, or they don't. If it is still not clear if your child has this signal or not, consider the following. Since children grow in spurts, their appetite increases a lot when they are growing and then diminishes when they aren't growing. If your child intermittently cleans up most of the food on their plate for a few weeks and then goes back to eating about half of their plate of food with no change in activity, then they probably have the satiety signal of fullness. Sometimes, after an episode of increased food consumption associated with growth has passed, you can recognize it because your child is taller. In addition, you might have also noted that their knees and ankles got larger right before the growth spurt started, as their bodies prepared to carry extra weight before growing.

The Second Satiety Signal of Loss of Savor

The question that I ask parents to determine if their children have the second signal of loss of savor is:

If you were to serve your child a favorite snack two hours after a substantial meal where they ate until they were satisfied, does your child usually:

A. Eat a little of the snack, but then not finish it before the next meal.

B. Eat the snack a little at a time until it's gone, usually before the next meal.

C. Eat the whole snack without stopping and then look for more.

If the answer is A, then your child has the satiety signal of loss of savor. If your answer is B or C, then your child doesn't have the satiety signal of loss of savor.

Some caution needs to be taken in answering this question. First, as emphasized above, this question must be answered for your child only after three days of inactivity. Second, children who have the satiety signal of loss of savor that are underfed at a meal will snack in the hours after the meal in an effort to make up for the calories that they didn't consume at the meal. The reasons that a child might be underfed at a meal could be:

1. The child got distracted by various forms of media, siblings, or friends and didn't finish their meal.

2. The child was served foods by their caregivers that were not their preferred foods, causing them to under eat.

3. There wasn't enough food for everyone at the table.

4. A toddler might have dumped their food off their highchair, or made a mess in their diaper, needed to be cleaned up, and didn't make it back to the table before the food was put away.

The Third Satiety Signal of Nausea in Response to Overeating

The presence of the third satiety signal, feeling nausea in response to overeating, is difficult to determine in children. Most children under twelve don't accurately verbalize that they feel nauseated. In response to nausea, they just quit eating and sometimes say they feel sick. When asked to eat more of the food on their plate by their caregivers, some children obediently try to eat more, but then either cry in frustration because they can't eat due to nausea or vomit after just a few extra bites. Children that are members of Muse Satiety Type 4 will eat a larger than expected amount of food for their age and body size at a meal and then will complain of feeling sick or, at times, will suddenly throw up.

Spitting up is not an indicator of nausea. Spitting up is the regurgitation of liquid out of the mouth of children under the age of one, usually in response to pressure on the stomach or to the tightening up of stomach muscles by the child, such as when trying to sit up. Spitting up almost always involves small amounts of liquid, and that liquid dribbles out of the mouth in a non-projectile fashion. Vomiting usually involves large amounts of liquid and is more explosive, since the vomit is forced out of the mouth by contractions of the stomach and esophagus.

Keeping the above in mind, try to answer the follow question for your child:

If your child were to eat too much at a meal, would your child:

A. Get sick to their stomach <u>most</u> of the time.
B. Get sick to their stomach <u>some</u> of the time.
C. <u>Rarely or never</u> get sick to their stomach.

If you answered A to this question, then your child has the signal of nausea and is a member of Muse Satiety Types 1, 2, or 4. If you answered B or C to this question, then your child doesn't have the signal of nausea and is either a member of Muse Satiety Type 3 or 5.

Of the three satiety signals, the signal of nausea in response to overeating is quite variable from child to child, just like in adults. In some children, the nausea triggers in response to eating just one to two bites past the full signal while in others, the signal of nausea triggers only with excessive and prolonged eating, such as at Thanksgiving dinner. To function as a signal with the strength to prevent overeating, the nausea must consistently trigger within just one or two bites after the full signal. If the nausea happens only after hundreds of calories of overconsumption and not every time, then it is weak in its ability to prevent weight gain and is considered not to be present in the child.

If it is still not clear to you what Muse Satiety Type your child belongs to, then here are a few additional helpful points:

1. If your pre-pubertal child is developing abdominal obesity, which can easily be identified by finding one or more inches of fat when gently pinching the skin next to the belly button up and down

while the child is standing, then they are not a Satiety Type 1 and are probably not members of Muse Satiety Types 2 and 3. That is because members of Muse Satiety Types 1, 2, and 3 all feel full at meals at the exact point where they have eaten enough to satisfy their calorie needs. Children in these Muse Satiety Types then ask to be excused from the table to go to play or just leave on their own to do the same, depending on family rules. If they are members of Muse Satiety Types 2 and 3, which means that they don't lose their savor, then they might circle back to the kitchen later to eat a few bites more, if palatable food has been left out to eat.

2. If your child breast fed every one to two hours when they were an infant and never seemed to get full, then your child is probably a Muse Satiety Type 4 or 5. Children that breast fed frequently that also ate so much that they threw up, and didn't just spit up, are members of Muse Satiety Type 4. Children that breast fed frequently and never threw up, no matter how much they ate, are members of Muse Satiety Type 5.

3. If, on a rainy day, when your child couldn't go outside to play and snacks were on the kitchen counter, your child returned to the kitchen to snack every 30-60 minutes, then they don't have the signal of loss of savor and are not members of Muse Satiety Type 1.

4. If a snack before dinner has typically and significantly ruined your child's appetite for dinner, then your child has the satiety signal of fullness and is either a Muse Satiety Type 1, 2, or 3, and is not a Muse Satiety Type 4 or 5.

5. And finally, if your child is thin and doesn't finish their snacks, but you are not sure they have the full signal or the nausea signal, then they might be a Muse Satiety Type 1a, 1b, 1c, or 1d, as discussed in the previous chapter.

If you still can't determine which Muse Satiety Type your child is in, your child might need to see a medical professional trained in the use of these questions to determine what your child's Muse Satiety Type is. That medical professional can help you by reviewing your responses to the questions above to clear up any misunderstandings and possibly to pierce through any denial that some parents might struggle with.

CHAPTER 5

SOCIAL IMPLICATIONS OF KNOWING YOUR MUSE SATIETY TYPE

IN ADDITION TO the adverse physical consequences of obesity, there are also negative social consequences. These negative social consequences range from discrimination at work, to lack of success in romance, and to a high cost of life and health insurance. Many individuals who are thinner now are at higher risk for long-term weight gain related to their Muse Satiety Type. As previously discussed, almost all members of Muse Satiety Types 4 and 5 will become obese, even if they are thinner now.

I hesitated to write this chapter for fear of putting derogatory ideas into people's heads about younger members of Muse Satiety Types 4 and 5 that are not yet obese. However, with the epidemic of obesity increasing so rapidly, it is best that we meet these problems head on and that I address them here.

At the root of discrimination against overweight people is a feeling of discomfort, and even disgust, for overweight people's bodies. This feeling is then extended to overweight people's personalities, with overweight people being assigned personality traits of laziness, lack of self-control, slovenliness, and self-indulgence. The overweight person is then treated differently, in a negative way, than other people who are not overweight. This discrimination could also extend to adults and children who are not yet obese but are in a Muse Satiety Type that will most likely lead to obesity later in life.

Let's look at an example of a potential employer that is faced with multiple thin, young, and equally qualified job applicants, but with different Muse Satiety Types. For this example, we'll assume that each applicant knows their correct Muse Satiety Type and that this information was divulged to the potential employer by the applicants. What would the potential employer do? An employer's priority is to hire employees that will be a long-term asset to the company since finding and training new employees is expensive. Obese employees are less productive at a number of different jobs and are unable to perform some jobs. If an employer is a modeling agency, a medical spa, a dance company, a TV news agency, a bar, a restaurant, etc., that is looking for employees that will be in front of the public, then it is clear that they will choose the applicant with the lowest Muse Satiety Type. Overweight individuals are also potentially problematic for employers in other areas. Significantly overweight individuals are more likely to be injured on the job and are more likely to need time off for illnesses related to their obesity, both of which are costly to the employer in terms of lost productivity and increased insurance costs. Without question, most employers will select applicants that have the lowest Muse Satiety Type.

Let's next consider a scenario related to long-term romantic relationships. A person who is not overweight and is a member of Muse Satiety Type 1 or 2 is seriously dating a person who is also not overweight but is a member of Muse Satiety Types 4 or 5. The first person becomes aware of the second person's higher Muse Satiety Type and realizes that their partner is more likely to be obese and that any children they might have together could also become obese. We will assume that the classification of Muse Satiety Type is accurate for both individuals and that they mutually agreed to disclose this information. What is the first person to do? Studies have indicated that women, and even more so men, prefer that their future mate not be obese.

In my insecurity related to my weight, I have proposed this very scenario to my sweetheart wife, Emily, multiple times. To remind you, Emily is a Muse Satiety Type 1, and I am a Muse Satiety Type 5, although neither of us knew anything about Muse Satiety Types when we were dating. We were

SOCIAL IMPLICATIONS OF KNOWING YOUR MUSE SATIETY TYPE

both young and thin, and the idea that I might be obese for most of my adult life never crossed either of our minds. What she didn't know, and what I never told her because I didn't think I was any different than anyone else, was that I had already repeatedly lost weight on multiple diets that totaled almost 150 pounds of cumulative weight loss by the time I first met her. I had lost 30 pounds just before we started dating. I stayed thin for the year that we dated, but then gained 25 pounds a year for the first two years that we were married.

At times I have asked Emily the question, "Would you have married me knowing that I was a Muse Satiety Type 5 and would be obese?" She has always answered, "Yes, I would have still married you, because I loved you then and I love you now, whether you are heavy or not." Of course, my angel wife has always given the perfect answer to that question. But I haven't been able to leave it alone because I am my own worst critic. Pressing the issue further, I have asked, "But would you have married me knowing that I was a Muse Satiety Type 5 and would pass those genes on to our children, condemning some of them to obesity?" Again, her answer has always been perfect, "I would have still married you. We are not personally responsible for the diseases that our parents pass on to us. We'll just have to teach our children to overcome this problem." Emily is amazing! For what it's worth, we have seven children, with three being Muse Satiety Type 1s, two being Muse Satiety Type 2s, one being a Muse Satiety Type 3, and one being a Muse Satiety Type 4.

I'm not so sure everyone would be as altruistic as my wife, especially when it comes to the men. It is true that women are more willing to date overweight males than men are to date overweight females (Lang, 1997). Since I am a man, you could turn the questions that I asked my wife around and you could ask them of me. And my answers would be the same as hers. I would have still married her. Even more, I would stay married to her if she ever became obese, which is pretty unlikely, since she is a Muse Satiety Type 1. There is one thing we have both agreed on: we would have been less likely to notice each other if either of us had been obese and had passed the other in the hallway at the university where we met. Luckily for both of us, our relationship started when a mutual friend asked me to help Emily with her physical chemistry homework. We became friends before we started dating.

There is no question that obese individuals find it harder to get into universities and into graduate education programs (Fowler-Brown, 2010). But, what about members of Muse Satiety Types 2 to 5 that have not yet gained weight? With the already significant obstacles of costly tuition on top of stringent grade-point average and test-score requirements to get into college, the last thing potential students need is to be threatened with rejection at an educational institution based on the knowledge that they have a higher chance of becoming obese during their time at the university.

Obese individuals have more health problems than their thin counterparts and are faced with higher health care costs, potentially including a higher cost of health insurance. In the past, people with obesity were sometimes unable to even get insurance, especially when they were self-employed, or their employer didn't provide health insurance. Under the new Affordable Care Act of 2013, overweight individuals can't be rejected when they apply for health insurance, but their rates can be higher through some insurers. Other insurers charge the same rate for everyone, heavy or thin, but then give cash discounts or bonuses to individuals based on weight and other parameters affected adversely by weight, such as high blood pressure, type 2 diabetes, and high cholesterol. Will insurers charge members of Muse Satiety Types 2 to 5 that are still thin, but probably won't be in the future, higher rates for their insurance? Time will only tell on this one.

If a thin grade schooler has a friend that becomes obese and that now obese friend becomes less popular on the playground because of their obesity, then will the thin grade schooler abandon their friend as well? We would all hope that this would not be true, but everyone knows that it happens all the time. Gratefully, social discrimination against established friends who become obese is less likely for teens and rare amongst adults.

I'm sure that I have not yet thought of all the ways that individuals who are not yet obese but have a higher chance of becoming obese due to their Muse Satiety Type, could be discriminated against at work, in relationships, and in the health and life insurance markets. While most would hope that society would become more accepting and less discriminating of people with obesity, we all know that it will take decades.

What is the best solution to end the discrimination I have described above? It is for the members of Muse Satiety Types 2 to 5 to never become obese in the first place. This sounds difficult, but it is doable. This will be explained further in later chapters.

CHAPTER 6

A BRIEF REVIEW OF THE BIOCHEMISTRY OF WEIGHT CONTROL

THE HUMAN BODY almost subconsciously controls hunger and satiety so meticulously that those with a completely intact system gain little to no weight over time, despite frequently living in a calorie-rich environment and often living a sedentary lifestyle. The body does this by the complex interaction of multiple hormones with the brain to modulate hunger and satiety. These hormones are secreted by various tissues throughout the body. In addition, there are nervous system signals that interact with the brain which also modulate hunger and satiety. Hunger is required to induce humans to start eating to replace the calories that have been used from the body's energy stores. Satiety is required to convince a human to stop eating once those energy stores have been refilled.

There are two types of appetite-controlling hormones produced by the body: orexigenic hormones and anorexigenic hormones. Orexigenic hormones increase hunger, and thereby increase food intake. Anorexigenic hormones decrease hunger, and thereby decrease food intake. These hormones are produced by the stomach, small intestine, pancreas, and fat cells, and then travel through the blood to the arcuate nucleus of the brain. The arcuate nucleus is a small part of the brain located in the upper portion of the brain stem. The blood-brain barrier is thinnest in the arcuate nucleus, allowing the orexigenic and anorexigenic hormones from the body to enter the arcuate nucleus and to stimulate, or inhibit, the hunger-and-satiety-related neurons in the arcuate nucleus.

Ghrelin is the body's main orexigenic hormone. It is produced mostly in the lining of the stomach and the first part of the small intestine. Higher ghrelin levels increase hunger and motivation to eat. Ghrelin levels increase when it is time for the body to eat, about three hours after the previous meal, and ghrelin levels rise higher and higher as food consumption is delayed, in an attempt to convince the conscious mind to eat. The higher the ghrelin rises, the individual first feels hungry, then really hungry, and then even hangry. Levels of ghrelin return to normal once the body consumes an adequate number of calories to meet its daily needs. Ghrelin is also increased by weight loss, lack of sleep (Taheri, 2004), and aging. Importantly, ghrelin levels are not higher in overweight individuals as compared to thin individuals (Cummings, 2002). Saying this differently, the disease of obesity is not due to excess hunger caused by higher-than-normal levels of ghrelin.

A number anorexigenic hormones are secreted by the body to counteract the hunger caused by ghrelin when the body has consumed the calories it needs. Some of these I have already mentioned in previous chapters. Glucagon-like peptide-1 (GLP-1), cholecystokinin (CCK), oxyntomodulin (OXM), and peptide YY (PYY) are produced by the small intestine. Insulin, amylin, and pancreatic polypeptide (PP) are produced by the pancreas. Leptin and adiponectin are produced by the fat cells. The vast majority of humans, whether overweight or not, have normal levels of these anorexigenic hormones. Studies in which giving higher-than-normal doses of these anorexigenic hormones to humans to induce weight loss have only been mildly successful or not successful at all. That is because the defect in satiety lies not in the lack of these anorexigenic hormones, but in the insensitivity of the nerve cells of the brain's arcuate nucleus to these anorexigenic hormones. These anorexigenic hormones bind properly to the receptors on the neurons in the arcuate nucleus, but the desired effect doesn't happen. This is called receptor resistance. The defects in the neurons of the arcuate nucleus, and possibly in other parts of the brain, that lead to receptor resistance to the anorexigenic hormones are not completely known, although many studies are underway to attempt to determine what those defects are.

The orexigenic and anorexigenic hormones discussed above bind to receptors on two key neurons in the arcuate nucleus: the POMC/CART neuron (an anorexigenic neuron) and the NPY/AgRP neuron (an orexigenic neuron). These neurons are large cells and have many receptors where hormones can bind and stimulate or suppress the actions of these neurons. For example, the anorexigenic hormone leptin from the fat cell stimulates the POMC/CART neuron and inhibits the NPY/AgRP neuron. The orexigenic hormone ghrelin from the stomach wall stimulates the NPY/AgRP neuron but doesn't stimulate or inhibit the POMC/CART neuron. The POMC/CART neuron takes the sum of the effect of all the hormones that are inhibiting or stimulating it at any given time and determines how much alpha-MSH (α-MSH) to produce to tell the next neuron deeper in the hypothalamus whether or not the person is hungry. The more α-MSH that is produced, the less hungry the person feels (Simpson, 2009). Some scientists are now calling obesity a disease of inadequate production of α-MSH. This is a limited overview of the complicated control system in controlling appetite in the human body.

Dozens of pharmaceutical compounds are in various stages of research in an effort to overcome the anorexigenic receptor resistance in the arcuate nucleus. In my opinion and based only on the known actions of the anorectic hormones mentioned above, the fullness signal that I have discussed in previous chapters is caused in part by the hormone CCK. The satiety signal of loss of savor that lasts for four hours is likely to be caused in part by leptin. From there, the nausea signal that results from attempts to eat past the full signal is likely to be caused in part by the hormones PYY and GLP-1.

In summary, receptor resistance to one or more anorexigenic hormones results in a steady weight gain throughout life. As indicated in my research study, the amount of weight gained over time can be predicted by the number of anorexigenic hormones to which a person is resistant.

CHAPTER 7

THE WEIGHT GAIN TRIPLE THREAT

NOW THAT I have introduced the Muse Satiety Types and the basic biochemistry surrounding hormonal control of weight, I can now present the second of the three disease processes that make up the triple threat that makes it so difficult for most of us to lose and maintain weight.

The first disease process is Muse's Satietopathy and has been presented previously, which leads about 85% of the population to experience weight gain throughout their lives. The second disease process in the triple threat is what I have come to term "maximum weight memory." After discussing maximum weight memory, I will end this chapter by discussing the role of the third member of the triple threat: the body's ability to become addicted, or to crave, certain foods.

Maximum weight memory describes the body's tendency to permanently remember an individual's previous maximum weight and then to defend against any effort at achieving and maintaining a lower weight. As an individual's maximum weight increases over time, which can be predicted by their Muse Satiety Type, the body incorrectly remembers the new higher weight as the weight that the person should now weigh for the rest of their life. This same process has also been described previously by other scientists, so what I call "maximum weight memory" they have called "body weight set point" (Yu, 2015). These scientists stated in their paper that the cause of the "body weight set point" was not fully understood, but it might be due to acquired leptin resistance (Arch, 2005), loss of synapses on regulatory neurons (Horvath, 2010), or diet-induced inflammation, and/or aging of the same regulatory neurons (Thaler, 2012).

We don't know how many people have the disease process of maximum weight memory. It isn't found in everyone, or so it seems to me, because there are few people who can lose weight and without much effort never gain it all back. I am calling maximum weight memory a disease process because the body should know that it is carrying a harmful amount of weight and it shouldn't fight against efforts to lower weight to a healthier level.

We also don't know how long an individual has to be a new maximum weight before the body increases its maximum weight memory to that new maximum weight, but I will make an estimate based on my observation that it is more than one year. We do know that many women can gain weight with pregnancy and then lose back to their pre-pregnancy weight and stay there without rigorous dieting. We also know that film and stage actors have gained weight for parts in movies and plays, and then have permanently lost the weight after their role in the presentation has ended. Because of maximum weight memory, there is a real urgency for all overweight individuals to not allow their weight to increase beyond their previous maximum weight, so that they don't get saddled with their body developing a maximum weight memory for their new and higher weight.

Once a new maximum weight memory has been established, the body resists any effort to reduce and then maintain a lower weight by using the human physiologic response to starvation. Any time an individual goes on a diet, what they are really doing is starving the body of calories. The body doesn't know whether the individual is trying to lose weight for better health or is lost on a deserted island with nothing to eat. The body responds to starvation by raising the level of the hunger hormone ghrelin and by lowering metabolism—all in an effort to conserve energy and force the individual to find and eat food, to regain the weight that was lost. In the case of dieting to lose weight for better health, the body does this even though the overweight body of the dieter already has an unhealthy amount of extra calories on it stored as fat.

As previously stated, ghrelin levels are the same in thin and overweight individuals. However, as an individual loses weight on a diet, ghrelin rises higher and higher with each pound lost. The first 10 pounds lost on any diet are lost relatively easily and hunger is mild. The next 10 pounds lost is harder as ghrelin increases, causing hunger to increase. Dieters find it harder to comply with their diet and weight loss slows. The third 10 pounds of weight loss causes even higher levels of ghrelin and, consequently, more hunger. The majority of dieters reach a plateau on their diets at around 10 to 15 pounds of weight loss. For those who try to lose more than 20 pounds, ghrelin continues to rise higher and higher with each 10 pounds of weight lost, until almost all dieters plateau in their weight-loss efforts.

Simultaneously, with more and more weight lost, the body responds by lowering the dieter's basal metabolic rate between 200 to 500 calories per day, which causes the dieter to feel tired and cold, and to suffer from constipation and hair loss. Lowering of the basal metabolic rate while dieting is called the metabolic response to starvation. When faced with rising hunger from increasing levels of ghrelin and increasing fatigue caused by a declining metabolism, most dieters almost subconsciously start to cheat on their diet and also start to decrease their physical activity, leading to a plateau, or a failure to lose further weight.

Elevated ghrelin and lower metabolism also undermine dieter's efforts to maintain their weight loss after a diet. Ghrelin stays elevated for more than a year after a diet, and probably much longer, and the metabolic rate stays low for up to six years after a diet, as the body tries to get the dieter to return to their pre-diet weight (Sumithran, 2011) (Nymo, 2018) (Fothergill, 2016). While research says that the effect of elevated ghrelin and low metabolism lasts for years, I personally have observed that the body never forgets the maximum weight that a dieter used to be and that the body never stops trying to get the dieter to gain weight back to that pre-diet weight. This frustrating problem with elevated ghrelin and depressed metabolism in weight maintenance is like attaching yourself to a wall with a bungee cord and then running away from the wall. Each time you try, the bungee cord tightens, and you get pulled back to the wall. The farther and faster you run, the faster you get snapped right back to where you started.

The third disease contributing to weight gain is food addiction. Food addiction is also known by the scientific terms, *food craving* and *hedonic feeding*. In the US, about two-thirds of the population reports having at least one food to which they are addicted. A food addiction is defined as a food that is so appealing that the person will knowingly overeat that food every time it is available to them. Food addiction will be discussed further in Chapter 12.

Obesity is caused by three separate diseases: Muse's Satietopathy, maximum weight memory, and food addiction. These diseases are genetically based and are inherited from an individual's parents. To those who suffer from the effects of these powerful diseases, it might appear that prevention of weight gain over time and permanent weight loss is just not possible. However, that is why I am writing this book, to teach what does work in the face of a particularly challenging problem.

CHAPTER 8

WHAT AM I SUPPOSED TO WEIGH?

A COMMON QUESTION asked by new adult weight-loss patients is what they should weigh. My answer to this question doesn't always make them happy. That is because they have convinced themselves that their ideal weight is 20 to 30 pounds over what it should be if they are an average-sized female and 30 to 40 pounds over what it should be if they are an average-sized male. Some of the possible reasons that they do this are because they can't imagine ever losing to below that weight, and that they might have never weighed less than that amount during their adult life. Even after I reassure them that their ideal weight is lower than what they think it is, many are still dubious, and a few are somewhat indignant that I'm suggesting that they are more overweight than they think they are.

There is not an exact ideal weight for anyone. There is instead an ideal weight range. There is no health risk to weighing any weight within a person's ideal weight range. An individual should feel no pressure to lose weight to the lower range of their ideal weight range, since there is no health benefit. It is completely a person's choice of where in their ideal weight range they want to be.

The most accurate way to determine a person's ideal weight range is to first determine their lean body mass. The lean body mass of a person is the weight of all the structures of their body minus the weight of the fat of their body. In my clinic, we determine the lean body mass of our patients with a DEXA (dual-energy x-ray absorptiometry). DEXA is reasonable in price in my office and is more accurate than most other methods of determining lean body mass. We also need to know the ideal fat mass for our patients. For women, the low end of the ideal fat mass range is about 18% and for men it is about 8%. The mathematical formula for the low end of the ideal weight range for women is the lean mass divided by 0.82, and the formula for men is the lean mass divided by 0.92. To next determine the high end of the ideal weight range, the low end for the ideal weight range for women is multiplied by 1.15 and for men it is multiplied by 1.13. For those wanting to know how this correlates to body mass index (BMI) and percent body fat, the resulting low and high end for ideal weight range approximately correlates with a BMI of 20 and 25, respectively. For body fat, this approximately correlates with 18% to 28%, respectively, for females, and 8% to 19%, respectively, for males (Halls, 2019).

Using the formulas above, a real-life example for a 5'7" tall woman with a medium frame and a lean body mass of 110 pounds is:

110 pounds / 0.82 = 134 pounds, which is her low end for her ideal weight range

134 pounds x 1.15 = 154 pounds, which is her high end for her ideal weight range.

A real-life example for a 5'11" tall man with a medium frame and a lean body mass of 154 pounds is:

154 pounds / 0.92 = 167 pounds, which is his low end for his ideal weight range

167 pounds x 1.13 = 189 pounds, which is his high end for his ideal weight range.

To determine the weight at which these people would be obese, the upper range for the ideal weight is multiplied again by 1.15 for women and 1.13 for men. In the examples above, the woman would be obese at 174 pounds and the man would be obese at 210 pounds. Again, for those wanting to know how this correlates with BMI and body fat percentages, the resulting weights for both would be approximately a BMI of 30. The percent body fat would be 34% for the woman and 26% for the man (Halls, 2019).

Once I have a person's ideal weight range and the weight at which the person is obese, I can then sit down with them and encourage them to set their weight-loss goal to be at least lower than the point at which they would no longer be obese. Since obesity has so many risks, I feel strongly that patients should try hard to lose weight into their non-obese weight range. If patients under age 40 want to set their weight-loss goal at the low end of their ideal weight range, which might have been what they weighed at age 20, then I am okay with that, as long as they know that it isn't needed for good health. I encourage my patients over 40 to not lose lower than five pounds over the lower end of their ideal weight range, since studies show that it makes them look older.

At the first visit for weight loss for an adult in my office, I don't have DEXA results for the patients to allow me to determine their ideal weight range. I have a method that I use to quickly estimate a patient's ideal weight range that is explained in Appendix 1 at the end of this book. In my experience, 90% of the time this method can determine a person's low end for their ideal weight range within five pounds for women and 10 pounds for men as compared to results from a DEXA. This can be especially important at the first weight-loss visit if a person's current weight is below the weight at which they would be obese by BMI and their current weight is the highest they have ever weighed while not pregnant. In this case, guidelines and state regulations would not recommend or allow treatment with weight-loss medication. Because BMI underestimates obesity, in cases like this I get the DEXA result before prescribing weight-loss medication. When the method explained in Appendix 1 is either known to be inaccurate, or just doesn't seem to fit the patient, but the patient is clearly obese, I don't require a DEXA before starting treatment with weight-loss medications. I do tell these patients for which the method explained in Appendix 1 is not applicable that they are welcome to get a DEXA to accurately determine their ideal weight range.

Besides DEXA, other machines can be used to measure lean body mass and fat mass. Air-displacement plethysmography (ADP), or as it is better known by its brand name, BOD POD, is only slightly less accurate than DEXA. Bioelectrical impedance analysis (BIA) is commonly used by machines at home and at commercial gyms. BIA machines involve the person standing on two conductive pads while simultaneously holding a separate conductive rod in each hand. Lean body mass and fat mass measurements by BIA are less accurate than DEXA and ADP. A computed tomography body scan (commonly known as a CT scan) and a magnetic resonance imaging body scan (commonly known as an MRI) are just as accurate as a DEXA in measuring lean body mass and fat mass but are too expensive to be used outside of medical research (Borga, 2018). A simple skin-fold caliper can give a less accurate but still helpful measurement of fat mass, and then by subtraction, lean body mass. Finally, there are a number of formulas proposed over the years that use height, weight, age, and gender to estimate fat mass. Multiple websites can be found that have body fat calculators that use these formulas. Lean body mass can then be calculated by subtracting the fat mass from the total body weight.

You have probably noticed that I have not said much about BMI, which is widely used in the medical industry to determine if a patient is obese at their current weight. The biggest problem with BMI is that it is based on an average human body frame, which is fine if you are an average frame. However, if you have a small frame, then BMI is too kind and indicates that a person is normal weight when they really have extra body fat. If a person has a large frame, BMI is unkind and indicates that a person is obese when they don't have extra body fat. In my experience, only about a third of the patients I see have a medium frame. That means, in my experience, that BMI can't accurately tell me if about two-thirds of my new weight-loss patients are truly obese or just overweight. Additional problems with BMI are that as older adults begin losing height due to increased curvature of the spine and compression of vertebra and disks of the spine, then BMI overestimates their fat mass. Also, as older people lose muscle mass, BMI underestimates their fat mass. BMI doesn't take into account abdominal fat, leading a thin male body builder with a heavy frame to have the same BMI as an overweight male with a small frame and a potbelly. For these reasons, I don't use BMI much in my weight-loss practice to determine my patients' ideal weight range and the weight at which they are obese.

Is it okay for people to weigh a little more as they age? We've all heard that it is okay to gain a little weight throughout your life. However, the answer is no, it is not okay to gain weight into the overweight range of body weight as you age. People in the overweight range have increases in many of the same risks obese people face, which can lead to huge health-care cost increases as well as increases in weight-related diseases and complications.

The ideal weight range for children is calculated differently than for adults. Using a child's age, sex, and height, a BMI is calculated and is then converted to a percentile to help determine where the child's weight stands in comparison to other children of the same age, sex, and height. Children in the 85th to 94th percentile range are overweight, and children who are in the 95th or greater percentile range are obese. Again, BMI can be less accurate in children with small and large frames. The same measurement techniques discussed above for adults can be used in children and teens to determine lean body mass and fat mass. The method for estimating the ideal weight range in Appendix 1 can't be used for children under 18.

An accurate assessment of a person's ideal weight range can be helpful in a number of ways. It can more accurately diagnose a person's weight as normal, overweight, and obese, which has implications for whether the person should begin efforts to lose weight and if they could be appropriately treated with medication to help with weight loss. In my weight-loss practice, I prefer to use the quick and easy-to-perform method that is presented in Appendix 1, and then to use DEXA only if the accuracy of the estimation is in question and if it would affect my decision to have the patient start a diet or not.

CHAPTER 9

WHEN SHOULD TREATMENT FOR OBESITY BEGIN?

THE SIMPLE ANSWER to this question is to start treatment as soon as a person gains 10 to 20 pounds of extra body weight for the first time in their life, no matter their age. If a young adult, or adult-sized child, has gained 20 pounds over their ideal weight, then they are most certainly not a Muse Satiety Type 1, and they will likely struggle with slowly increasing body weight for their whole life. The same applies to smaller children who have gained 10 more pounds over their ideal weight.

In this era of highly palatable, addictive, and ever-present snacks, and larger portions of highly palatable food at meals, Muse Satiety Type 4s and 5s will become overweight at a younger age as compared to previous decades, with many developing obesity as toddlers. For children under 12 years of age that are members of Muse Satiety Types 4 and 5 and have gained 10 pounds or more over their ideal weight, careful attention to a lower-calorie diet is critical and can be quite successful, since children under 12 typically don't prepare food for themselves and likely obey family rules about not opening the fridge and pantry to snack between meals. If children under 12 have a weight above the 95th percentile, medication might be considered to prevent additional weight gain. It is important to stress that no prescription weight-loss medication is approved by the FDA for treatment of children under age 12, so the younger child's medical provider will need to determine the appropriateness of the use of off-label medication to prevent long-term weight gain. Medication for weight loss and weight maintenance for children who are overweight and obese will be discussed in greater detail in Chapter 10.

For adults and children 12 and over that are members of Muse Satiety Types 4 and 5, maintenance therapy with medication should be started as soon as difficulty with weight maintenance appears. Deciding to try diet and exercise as the only treatment modality for these individuals is often futile, especially for teens. These individuals often have already gained 20 pounds and have done so at an early age. They never will be able to sense that they are full at the exact moment they have consumed enough calories to meet their calorie needs at meals and they will eat past that point at every meal. Additional weight gain is inevitable. Please help them! Don't assume that they will remain thin if they just exercise and diet. It is true that the use of weight-loss medications for long-term weight maintenance is not commonly recommended by many medical providers. The medications that are used by obesity specialists for weight maintenance are often not FDA approved for weight maintenance and often have to be prescribed off-label.

As I write this chapter, I am very aware that I am blazing new ground by recommending treatment of individuals to prevent obesity before they ever become obese for the first time. Sure, we could wait until these individuals become obese, and then start treatment to lose the weight they have gained, followed by treatment for weight maintenance. But the average person struggles to lose more than 20-30 pounds on any diet, which then often leaves the person still overweight, if not still obese. If members of Muse Satiety Type 4 and 5 have nearly a 100% chance of becoming obese and are already over halfway to becoming obese, or are above a BMI of 25, then I recommend starting medication for weight maintenance for them now. I don't have a study to support this recommendation. But do I believe that people who are members of Muse Satiety Types 4 and 5 that start and continue medication for weight maintenance early in life at the first sign of a significant weight gain will be significantly thinner long term than their counterparts.

It is well-known that children who began dieting early in life have been found to be heavier than other children who didn't diet at an early age (Field A. , 2003) (Neumark-Sztainer, 2007). The conclusion of some researchers has been that we should teach children not to diet so that they would remain thin like their counterparts. I believe that these researchers have misunderstood the disease of Muse's Satietopathy. Most likely, most of their subjects that were dieting as children were members of Muse Satiety Types 4 and 5 that were already gaining weight as children and were trying to correct the problem. We owe it to our children who are Muse Satiety Type 4s and Type 5s to allow them to reach adulthood without being obese, since obesity in our children has so many negative physical and social ramifications. We also owe it to the young adults in society that are Muse Type 4s and Type 5s to increase access to medication to prevent weight gain over the years.

The same message applies to children and adults who are members of Muse Satiety Types 2 and 3 that have gained 20 pounds or more, or are at a BMI above 25, although treatment with medication doesn't need to be started as early and not with the same urgency. Despite the unfavorable food environment that we live in, most members of Muse Satiety Types 2 and 3 don't start gaining weight as children or teens, since at those younger ages they feel full at meals and leave the table. Once a member of Muse Satiety Types 2 or 3 has gained 20 pounds in either childhood or adulthood, or their BMI is above 25, they should lose the weight with a diet and they should try to diet and exercise for maintenance. If that fails, they should then be considered by their medical provider for treatment with medication to prevent additional weight gain.

I envision a future when individuals who have been identified as members of Muse Satiety Types 2 to 5 will be treated at the first sign of difficulty maintaining weight with medication and exercise to help to keep them from gaining weight. A huge amount of work needs to be done between now and then to produce more effective and better tolerated medications, as well as better education for medical providers, parents, and individuals on the importance of early and aggressive treatment of weight gain to prevent subsequent obesity.

CHAPTER 10
WHAT IS THE BEST WAY TO LOSE WEIGHT?

THE SIMPLE ANSWER to this frequently asked question is that all diets work as long as they keep calories burned per day at a greater level than calories consumed per day. Even the craziest and zaniest diets can result in significant weight loss, at least for a short time. However, when the enemies of all diets rear their ugly heads—namely hunger, fatigue, and boredom—then diet efforts weaken, and the weight loss stops. I call this time limit that each of us have on how much suffering we can tolerate before giving up on a diet our "diet attention span."

In studies of individuals who have been successful at weight loss, the methods that each individual used to lose weight have varied significantly (Wien, 2003). There are a lot of diets because no one diet fits everyone's food preferences, food environments, eating triggers, social environments, food addictions, and Muse Satiety Types. At the same time, there is a small list of diets that have distinguished themselves from the rest by having three important characteristics. These characteristics are that these diets are safer, cost less per pound lost, and are effective for a larger group of participants. My goal in this chapter is to point out the diets that best embody these three traits. As an obesity specialist with decades of experience, I have my favorites because they meet these characteristics. Although it is not my intent to discredit any diet besides my favorites, I will also mention the diets that in my opinion should be avoided due to their being unsafe. I will also try to address the key questions that dieters ask as they begin a diet, namely:

1. Is the average weight loss on this diet enough to help me meet my weight-loss goals?

2. How long will it take on this diet to lose to my goal weight?

3. Will I be hungry on this diet?

4. Will I be tired on this diet?

5. Does the food I am allowed to eat on this diet taste good?

6. Will this diet require more time than I have available? (in support meetings and in food preparation)

7. What are the side effects of this diet?

8. Can I afford this diet?

Getting answers to these questions, especially from research studies about individual diets, can range from difficult to almost impossible. That is because research on diets in humans is significantly biased toward the beliefs of the researchers. If a researcher who believes in a certain diet sets out to prove that the diet is superior to other diets, then his research will be biased in favor of the diet he believes in. If another researcher sets out to prove that the same diet is inferior to other diets, then his research will be biased against the diet he believes is inferior to other diets. This bias even happens in randomized controlled trials. This bias results in widely different ranges of weight lost in studies on the same diet.

Comparing weight-loss results from studies is fraught with inaccuracy. We all wish that we had multiple reliable studies that have compared each of the diets and medications listed in the rest of this chapter head to head against each other. Sadly, we just don't have those studies. Instead, we are left to compare results from studies done at different research sites, on different populations, with different inclusion and exclusion criteria for the studies, with different diet and exercise recommendations, and with different result-reporting methods.

In regard to the different result-reporting methods, it is important to know that results from some weight-loss studies have been reported by using completer results and that other weight-loss studies have been reported as intent-to-treat last-observation-carried-forward (ITT-LOCF) results. Completer results refer to the weight-loss results of only the patients who completed the study, no matter how many patients dropped out of the study before it was completed. ITT-LOCF results refer to weight-loss results of all the subjects that started the study, whether they dropped out before the end of the study or not. The final weight of the patients who dropped out early is inferred from the last measured weight of a subject at the study clinic, or the last observation carried forward. Completer results from weight-loss studies are always higher than ITT-LOCF results. The biggest reason for this difference is because the dropout rate for most weight-loss trials runs about 50%. In the figures below, I have listed percentages of weight lost as completer or ITT-LOCF study results when they are available. For comparison purposes within a single figure, I have reduced completer study results by an estimated 40% in an effort to make them somewhat comparable to the ITT-LOCF study results. For comparison of completer results and ITT-LOCF results between two different figures, I recommend reducing the completer results by about 40% in an effort to make the results somewhat comparable.

A question that I am often asked is what foods are best to eat while losing weight. While every proponent of every diet will go on forever on why the food on their diet is best, I would like to cut through it all and say the following: The best food to consume while on a diet is heart-healthy food. That is because almost half of us will ultimately die from heart disease. In addition, since the other half of us will die from cancer, the very diets that are heart healthy are also good for cancer prevention. What are the foods that are the healthiest for your heart and also help to prevent cancer? They are the foods used in the Mediterranean diet, a generic blend of the diets from multiple Mediterranean countries that has been proven to reduce cardiovascular risk and cancer risk. The Mediterranean diet is defined as a diet that is high in starchy vegetables, whole grains, beans, nuts, seeds, and whole fruits. Olive oil is the main source of fat. The diet contains low to moderate amounts of protein from fish, poultry, and dairy, with only rare consumption of red meat (Mediterranean Diet, 2018). Every effort should be made by dieters to be sure that foods that they eat while dieting are from the Mediterranean diet. If a dieter is looking for recipes that are compliant with the Mediterranean diet, there are many cookbooks online that can be found by searching "Mediterranean diet."

As I discuss various dietary options below, I want to stress that the list is not all inclusive and that the observations that I make are based on training I have received from the Obesity Medicine Association, my review of the medical literature, my experience as an obesity medicine specialist, and my personal weight-loss experience. I will present the many available diets in the following main categories: Self-directed diets, do-it-yourself commercial diets, supervised diets by a non-medical provider, and supervised diets by a medical provider. Weight-loss surgery will be discussed in Chapter 16.

SELF-DIRECTED DIETS

A self-directed diet is a diet where the dieter follows a weight-loss plan of their choosing with little or no outside support. Use of support groups in person or online is uncommon. Exercise is often part of this weight-loss effort, but a personal trainer is most often not used. Many who do this kind of diet, and there are many, succeed at losing for only a few months, at which time increasing hunger from rising ghrelin levels and worsening fatigue from dropping metabolism result first in a plateau in weight loss and then a regain of most of the weight that was lost. As a word of caution, no self-directed diet should ever supply less than 1,000 calories per day, due to the risk of life-threatening mineral deficiencies. I will discuss the following general categories of self-directed diets as are noted in Figure 4: Eating less per day, food-elimination diets, calorie-counting diets, single-food diets, intermittent diets, and intermittent fasting.

Self-Directed Diets	Eating Less Per Day	Food-Elimination Diets	Calorie-Counting Diets	Single-Food Diets	Intermittent Diets	Intermittent Fasting	Colon Cleansing Diets
Average weight loss in 6 months (pounds) (completers)	8	18	20		?	15	
Cost to participate for 6 months (dollars)	$0	$0	$0		$0	$0	
Estimated cost of food per month above usual cost (dollars)	$0	$200	$0	Not Recommend	$0	$0	Not Recommend
Estimated time required per week in meetings and meal preparation (hours)	0	0-4	0		0	0	
Helps to reduce hunger while dieting	No	No	No		No	No	
Helps to reduce fatigue while dieting	No	No	No		No	No	

Figure 4 - Self-Directed Diets

Eating Less Per Day

This is the no-frills kind of dieting where an individual attempts to lose weight on their own, with minimal help from others and without medication. This is the most common diet and all but the thinnest of adult humans have tried this type of diet by determining to "eat less," even if just for a few days or weeks. Calories are not counted. Examples of what patients have told me they have done in the past to lose weight by this type of diet are to skip breakfast, to not eat after 5 p.m., to cut back on sweets, to stop taking seconds at meals and to just eat less food in general. Weight loss on this type of diet averages about eight pounds six months for completers (Painter, 2017) and three pounds in six months for the ITT-LOCF results (Hartmann-Boyce, 2015). The ITT-LOCF is lower due to the high dropout rate in most weight-loss studies. I know that this is a discouraging small amount of weight loss for both methods of study analysis. The results of these studies include study participants that try harder and lose more than the average and others that don't try very hard and lose little or nothing. Some subjects might even gain weight while on a weight-loss study. For most people who do this type of diet, it doesn't take long to gain back the weight that was lost. This type of dieting is free of cost, doesn't require the purchase of expensive food ingredients and takes no extra time, but it doesn't offer any help with mounting hunger and fatigue caused by weight loss.

Food-Elimination Diets

Food-elimination diets are self-directed diets that prohibit the intake of one or more foods, or food types, in an effort to decrease daily food intake and thereby induce weight loss. Calories are not counted in food-elimination diets. Central to the theme of food-elimination diets is that certain foods, or food groups, make people gain weight, so they should not be consumed. This concept is true to a degree, since highly processed foods—with the fiber removed or destroyed by cooking, and with added fat, salt, sugar, and spices—promote overconsumption (Louzada, 2015).

There are more than a hundred food-elimination diets, and I can't address them all here. Most of these diets are based on a book or website. While there are few that offer online support groups, most often the dieter alone monitors their own compliance and progress. Some of the more popular diets in this category are the original Atkins diet, new Atkins diet, Ornish Diet, Paleo Diet, Wheat-Belly Diet, Real-Food Diet, Acid-Alkaline Diet, and Keto diet. The original Atkins diet eliminated all sugars and grains and promoted the consumption of a high-animal-fat diet with low-glycemic vegetables. The new Atkins diet eliminates all sugars and grains and promotes the consumption of a high-protein diet with low-glycemic vegetables. The

Ornish diet reduces fat intake to no more than 10% of total calories per day; doesn't allow meat, fish, or chicken; and encourages intake of fruits, vegetables, whole grains, and legumes. The Paleo Diet promotes the consumption of a meat-based diet with added fruits and vegetables and the avoidance of all manufactured foods. The Wheat-Belly Diet primarily promotes avoidance of wheat and gluten-containing products, along with reducing sugars. The Real-Food Diet promotes avoidance of all manufactured and processed foods. The Acid-Alkaline Diet promotes the avoidance of acidic foods, such as meats, most grains, and dairy. The Keto diet in all its varieties is similar the Atkins and Paleo diet, but with a different name.

For completers, or the dieters who don't stop following the diet, the average person on most elimination diets loses 10 to 25 pounds in six months, or a rough average of 18 pounds, depending on the study and the diet studied (Shai, 2008) (Brinkworth, 2009). Elimination diets often involve changing the dieter's foods to a higher intake of protein, which costs more to purchase than carbohydrate, so elimination diets can cost more per month for this reason. Elimination diets are generally safe, especially as long as the dieter never consumes less than 1,000 calories per day without a medical provider's close supervision, and as long as the Mediterranean diet is used to guide the foods that will be consumed on the diet. Elimination diets can take more time in food preparation as well.

Although it is a hot bed of debate, there still is not enough evidence to state with certainty that low-fat diets and low-carbohydrate diets are any different from each other with respect to weight loss at six months. Studies of individuals on low-carbohydrate diets versus low-fat diets have demonstrated that the types of foods eaten on a diet doesn't affect the amount of weight lost on the diet (Hu T. , 2012). Low-carbohydrate diets do have side effects of muscle cramping, flu-like symptoms at the beginning of the diet, diarrhea, and bad breath, and some experts believe that they are harder to stay on long term.

Why is the weight loss not larger on food-elimination diets for most people? There are a number of reasons, with some applying to most dieters and others applying to just some dieters:

1. Mounting hunger and fatigue cause weight loss to cease after the dieter has lost about 10 pounds. This is called a weight-loss plateau. A plateau in a diet occurs when calories consumed equal calories burned. For example, let's take an individual who is burning an average of 2,000 calories per day that starts a food-elimination diet that supplies about 1,200 calories per day. The dieter assumes that he or she will continue to burn 2,000 calories per day throughout the diet, but that is not what happens. Three processes occur during the diet that steadily decrease the individual's daily calorie burn. First, a dieter's basal metabolic rate drops about 200 calories a day while dieting. Second, with increasing fatigue from dieting, non-exercise activity drops by about 200-plus calories per day by the second month. Non-exercise activity is the amount of energy spent completing tasks throughout the day, such as taking out the garbage, moving the lawn, and vacuuming the carpet. Third, with the loss of the first 10 pounds on the diet, calories burned from both non-exercise activity and from exercise drop 100-200 calories per day because the dieter is 10 pounds lighter, and it takes less energy to complete the same activities each day. As a result of these three processes, the amount of daily calories burned by a dieter drops from 2,000 calories per day to about 1,600 calories per day. On the food intake side, increasing hunger as the diet goes along causes the dieter to begin to consume more food. This can happen overtly with outright cheating on the diet, or more subtly with increasing portion sizes of allowed foods. Studies have established that humans underestimate how much they eat per day by 40%-60% (Lansky, 1982) (Lichtman, 1992). The dieter gradually begins consuming about 400 calories more per day, making their daily intake of food about 1,600 calories, which is still less that what the dieter was eating before the start of the diet. The dieter feels like they are still dieting. However, the end result is that the dieter's daily calories burned, and calories consumed, are equal at about 1,600 calories per day. Weight loss stops.

2. Pressure to eat socially increases over time and causes a dieter to begin cheating on the diet, both with larger portion sizes and with eating prohibited foods. Pressure to eat socially comes with many faces. Just some of them are:

    a. The perceived need to dine on a similar meal with clients at work-related events.

    b. The urge to eat meals with family where the dieter's favorite foods are right in front of them.

    c. The insistence by family and friends that the dieter needs to try foods cooked by friends and family or their feelings will be hurt.

    d. Negative talk about the dieter's current diet by family, friends, and co-workers that is designed to get the dieter to break their diet and enjoy eating with them.

3. With no one monitoring the progress of the diet, the dieters commonly cheat while on the diet. I'm not saying this to make people feel guilty. The drive to eat and enjoy food is strong and awfully hard to resist.

4. As the diet progresses, the dieter misses their favorite foods more and more, and often those favorite foods are foods that are addictive to the dieter. Once the dieter restarts consumption of their addictive foods, it is hard to stop.

5. Elimination diets often discourage counting calories, and dieters are encouraged to eat until they are satisfied on the allowed foods. However, the body is designed to feel hungry until it consumes the same number of calories that were burned in the previous day. Within about a month, the initial calorie deficit caused by drastically reducing overall food intake is lost by increasing intake of allowed foods. Since Muse Satiety Type 4s and Type 5s don't have the fullness and loss of savor signals, they are especially prone to overconsume the allowed foods on these diets.

Food-elimination diets will often be less effective than desired because they don't control calorie intake, don't address mounting hunger and fatigue as the diet goes along, don't include support groups, don't require strict journaling, and don't involve monitoring by a third party. Food-elimination diets are more effective for Muse Satiety Type 1s and 2s, are less effective for Muse Satiety Type 3s, and don't work well for Muse Satiety Type 4s and 5s.

Calorie-Counting Diets

With this type of self-directed diet, a person selects a certain number of calories to consume per day and then the person attempts to keep their calorie intake at that level for the length of the diet. Some of these diets combine calorie counting with a food-elimination diet. There are too many of these types of diets to list, but some of the more popular are the MyFitnessPal app, the Lose It! app, the FatSecret app and the South Beach Diet. MyFitnessPal, Lose It!, and FatSecret are websites and smart-phone applications through which a person tracks both calories consumed and calories burned per day. South Beach is a website diet that promotes a low-carbohydrate diet, along with keeping calories between 1,200 to 1,500 per day (What is the South Beach Diet, n.d.).

As an example, let's take a person who burns 2,000 calories per day. Let's assume this individual has selected to aggressively reduce their calorie intake to 1,200 calories per day. The dieter will then have an 800-calorie deficit per day and a 24,000-calorie deficit in 30 days. Using 3,500 calories per pound of fat (Counting Calories: Get Back to Weight-Loss Basics, 2018), that will be about a seven-pound weight loss in 30 days. That sounds small, but most dieters assume they will keep dieting for six and even 12 months and that their diet will result in 42 to 84 pounds lost, respectively. Unfortunately, that is rarely what the dieter will actually lose.

With calorie counting, the first month is often pretty successful, since most humans can stay faithful on a diet for about a month (Kirkova, 2013). Also, the amount of weight lost in the first month is enhanced by water-weight loss. The amount of water weight that a person loses in the first month of dieting can vary widely, from a few pounds to more than 30 pounds, depending on the starting weight of the dieter and on how much fluid the dieter is retaining at the beginning of the diet. However, as the months progress, many of the same processes that undermine the food-elimination diets begin to occur:

1. Mounting hunger that increases cheating, growing fatigue that decreases activity, and a decrease in calories burned per day due falling metabolism results in a weight-loss plateau at around the fourth week.

2. Overconfidence by the dieter in their ability to monitor the calorie content of foods results in increasing portion sizes. Individuals start calorie-counted diets by measuring everything, but within weeks, they tire of measuring everything and begin to eyeball their portion sizes. They assume that what looks like a cup of food is a cup of food, when in reality it is more like one and one-half cups of food.

3. Pressure to eat socially increases over time and causes a dieter to begin cheating on their diet.

4. With no one monitoring the progress of the diet, cheating while on the diet is common.

5. As the diet progresses, the dieter misses their favorite foods more and more, and often those favorite foods are foods that are addictive to the dieter. Once the dieter restarts consumption of these foods, it is hard to stop overeating them, even though they are counting calories.

The average weight lost on a calorie-counting diet is about 20 pounds in six months for completers (Clifton, 2017). Calorie-counting diets are safe, cost free, and have no side effects. The average weight loss on self-directed calorie-counted diets will be smaller than some diets, since they lack support groups, lack monitoring by a third party, and don't address the problems of mounting hunger and fatigue as the diet progresses.

Single-Food Diets

I am not going to address self-directed single-food diets, such as juice diets, grapefruit diets, and protein-only diets, since they are dangerous due to protein deficiency on some of these diets and life-threatening mineral deficiency that can occur on others, if they are continued for more than a few days. In addition, these diets often supply less than 1,000 calories per day, which is also not safe. Since these diets can't be continued safely for very long, the true fat loss is limited and is regained quickly. Any claims that consuming these single-food diets results in more calories burned than on other diets are not supported by good-quality studies. I don't recommend single-food diets for anyone.

Intermittent Diets

I am also not going to spend a lot of time addressing diets that promote dieting for a number of days, returning to normal eating for a number of days, and then repeating until a weight-loss target is reached. Over the years, I've heard about people who would diet on about 1,200 calories per day for five days a week, would return to eating whatever they wanted for the last two days of the week and then would repeat. More recently, I have learned of a small study on males doing the same thing, but for two weeks on 1,200 calories a day, two weeks back to normal eating, and then repeat for seven cycles. The participants did go to the weight-loss research clinic every month to be weighed while they were on the study, so it wasn't a self-directed diet. At the end of seven months, the intermittent dieting group lost 31 pounds, which was about 11 pounds more than the continuous dieting group that they were compared to (Byrne, 2018). The theory is that the two weeks off the diet may convince your body that you're not really starving and that it doesn't need to raise ghrelin and lower metabolism. Further studies are needed to prove this hypothesis. The higher weight loss than expected for a self-directed diet was probably because this wasn't a self-directed diet. It was a medical-provider-supervised diet with monthly follow-up visits. It is also important to point out that the men ate a weight-maintenance diet for the two weeks that they were not dieting. They didn't get to eat whatever they wanted.

I do have reservations about intermittent dieting. A hypothetical person who burns 2,000 calories per day that then diets on 1,200 calories of food per day for five days will build up a 4,000-calorie deficit for the first five days of the week. Muse Satiety Type 1s, 2s, and 3s can't overeat as easily at the meals on the next two diet-holiday days, due to feeling full and/or feeling nausea if they attempt to overeat. This kind of diet probably works well for them. However, for the Muse Satiety Type 4s and 5s, the two days of diet holiday each week are enough time to completely eat back all of the 4,000-calorie deficit that was generated for the five days of dieting earlier in the week, and even more.

In my opinion, intermittent diets just don't work well for Muse Satiety Types 4 and 5. However, these diets are safe, cost free, and side-effect free.

Intermittent Fasting

Intermittent fasting has been around for a long time. It has been recently revived as a "new" way to lose weight. The idea behind intermittent fasting is to consume 0% to 25% of a person's usual calorie intake for a time period, then eat in an unrestricted fashion for a time period and then repeat until weight-loss goals are achieved. There are three main types of intermittent fasting (Stockman, 2018):

1. Alternative day fasting, where a person consumes less than 25% of their energy needs for one day, feasts for one day, and then repeats.

2. Time-restricted fasting, where a person eats only during certain time periods each day, such as only eating between 8 a.m. and 5 p.m. each day.

3. Periodic fasting, where a person completely fasts for 24 hours once or twice a week.

There is insufficient evidence that any of these three types of intermittent fasting causes more weight loss or is better tolerated than the others.

Some studies have shown slightly greater weight loss with intermittent fasting versus reduced calorie diets, but others have not. Some studies have shown that patients don't tolerate intermittent-fasting diets as well as calorie-counted diets (Trepanowski, 2017) (Stockman, 2018). All these studies were done with frequent follow-ups at the research clinics, which makes it hard to apply these findings to people doing intermittent fasting on their own without seeing a medical provider. Plus, the studies could have been biased due to the researchers and investigators knowing which group each subject was in. Intermittent fasting is safe, side-effect free, and cost free. The average weight loss is about 15 pounds in six months (Trepanowski, 2017).

In my opinion, intermittent fasting doesn't work well for members of Muse Satiety Types 4 and 5, since they can eat so much on the non-fasting days.

Colon Cleansing Diets

I'm not going to address the diets that use colon cleansing. There is no body fat lost with cleaning out the colon, whether by natural laxatives or by doing enemas. Any weight that is lost is related to temporarily cleaning out the stool from the colon, to body-fluid loss related to the enemas, and to the severe food-elimination diets or single-food diets that are often prescribed with the colon cleansing. I don't recommend any self-directed diet that severely limits intake of most foods, such as eating fruit only for days to weeks, due to the risk of protein-calorie malnutrition and the risk of dangerous electrolyte imbalance. There is also the rare possibility of perforation of the colon if enemas are part of the colon cleansing.

Most self-directed diets are safe, side-effect free, and inexpensive, but don't result in a lot of weight loss for the average person. The weight-loss numbers in Figure 4 are all based on completer study results and should be reduced by about 40% before comparing them to other diets that are reported with ITT-LOCF results that I will discuss later in this chapter. Self-directed diets don't help with the increasing hunger and fatigue that worsen as weight is lost. They don't provide help with long-term weight maintenance.

DO-IT-YOURSELF COMMERCIAL DIETS

Do-it-yourself commercial diets are where commercial products are consumed along with a diet. The types of diets in this category, as listed in Figure 5, are herbal supplement diets and Nutrisystem.

Do-It-Yourself Commercial Diets	Herbal supplement diets	Nutrisystem
Average weight loss in 6 months (pounds) (completers)		12
Average cost to participate for 6 months (dollars)		$0
Estimated cost of food per month (dollars)	Not Recommend	$300
Estimated time required per week in meetings and meal preparation (hours)		0
Helps to reduce hunger while dieting		No
Helps to reduce fatigue while dieting		No

Figure 5 - Do-It-Yourself Commercial Diets

Herbal supplement diets

This is such a frustrating area of weight-loss medicine to discuss. That is because, in my opinion, there isn't a segment of the medical industry that is as corrupt and as dishonest as the herbal supplement industry. Multiple recent studies have indicated that only 15% to 25% of bottles of herbal supplements available in pharmacies and online contain what is supposed to be in them per the label on the bottle. About another 50% of the bottles of herbal supplements available in pharmacies and online contain lesser quantities of the ingredients listed on the label, and they are contaminated with plants and chemicals that are not listed on the label. Up to 25% of the bottles of herbal supplements contain nothing that is listed on the label and contain only plants and chemicals that are not listed on the label. Interestingly, some of the plant contaminants include asparagus, rice, pea, alfalfa, echinacea, and houseplants. Some of the chemical contaminants include dangerous levels of heavy metals and pesticides. Additionally, as many as half of all the herbal products in pharmacies and online illegally contain prescription medications from other countries, many of which are not approved by the FDA and are considered to be dangerous. The problem with the contamination of herbal products is worse for weight-loss herbal products. Up to 80% of herbal weight-loss medications in pharmacies and online contain one or more prescription weight-loss medications, many which have been banned in US by the FDA due to dangerous side effects (Newmaster, 2013) (Schneiderman, 2015) (Tucker, 2018). How can this happen you might ask? The answer is complex:

1. Herbal products are protected from direct FDA oversight due to the Dietary Supplement Health and Education Act (DSHEA) of 1994. As long as herbal products have the boxed statement somewhere on the bottle, "These statements have not been evaluated by the Food & Drug Administration. This product is not intended to diagnose, treat, cure or prevent any disease." (FDA, 2005), then the herbal company can combine as many herbs they want in the bottle and make any general health claim that they desire about the herbal product. The way I understand it, herbal products are considered by the government to be like fruits and vegetables. And yet, you can request the produce person in the grocery store to cut open fruits and vegetables to see if they are really what they say they are. But, when you have a capsule or tablet of an herbal product in your hand, you have no way of knowing what is in the capsule or tablet. The FDA can't do a lot to protect you due to the DSHEA, unless the herbal product is known to harm humans, or unless the herbal product contains generic prescription medications, which is a common occurrence. The FDA can then issue a safety warning, but

most products remain in the market after FDA warnings. For the most potentially dangerous herbal supplements, the FDA can issue a Class I recall and take the drug off the market (Recalls Background and Definitions, 2014). Even when the FDA forces a product off of the market that contains dangerous herbs or generic prescription medications, the product often just makes its way back to the market under a different name (Avigan, 2016). A recent study indicated that 30% of the herbal products containing potentially dangerous ingredients that have been given FDA Class 1 recalls are still on the market (Starr, 2015).

2. Most of the individual components of herbal products are grown and processed overseas. As far as I know, there is no US government agency that is regularly inspecting the fields and factories where these products are being grown and prepared for shipment to the US. With no one watching, this must be where most of the dishonesty is occurring. The products are watered down with, adulterated with, or completely replaced with other ingredients. Illegal generic prescription medications are added to increase sales by increasing the effectiveness of the product. In virtually every therapeutic area where there is an herbal product with a supposed medicinal effect, there is a prescription drug that is more efficacious. Many of those prescription drugs are very inexpensive, especially when bought in bulk. If you're a dishonest person, then why not increase sales by adding a few penny's worth of a generic prescription medication to enhance the medicinal effects as your herbal ingredient.

3. The US companies that buy the ingredients for their herbal products are most often not required to check the purity of the components of the products they sell. It's a difficult and expensive task to set up the laboratories to test every batch of ingredients coming in from all over the world for purity. Each batch of flower, root, stem, or leaf from a single plant can have dozens of different chemicals in it, and the levels of each of those chemicals can vary from season to season, from location to location, from wet year to dry year, by time of harvest,

etc. The process to check for the presence of the desired chemicals and the absence of undesired contaminants is very involved and includes needing to remove the chemicals from the herbal products without destroying them, which can require multiple steps and a number of solvents. Then, the dissolved chemicals are run through large columns of ionized resin to slow down the flow of some of the chemicals through the column and allow others to proceed through the column more quickly. The fluid exiting the columns drips into test tubes in a large rotating rack, with each test tube collecting a half ounce or so of the fluid. Then, each test tube is analyzed by special machinery to see if the chemicals that are supposed to be there are there. Again, this would have to be done for every shipment of each ingredient in the US company's herbal product. Many of the herbal products sold in the US have 10-30 different ingredients. Needless to say, the US manufacturers are not checking for confirmation and purity of the samples they receive, especially when they are most often not required to do so.

If the gross lack of purity of herbal products is not bad enough, the lack of proof for the claims made by herbal products is just as bad of a problem. If an herbal product is touted to treat symptoms and it really doesn't, then it doesn't really matter if it is pure or not. How did we ever get to the point that products can be sold in a pharmacy that have never been proven adequately to have the medicinal properties that they claim to have? Never mind the disclaimer label on the back that says, "These statements have not been evaluated by the Food and Drug Administration. This product is not intended to diagnose, treat, cure, or prevent any disease." No one even notices that label anymore. At least, my patients don't. How did we end up with herbal-product manufacturers making general health claims about their products that have not been proven?

4. The government passed the DSHEA, which largely protected herbal products from FDA oversight. The herbal manufacturers were not required to prove the general health claims on their bottles and in

their websites. To me, this sounds very much like the US pharmaceutical industry before the FDA was created.

5. Many of the herbal products in the US are touted as having been proven to work in clinical research studies. However, careful analysis of the supposed studies often results in finding that there were no studies, poorly done studies designed to show the product in question in a good light, and/or studies cherry-picked from a group of studies with a mix of positive and negative results because they showed the product in question in a good light. It's hard to believe that companies would say there are studies that prove their products work, when in fact there are none that are scientifically sound. For example, a manufacturer of an antioxidant might have a study that shows that their product is an antioxidant in a chemical reaction in a petri dish, which might be true, but virtually all well-done studies on all antioxidants have failed to show that they reduce heart attacks. Yet, the label on the product will state it is for heart health. Studies can be poorly done in so many ways, such as not using a placebo group, making studies short so that the placebo effect of the herbal product is still high when the study ends, excluding patients that might show the product in a bad light, and bias entering into the study due to an inability to keep the study staff and study subjects from knowing who is and is not on the study drug. Cherry-picking of study results can occur when a company starts multiple studies on a product and then only publishes the one that shows their product in the best light.

6. There is big money in the herbal industry. US citizens spend more than $12 billion a year on herbal products, including herbal weight-loss products (HCCIH, 2017). Since the FDA is prevented from forcing the herbal industry to prove its general health claims, the scene is ripe for advertising that lacks integrity. Big name stars and famous doctors promote the general health benefits of herbal products. People innocently believe what they say and buy the products. Testimonials are given by paid actors and by individuals who have

had supposed success on the herbal products. And yet, there is little to no proof of the claims. The paid actors jump from product to product as new weight-loss herbal products come along, seeming to completely forget about the products that they touted so convincingly just months earlier. Have raspberry ketones, bitter orange, garcinia cambogia, hoodia, and forskolin been proven to cause clinically significantly greater weight loss than placebo in large properly performed trials? No, they haven't (Dietary Supplements for Weight Loss, 2019).

For all these reasons, I can't recommend any herbal weight-loss product to help with weight loss. And I won't be able to recommend herbal weight-loss products until the makers of these products are forced to prove their product's efficacy with the same degree of precision that the FDA requires for prescription medications. I am not alone in calling on the US government to change the DSHEA to protect the US consumer from unscrupulous efficacy claims, faulty supporting research, and significant problems with product purity in the herbal industry.

Nutrisystem

Nutrisystem is a modestly effective diet program. Participants consume low-glycemic food comprised of delivered meals and grocery food purchased by the participant. Various menu plans exist that provide between 1,300 and 1,500 calories per day, which, if followed perfectly, would result in about six pounds of weight loss per month. Online and phone counseling is provided.

In studies, participants in a Nutrisystem diet lose 7% of their body weight in six months, which would be about 12 pounds for a 200-pound person. The cost per pound lost is about $35 (Lee J. , 2010).

SUPERVISED DIETS – NOT SUPERVISED BY A MEDICAL PROVIDER

This section discusses diets that are supervised by an outside professional or professional company. These diets include, as listed in Figure 6, Weight Watchers (WW) and Jenny Craig.

Supervised Diets – Not Supervised by a Medical Provider	WW© (formerly Weight Watchers©)	Jenny Craig
Average weight loss in 6 months (pounds) (completers)	20	15
Average cost to participate for 6 months (dollars)	$200	$120
Estimated cost of food per month above usual food cost (dollars)	$200	$300
Estimated time required per week in meetings and meal preparation (hours)	8	8
Helps to reduce hunger while dieting	No	No
Helps to reduce fatigue while dieting	No	No

Figure 6 - Supervised Diets - Not Supervised by a Medical Provider

WW© (formerly Weight Watchers©)

WW©, formerly known as Weight Watchers©, has been a valuable tool for weight-loss for many years. The new myWW© plans allow dieters to choose the foods they will eat, either from foods prepared at home or from food purchased from WW©. Foods that might be more difficult to control while dieting, such as fast food, desserts, and treats, are assigned points and the points of those foods are kept under a certain level. Other foods that are not as likely to be overconsumed during a diet, such as vegetables, lean proteins and fruits, are lower in points or point-free. The three levels of myWW© are still mostly based on a point system, which still makes myWW© a cal-orie-counted diet. Weekly support meetings, either online or on-site, are an optional part of the program and add additional cost to the diet. Internet support programs have been shown to result in less weight loss during a diet than face-to-face support programs (Wing R. , 2006).

The newer myWW© diet plan has not been around long enough for a lot of efficacy studies to have been completed. In a study that was funded by WW© and performed by a research group in North Carolina, study partici-pants lost 8% of their body weight in six months. That would be 16 pounds for a person who started at 200 pounds and 24 pounds for a person who started at 300 pounds. The cost of participating in WW© is higher than self-directed diets and ranges from about $20 per month to about $60 per month as of 2019, depending on the support group chosen (Mikstas, 2019). WW© can cost more if the dieter chooses to purchase WW© food. There is no data on long-term weight maintenance for participants in the new WW© diet.

Jenny Craig

Jenny Craig is a modestly effective way of losing weight. Participants attend private counseling sessions with program consultants and consume pre-pack-aged food purchased from a local Jenny Craig office. Online purchasing of the pre-packaged food is available. Participants are given pre-prepared menus to follow that consist of both the food purchased from Jenny Craig and grocery foods.

Participants in the Jenny Craig diet lose about 6% of their body weight in 52 weeks based on ITT-LOCF results, which would be 12 pounds for a 200-pound person and 18 pounds for a 300-pound person (Martin C. , 2010). The cost per pound lost on the program is $54 to $106, depending on the types of foods purchased (Lee J. , 2010).

SUPERVISED DIETS – MEDICAL PROVIDER SUPERVISED

There are two main types of medical-provider-supervised diets that are noted in Figure 7. They are medication-assisted diets and very-low-calorie diets, or VLCDs.

Supervised Diets – Medical-Provider Supervised	Medication-Assisted Diets	Very-Low-Calorie Diets (VLCDs)
Average weight loss in 6 months (pounds) (completers)	30	50
Average cost to participate for 6 months (dollars)[1]	$600	$1,800
Estimated cost of food per month above usual food cost (dollars)	$300	$450
Estimated time required per week in meetings and meal preparation (hours)	0.5	1
Helps to reduce hunger while dieting	Yes	Yes
Helps to reduce fatigue while dieting	Yes	Yes

Figure 7 - Supervised Diets - Medical Provider Supervised

[1]*Cost of medication is not included; see Figure 8 for the monthly costs of different medications.*

Medication-Assisted Diets

Weight-loss medications to assist with dietary compliance have been on the market for more than 50 years. Some have been taken off the market, some have withstood the test of time, and others are new to the market in the recent years. Most of these medications help with reducing savor and are especially helpful when the satiety signal of loss of savor is absent. When savor is reduced, dieters have less urge to snack in between meals, both short and long term. Most weight-loss medications also help with increasing fullness, especially when the satiety signal of feeling fullness is absent, which results in a decrease of food intake at meals. This effect is short lived for most weight-loss medications but can persist long term with some of the weight-loss medications. Finally, some of these weight-loss medications either reduce absorption of fat or cause a loss of glucose in the urine, thereby causing a decrease in the calories available to the body per day, but not an increase in fullness or a loss of savor.

It is important to stress that weight-loss medications that increase fullness and decrease savor aren't very effective for weight loss, unless they are accompanied by a calorie-reduced diet. It is the diet that causes the weight loss. The weight-loss medications simply improve compliance on the diet. Most dieters can last three to six weeks on a diet, and then will reach a weight-loss plateau due to cheating caused by increasing hunger, fatigue, and boredom. With the help of weight-loss medications that increase fullness and decrease savor, most dieters will be compliant on their diets for much longer, resulting in greater weight loss before reaching a diet plateau. This can result in an average of two to three times more weight lost by patients on these medications versus patients dieting without these medications.

I put almost all my medication-assisted diet patients on a diet of 1,000 calories per day. While on this diet, I ask them to also shoot for about 80 grams of healthy protein per day. I don't ask them track carbohydrate intake per day, since studies have not convincingly proved that tracking intake of carbs on top of counting calories adds significant benefit. The use of protein bars and protein shakes is usually needed to be able to get the protein up to 80 grams per day while on a 1,000-calorie-per-day diet. I encourage patients to have about four small mostly-protein meals throughout the day and then to eat a small dinner in the evenings. If patients want to cook food for their diet, I ask them to use the recipes from books on the Mediterranean diet that are available at most bookstores and online. Why do I choose these dietary instructions for my patients?

1. They are simple.

2. I want my patients to lose about 10 pounds a month while they are dieting, which is what an average person who burns 2,000 calories per day will lose per month on a 1,000-calorie-per-day diet.

3. 1,000 calories per day is as low as people can safely go without needing to supplement their diets with prescription potassium and without needing to regularly monitor blood levels of potassium and sodium.

4. The average person will eat about 1,400 calories per day when I tell them to eat 1,000 calories per day, which will result in six pounds of weight lost per month for the average person who burns 2,000 calories per day. That is an acceptable monthly weight loss. If I asked my patients to eat 1,200 calories per day while dieting, then they would consume about 1,600 calories per day, and only lose four pounds a month. Four pounds per month of weight loss is slow enough that most patients get discouraged and quit dieting before reaching their weight-loss goals.

5. Since I know that the average dieter starts to plateau at about three to four months into a diet, then I want my dieters to lose about 10 pounds a month for the first three to four months on the diet until they reach that plateau. That way they will lose at least 30 pounds. That is a meaningfully visible weight loss that my patients can be proud of. Also, a 30-pounds weight loss has many health benefits.

6. Multiple studies have indicated that it is not what you eat that causes weight loss, it is just the calories (Hu T. , 2012) (Sacks F. , 2009). One thousand calories a day of a low-fat diet for six months results in about the same weight loss as 1,000 calories a day of a low-carbohydrate diet.

The average weight loss for a medication-assisted diet in my weight-loss clinic is about 30 pounds in six months. That means that half the dieters will lose more than 30 pounds and half will lose less than 30 pounds. For dieters who need to lose 50 to 100 pounds, a 30-pound weight loss is disappointing from a cosmetic standpoint. However, there are significant health benefits that result from a 30-pound weight loss, such as reductions of blood pressure in patients with high blood pressure, blood sugar in type 2 diabetes, knee pain in patients with knee arthritis, and sleep apnea.

As I present the way that I use prescription weight-loss medications in my practice, I will at times describe the uses of prescription medications that are off-label, or, in other words, not indicated in the FDA-approved package insert for these medications. However, off-label prescribing of medications by medical providers is allowed by the FDA, as long as the medical provider bases their decision to prescribe off-label on reliable study data, results of studies on other similar medications, guidelines for the use of the medications published by a specialty society, positive experience of the provider's colleagues with the medications, and positive personal experience with the medications. When prescribing off-label, the provider must also assess the risk-benefit ratio of prescribing off-label medications for each individual patient. The use of weight-loss medications as discussed below is the way that I use weight-loss medications in my practice and are, to the best of my knowledge, in accordance with the guidelines of the Obesity Medicine Association (OMA). The ways that I use weight-loss medications in my office are suggestions that other providers might consider following, although each provider needs to determine for themselves what medications they will prescribe off-label and to whom and how they will prescribe them. If a patient is not satisfied with the way that their provider is practicing weight-loss medication, they might consider searching for another local provider that is a member of the OMA at obesitymedicine.org.

No prescription weight-loss medication should be used by females when there is any chance of pregnancy. Female patients should see their gynecologic provider to ensure they are adequately preventing pregnancy before starting any prescription weight-loss medication. If pregnancy is suspected at any time while taking a weight-loss medication, then the prescription or over-the-counter weight-loss medication should be stopped immediately, and the patient should consult with both their weight-loss provider and their gynecologic provider as soon as possible.

The prescription medications that weight-loss providers use to help patients lose weight are generally safe, but each does have risks. The patient and the prescribing provider should consider all the risks and benefits of prescribing weight-loss medications for that patient and then make a decision unique to that patient as to whether the medications discussed below are appropriate. On one hand, the benefit of weight loss from the use of these medications is often life changing and health improving. On the other hand, care must be taken to keep adverse side effects to as low of a level as possible. Multiple weight-loss medications have been removed from the market by the FDA in the US in the past 30 years for the harm they were causing some patients, despite their benefits for other patients. Fenfluramine, from the fen-phen combination, was removed from the market in 1997 for heart valve damage. Phenylpropanolamine, a main ingredient in some over-the-counter weight-loss medications, was removed in 2000 due to an association with intracranial hemorrhage. Ephedrine-containing products were removed in 2004 due to cardiovascular concerns. Sibutramine (Meridia) was removed from the market in 2010 due to concern for cardiovascular events (Steffen, 2012). Lorcaserin (Belviq, Belviq XR) was removed from the market in 2020 due to concern for an increased risk of various cancers. I am grateful that the FDA is vigilant in allowing carefully studied and relatively safe medications on the market and in removing those medications that are found, after approval, not to be safe from the market.

Finally, I want to stress now, and throughout this book, that weight-loss medications are effective for both weight loss and long-term weight maintenance. I will discuss their benefit for long-term weight maintenance later in this book.

Below are presented the different single-agent weight-loss medications and weight-loss-medication combinations that are available in the US as of the publication of this book. The single-agent weight-loss medications are presented in Figure 8 below and the combination weight-loss medications are presented in Figure 9.

Single-Agent Weight-Loss Medications

Single-Agent Weight-Loss Medication Comparison	Phentermine	Topiramate	Liraglutide	Orlistat, Rx/OTC	Bupropion	Canagliflozin	Zonisamide	Metformin	Plenity
Percent weight loss in 12 months (ITT-LOCF results)	9[1]	7	9	4/4[2]	5	4	7	3	7
Average weight loss in 12 months for a 250-pound person (pounds)	23	18	24	10/10	13	10	18	8	18
Average cost per month	$23	$11	$1,288	$760/$60	$28	$576	$33	$10	$100
Drop-out rate due to side effects in studies	14%	21%	10%	9%/9%[2]	7%	3%	6%	12%	4%
Helps to reduce hunger while dieting	Yes	Yes	Yes	No	Yes	No	Yes	No	No
Helps to reduce fatigue while dieting	Yes	No	No	No	No	No	No	No	No

Figure 8 - Single-Agent Weight-Loss Medication Comparison

[1]*Completer data that has been reduced by 40% to make the result somewhat comparable to the other studies in this figure that were all reported using ITT-LOCF results*
[2]*Percent weight lost and dropout rate on the OTC dose was presumed to be similar to the Rx dose*

As previously mentioned, comparing weight-loss results from use of these medications from studies is fraught with inaccuracy. I wish again that we had multiple studies comparing each of the single-agent medications listed above against each other, head to head. Sadly, we just don't have those studies. All of the weight-loss percentages in Figure 8 are reported as ITT-LOCF, which is always lower than the weight-loss percentages of only the patients who completed each study. ITT-LOCF results are used to give a better understanding on what happens weight-loss-wise with all the study participants and not just those who complete the study.

In Figure 8, the average weight loss for a 250-pound person was obtained by taking the percent weight lost at 12 months from the package insert, from available studies and from my clinical experience and then multiplying that times 250 pounds. When the only data I could find was from studies that were shorter than one year, then that data was used in place of one-year data. This is a reasonable option since most weight loss in studies occurs in the first six months of the study with only a small amount of additional weight loss occurring between the sixth and twelfth months. The average cost for each medication was obtained from online resources as of January 2020 and is an estimation at best. The prices listed are after the use of manufacturer coupon cards, if available. Some of the medications can be covered by insurance, if a person has insurance, and could cost less per month than the prices I have listed. I didn't list the cost of brand-name combination medications when there were separate generic medications available; I instead listed the combined cost of the separate generic components in the doses that I prescribe in my clinic.

When I prescribe any of the medications I will present below, I see my patients monthly for follow-up visits. In my experience, monthly visits are needed during weight loss in order for patients to successfully reach their weight-loss goals. Follow-up visits for weight-loss patients in my office that occur less than once a month are associated with less weight lost from visit to visit. If a patient has been dieting and using any of the medications presented below for a month and has not lost weight, I carefully evaluate the patient's reported diet to be certain that the patient is adhering to the prescribed diet. Consideration is given for increasing the dose of the current weight-loss medication or adding a second weight-loss medication in an attempt to improve weight loss. If a patient has been using any of the weight-loss medications below for more than 12 weeks and has not lost weight, then the medication(s) should be stopped, and consideration should be given to starting a trial of a different weight-loss medication.

Phentermine

In this section, I will discuss the prescription stimulant weight-loss medication phentermine (Adipex). Phentermine belongs to a class of adrenaline-like medications called sympathomimetics. There are three other medications in this class, diethylpropion (Tenuate), benzphetamine (Didrex), and phendimetrazine (Bontril). Since many people ask, these medications are not amphetamines. They are similar in effect, generic, inexpensive, and are controlled medications per the Controlled Substances Act in the US. Phentermine and diethylpropion are Schedule IV drugs, and benzphetamine and phendimetrazine are Schedule III drugs. State laws vary on the allowed use of these medications, with some states not allowing the prescribing of benzphetamine and phendimetrazine at all, and other states limiting the prescribing of these four weight-loss medications to no more than 30 pills in 60 days.

Since these four medications are similar in effect and in side effects, since phentermine is the most widely used of the four, and since I have the most experience with phentermine, I will continue by discussing only phentermine. Further information on the other three medications can be found in their FDA-approved package inserts and can be had by discussion with medical providers that are experienced with prescribing these medications.

In discussing the use of phentermine for weight loss and weight maintenance, I want to be clear again that what I am discussing is based on my personal experience with prescribing phentermine to my patients, on the FDA-approved package insert and on the guidelines of the OMA. My discussion of how I prescribe phentermine to my patients is meant to be advice only and is not meant to replace or supplant the FDA-approved package insert, the OMA guidelines, and the advice of a patient's prescribing providers.

It is important to know that phentermine is only approved by the FDA for weight loss for a "few weeks" per its package insert (Adipex-P, 1959). Many medical providers erroneously think that the package insert for phentermine allows use for three months. The FDA has approved a phentermine-containing drug, Qsymia, for "chronic weight management" in appropriate patients (Qsymia, Full Prescribing Information, n.d.), with no time limit and with no upper age limit. The FDA's approval of Qsymia in 2012 for "chronic weight management" has given me further confidence in prescribing single-agent off-label phentermine for longer than a few weeks.

As a single agent, generic phentermine comes in 15 and 30 mg capsules, and in 37.5 mg tablets. While the phentermine 30 mg capsules and the 37.5 mg tablets are considered to work about the same for weight loss, most of my patients prefer the 37.5 mg tablet.

Phentermine is taken once a day in the morning, about one to four hours after arising. Most patients are faster metabolizers of phentermine, in my opinion, and find that phentermine doesn't suppress their appetite long enough into the evening if they take it too early in the day. I have these patients move the phentermine dosing time to 10 a.m. for patients who arise at 7 a.m. and sometimes as late as 1 p.m., so that they won't be hungry in the evenings. If phentermine is taken too late in the day, it can cause insomnia. For some patients who are slower metabolizers of phentermine, the 7 a.m. dosing time is best, because if it is taken later, then these patients have trouble sleeping. Some patients find that taking a half a phentermine in the morning upon arising and another half about four hours later works best for them.

Phentermine mainly works by causing a reduction in savor, or the pleasure of eating. In my practice, I have observed that for the first three weeks or so, it also increases a sense of fullness at mealtimes, making it easier for a dieter to eat less at meals because they feel full sooner. Unfortunately, this second effect fades after about three weeks and the dieter can then easily eat a full meal. If the dieter is not carefully following a calorie-restricted diet, then their weight loss can plateau as mealtime portions increase. On the other hand, if a patient is following a calorie-restricted diet and can grit their teeth a little and keep on going with the diet, they will continue to lose weight. It will be a little harder each month as the effects of the phentermine fade but will be much easier than trying to comply with a diet without the phentermine. In most studies of weight loss with the use of phentermine, the weight loss for the average patient plateaus at about the sixth month.

Phentermine's other effect of reducing savor leads to reduced snacking and eating in between meals. This effect fades a little over time, but not to the point where the effect is completely gone. For most patients, this effect will persist for years, which assists patients by helping to prevent weight regain after a diet.

As previously mentioned, phentermine is in the medication class of sympathomimetics, or medications that stimulate the sympathetic nervous system. Adrenaline is an example of a naturally occurring agent that stimulates the sympathetic nervous system. Therefore, phentermine is possibly better understood as being an adrenaline-like medication. Phentermine is thought to work by stimulating receptors on the POMC-CART neuron in the arcuate nucleus of the brain that result in the suppression of appetite.

Phentermine, when used as a single agent in my practice, results in about a 9% weight loss over a six-month period, when used in combination with a 1,000-calorie-per-day diet, with strict journaling of all calories consumed, and with monthly weight-loss visits. There isn't much additional weight loss after the initial six months for most patients. The 9% weight-loss from the use of phentermine would be about 18 pounds for a 200-pound person and 27 pounds for a 300-pound person. This degree of weight loss is roughly similar to what has been reported in two studies, namely 13% (Munro, 1968) and 17.5% (Hendricks, 2011). Both studies were based on completer results and not ITT results, so the ITT results would be about 40% less, by my estimate, mostly due to a dropout rate of about 50% in each trial. In the Munro study, the dropout rate from the most common side effect of phentermine, overstimulation, was 14%.

As the weight-loss effect of a single tablet of phentermine fades, there is a tendency for both the medical provider and patient to desire to try a higher dose of phentermine in an effort to increase weight loss. A study has indicated that there is an increase in weight lost on higher doses of phentermine that were used later in a phentermine-assisted diet. In this study, dieters on 37.5 mg a day of phentermine for three years lost about 10% of their body weight and dieters who ended up on 75 mg of phentermine at the end of their diet lost about 12% of their body weight (Hendricks, 2011). That 2% difference would be an additional four-pound weight loss for a 200-pound person. There were no serious side effects by using phentermine at up to 75 mg per day in this study. For some of my patients, I have increased the dose of phentermine to 56.25 mg per day (1.5 tablets of phentermine 37.5 mg per day) in divided doses and rarely I have increased the dose to 75 mg per day (two tablets of phentermine 37.5 per day) in divided doses. I do recommend that patients on phentermine doses higher than 37.5 mg a day split the dose with the first part of the daily dose being taken upon arising and rest of the daily dose being taken about four hours later, depending on the patient's metabolism of phentermine, as discussed above. I don't recommend phentermine doses higher than 75 mg per day.

Phentermine is helpful for long-term weight maintenance when continued at the same dose that was used for the initial diet. In a five-year study by Dr. Allen Rader on 10,000 patients in his weight-loss clinics indicated that the average patient lost 20 pounds in the first six months on a phentermine-assisted diet, and then had gained back only two pounds of those 20 pounds at the end of five years of phentermine use (Rader, About 2014). For those of us that have dieted and then gained most of it back, repeatedly throughout our lives, the result of this study is astounding.

Some patients who take phentermine have side effects of dry mouth, insomnia, constipation, irritability, impotence, and urinary hesitance. Dry mouth is common and is addressed by drinking more water and by a limited use of sugar-free breath mints. The reason that I say a limited use of sugar-free breath mints is that sugar-free breath mints are often sweetened with sugar alcohols, and sugar alcohols in larger quantities are laxatives and can cause diarrhea. Insomnia is frequent in phentermine users. When a phentermine user is getting less than six and a half hours of sleep a night, I recommend that they first try over-the-counter sleep aids, and then, if they are still not sleeping seven hours per night, they should call their medical provider to discuss other solutions to their insomnia.

Constipation is a less common side effect of phentermine and can be prevented with over-the-counter fiber products. If constipation occurs despite the use of fiber products, it can be treated with over-the-counter laxatives, glycerin suppositories, and enemas. Irritability can occasionally occur in patients who take phentermine. If the irritability is any more than mild, the phentermine should be stopped, and the prescribing medical provider called for advice. With regards to the irritability, I have found a strong correlation between patients who can't tolerate other stimulants (such as decongestants) and patients who may have irritability with phentermine. I most often pre-treat these patients off-label with a low dose of one of the prescription medications from the beta-blocker drug class that doesn't cause fatigue or weight gain. With the help of these beta-blockers, most patients who are otherwise irritable on phentermine can safely tolerate the phentermine and still lose weight.

Impotence and urinary hesitance in males occur less commonly. Urinary hesitance in females on phentermine is rare. When these symptoms occur, and when they are more than mild, the phentermine should be stopped, and the prescribing medical provider called for advice. When my patients have these symptoms, I see them in my office to discuss either changing to another weight-loss medication, or to discuss adding prescription medications to improve urinary flow for both men and women.

The package insert for phentermine lists a number of contraindications to the use of phentermine, which I take very seriously. Phentermine should not be taken by anyone with a history of coronary heart disease, stroke, arrhythmia, congestive heart failure, or uncontrolled hypertension. It shouldn't be used by anyone who has taken a monoamine oxidase inhibitor (such as rasagiline, selegiline, phenelzine, isocarboxazid, or tranylcypromine) in the previous 14 days, has high thyroid, glaucoma, agitation, a history of drug abuse, or is intolerant of stimulant medications. It is important to be aware that the package insert states that rare cases of pulmonary hypertension and leaky heart valves have been reported in phentermine users. These effects are not proven to be caused by phentermine in studies and are based only on case reports to the FDA. See the package insert for the full listing of all contraindications, warnings, and adverse reactions with the use of phenter-mine (Adipex-P, 1959). Again, the final decision to prescribe phentermine off-label to a patient is the responsibility of the prescribing provider and should be made carefully after the provider considers the contents of the package insert, the current regulations of the state where the prescriber is working, and the patient's medical history.

Phentermine is not approved by the FDA to be taken safely during pregnancy, and strict compliance with adequate birth control for female patients is necessary. Adequate birth control must be discussed with the female patient's medical or gynecologic provider before starting phentermine. Phentermine should be stopped immediately if there is ever any suspicion of pregnancy and the patient should contact their gynecologic provider as soon as possible for advice.

Topiramate

The inexpensive generic prescription medication topiramate, also known by its brand name, Topamax, is approved by the FDA for the treatment of partial and grand-mal seizures and for the prevention of migraines. Topiramate is not approved as a single agent by the FDA for weight loss and weight maintenance. However, the FDA has approved a topiramate-containing drug, Qsymia, for the "chronic management of obesity" in appropriate patients (Qsymia, Full Prescribing Information, n.d.). The FDA's approval of Qsymia for "chronic management of obesity" gives me further confidence in prescribing single-agent topiramate off-label for weight loss and weight maintenance.

In discussing the use of topiramate for weight loss and weight maintenance, I want to be clear that what I am discussing is based on my personal experience with prescribing topiramate to my patients, as well as the FDA-approved package insert and on the guidelines of the OMA. My discussion of how I prescribe topiramate to my patients is meant to be advice only and is not meant to replace or supplant the FDA-approved package insert, the OMA guidelines, and the advice of a patient's prescribing provider.

Topiramate comes in 25, 50, 100, and 200 mg tablets. I prescribe topiramate to be taken at night before bed, since it is sedating for most patients. To allow patients to become tolerant of the side effects of topiramate, I start my patients on topiramate at 25 mg at bedtime for a week, then I increase it to 50 mg at bedtime for a week, then 75 mg at bedtime for a week, and then finally to 100 mg at bedtime. I only rarely use topiramate at a dose over 100 mg at bedtime, because higher doses are associated with a higher rate of side effects. However, doses up to 300 mg a day of topiramate have provided a modest additional weight loss over the 100 mg per day dose (Wilding, 2004). Some patients don't tolerate the steadily higher doses of topiramate during the upward taper and should reduce the dose back to the largest dose that they tolerated without any more than mild side effects. At any time that a patient has more than mild side effects, they should stop the topiramate and should call their medical provider immediately, or they should go to an urgent care or ER. In a 60-week study of 1,282 subjects in 2004, the ITT-LOCF weight loss was 7% for the 96 mg per day dose and 9% for the 192 mg per day dose. The dropout rate for adverse events was 21% (Wilding, 2004).

Topiramate is in the medication class of seizure medications. It is not known how topiramate use results in weight loss.

There are no black box warnings or contraindications listed for topiramate in the package insert. Side effects that occur commonly on topiramate are sedation, nausea, mental slowness, short-term memory loss, taste perversion, and tingling of the fingers. If any of these side effects occur and are more than mild, the topiramate should be stopped and the prescribing medical provider should be called as soon as possible. For mild morning sedation, taking the topiramate two hours before bedtime should give more time for the drug to get out of the patient's system before the patient awakens in the morning, and hence resulting in less morning sedation. If the patient's provider choses to do so, prescribing phentermine in the morning with topiramate can help with morning sedation and enhanced appetite suppression.

Nausea with the use of topiramate is dose dependent and is often the cause for a patient's inability to taper all the way up to a dose of 100 mg at bedtime. The nausea usually fades with time, but not always. If the nausea is persistent, the patient should notify their medical provider. Mental slowness and short-term memory loss are also significant problems with topiramate. I have had to write letters requesting to reinstate scholarships and to retry court cases for patients who have had these side effects with topiramate. About half of my patients are unable to tolerate topiramate due to short-term memory loss and cognitive side effects. Lower doses do cause less side effects, but also cause less weight loss. The side effect of numbness in the fingertips is bothersome but is not permanent and goes away as soon as the drug is stopped. It also tends to fade away over time in those who continue taking topiramate. Taste perversion with use of topiramate is easily treated by stopping the foods that don't taste good because of the topiramate.

Less common, but more serious side effects, can occur in patients who take topiramate, such as visual changes, decreased sweating, increased body temperature, increased acid levels in the blood (metabolic acidosis), suicidal thoughts and suicide attempts, changes in mood, depression, significant confusion, difficulty speaking, anxiety, fever, rash, and kidney stones. In case of these side effects, the topiramate should be stopped immediately and the patient should immediately call their medical provider or go to an urgent care/ER. Once a patient has been taking topiramate for more than a few weeks, some medical providers feel it should not be stopped suddenly. Patients should discuss in advance with their medical provider how to stop the topiramate when the time comes to stop it.

The final decision to prescribe topiramate off-label to a patient is the responsibility of the prescribing provider and should be made carefully after the provider considers the contents of the package insert (Topamax Package Insert, 2012) and the patient's medical history.

Topiramate is known to cause birth defects in humans and strict compliance with highly effective birth control for female patients is necessary. Highly effective birth control must be discussed with the female patient's primary care or gynecologic provider before starting topiramate. In my weight-loss practice, patients are required to be on a birth-control method that has a yearly pregnancy rate of less than 1% to be prescribed topiramate. Hormonal methods of birth control are the only methods of birth control that have yearly pregnancy rates of less than 1%. Topiramate should be stopped immediately if there is ever any suspicion of pregnancy and the patient should contact their gynecologic provider as soon as possible for advice.

Liraglutide

The single-agent prescription-medication liraglutide, also known by the brand name Saxenda, is approved by the FDA for "chronic weight management" in patients with an initial body-mass index (BMI) of 30 kg/m² or greater, or a BMI of 27 or greater in patients with at least one weight-related medical problem. In discussing the use of liraglutide for weight loss and weight maintenance, I want to be clear that what I am discussing is based on my personal experience with prescribing liraglutide as the diabetic drug Victoza to my patients, on the FDA-approved package insert, and on the guidelines of the OMA. My discussion of how I might prescribe liraglutide to my patients is meant to be advice only and is not meant to replace or supplant the FDA-approved package insert, the OMA guidelines, and the advice of patient's prescribing providers.

Liraglutide (Saxenda) comes in a multi-dose pre-filled pen device that delivers 0.6 mg, 1.2 mg, 1.8 mg, 2.4 mg, and 3.0 mg per dose. It is to be used once a day, at any time of day, by injection into the fatty layer beneath the skin and above the muscle in the abdomen, thigh, or outer arm. After an initial daily dose of 0.6 mg for a week, the dose is then increased weekly by 0.6 mg until a dose of 3.0 mg a day is reached. The upward taper can be delayed at each dose level for an extra week, if needed, due to side effects. I have limited experience with the higher weight-loss dose of liraglutide (Saxenda) in my practice as of writing this book, due to its high cost and limited insurance coverage. In the study that was submitted to the FDA for approval of liraglutide (Saxenda), non-diabetic subjects that completed the study lost about 9% of their initial body weight in about nine months, and then maintained the weight lost for the rest of the one-year study. Subjects in this study were placed on a diet that was 500 calories less than their estimated energy requirement and were asked to exercise 150 minutes per week (Saxenda, Full Prescribing Information, n.d.).

Liraglutide is a glucagon-like peptide-1 (GLP-1) agonist and works for weight loss by binding to the GLP-1 receptors in the brain and causing a reduction of appetite.

Common side effects of liraglutide (Saxenda) include the gastrointestinal side effects of nausea, diarrhea, constipation, vomiting, indigestion, abdominal pain, and elevated lipase, as well as headache, fatigue, and dizziness. Up to 40% of patients have nausea with the use of liraglutide (Saxenda). Due to side effects, 9.8% of patients using liraglutide in the study mentioned above.

If side effects are more than mild, then the liraglutide should be stopped and the prescribing medical provider notified. Less common side effects can occur and can be serious. A full listing of those side effects can be found in the package insert for liraglutide.

The package insert for liraglutide does contain a black box warning about liraglutide causing thyroid C-cell tumors at clinically relevant doses in male and female rats and mice. It is unknown whether liraglutide causes thyroid C-cell tumors in humans. Liraglutide is contraindicated in patients with medullary thyroid cancer and in patients with Multiple Endocrine Neoplasia (MEN) syndrome.

Liraglutide (Saxenda) is not approved by the FDA to be taken safely during pregnancy, and strict compliance with adequate birth control for female patients is necessary. Adequate birth control must be discussed with the female patient's primary care or gynecologic provider before being prescribed liraglutide (Saxenda). Liraglutide (Saxenda) should be stopped immediately if there is ever any suspicion of pregnancy and the patient should contact their gynecologic provider as soon as possible for advice.

Other medications in the same drug class as liraglutide, the GLP-1 drug class, have also been studied for weight loss. These GLP-1 medications are exenatide (Byetta, Bydureon), dulaglutide (Trulicity), lixisenatide (Adlyxin), and semaglutide (Ozempic). These four additional GLP-1 medications are given by injection, are expensive, and are not approved by the FDA for weight loss. There are no manufacturer coupon cards to reduce their price if they are used for weight loss, and I doubt that health insurance companies will cover them for weight loss. They are similar enough in weight-loss efficacy and side effects to liraglutide (Apovian, 2010) (Smith L. , 2016) (Anderson S. , 2016) (O'Neil, 2018), so I have decided not to include them as separate medications in Figure 8. Of note, exenatide is expected to be available as a generic in mid-2020 and will hopefully drop in price quickly over the following year so that weight-loss providers can begin to use it off-label for weight loss. Of note, semaglutide was found to have an impressive weight-loss of almost 14% in one study at a dose that is 2.8 times higher than the maximum dose approved by the FDA for the treatment of type 2 diabetes (O'Neil, 2018). However, at this dose, the monthly cost of semaglutide as of January 2020 would be a prohibitive $4,000. Last, an oral form of semaglutide was approved for the treatment of type 2 diabetes in 2019 (FDA approves first oral GLP-1 treatment for type 2 diabetes, 2019), which, when it goes generic and the price drops, could provide an easier way to dose our weight-loss patients off-label with semaglutide.

Orlistat

The single-agent prescription-medication orlistat is also known by the brand name Xenical. It is approved by the FDA for "obesity management including weight loss and weight maintenance when used in conjunction with a reduced-calorie diet" (Xenical Package Insert, 2012). Per the FDA, orlistat is for patients with an initial body-mass index (BMI) of 30 kg/m² or greater, or a BMI of 27 or greater in patients with at least one weight-related medical problem. In discussing the use of orlistat for weight loss and weight maintenance, I want to be clear that what I am discussing is based on my personal experience with prescribing orlistat, on the FDA-approved package insert, and on the guidelines of the OMA. My discussion of how I might prescribe orlistat to my patients is meant to be advice only and is not meant to replace or supplant the FDA-approved package insert, the OMA guidelines, and the advice of patient's prescribing providers.

Prescription orlistat comes as a 120-mg capsule that is taken three times a day, either with the main meals, or within one hour of meals. Over-the-counter orlistat comes as a 60-mg capsule, also to be taken three times a day with the main meals. Daily fat intake should be limited to no more than 30% of total calories per day and the fat intake should be evenly distributed between the main meals. A daily multivitamin containing fat-soluble vitamins is advised to prevent fat-soluble vitamin deficiency. The daily multivitamin should be taken at least two hours before or after the orlistat.

In XENDOS, a four-year study of 3,304 subjects that was submitted to the FDA for approval of prescription-dose of orlistat, subjects that completed the study lost about 10.5% of their initial body weight in about 12 months, compared to placebo patients who lost about 6.5% (Xenical Package Insert, 2012). Forty-eight percent of the orlistat subjects and 66% of the placebo subjects dropped out of the study by the end of four years. Those who dropped out did so for various reasons, including lack of response, side effects, and plain refusal to continue participation. Subjects in this study were placed on a diet that contained about 800 less calories per day than their usual diet and they were encouraged to walk an additional kilometer per day. The results from this study were based only on the patients who finished the study and didn't include the results from those who dropped out. From the completer results of this study, the weight loss on the orlistat would be about 21 pounds for a person who started the study at 200 pounds and 32 pounds for a person who started the study at 300 pounds. The ITT-LOCF weight-loss result from the study, which can then be used to compare orlistat more fairly to the other weight-loss medications that I have already presented, was 3.6% in the subjects taking orlistat and 1.4% in the subjects on placebo. These percentages of weight loss are much lower than the completer results due to the high dropout rate in the study. Using these ITT results, a 200-pound subject would have lost seven pounds in one year and a 300-pound subject would have lost three pounds in one year. Study subjects then continued the orlistat for three additional years and were found to have gained back about 43% of the weight that they had originally lost by the end of the study. It should be remembered that the subjects in this study were still on the orlistat for the full four-year study. They were still being seen in the research clinics on a monthly basis and were still being encouraged to lose weight during the whole four-year study. Weight loss on the over-the-counter version of orlistat, or Alli, has been stated by some to be about the same as the higher dose prescription orlistat, although I have not been able to find a reference to confirm this.

Orlistat works by blocking about 30% of the absorption of fat from the diet, thereby reducing absorption of calories from the food that a person consumes, resulting in weight loss. It does not reduce appetite or help with the fatigue associated with increasing weight loss. Common side effects of orlistat include the gastrointestinal (GI) side effects of oily stools (ranging from clear to orange in color), increased flatus, oily spotting from the rectum, increased defecation, fecal urgency, and fecal incontinence. These GI side effects are all related to the orlistat blocking absorption of fat by the small intestine. The unabsorbed fat is then passed out the GI tract in the stool. These GI side effects do lessen over time. In the studies submitted to the FDA for drug approval, 8.8% of patients using orlistat stopped study participation due to GI side effects. If side effects occur while on orlistat that are more than mild, then the orlistat should be stopped, and the prescribing medical provider notified. If the orlistat was purchased over the counter, then it should be stopped, and the patient's primary care provider notified if the side effects persist. Less common side effects can occur and can be serious. A full listing of those side effects can be found in the package insert for orlistat (Xenical Package Insert, 2012).

My experience with orlistat in my patients has been limited by the GI side effects and lack of efficacy. I can't recall a patient in my weight-loss clinic, or in my medical clinic, that has lost more than 10 pounds on orlistat. Of course, my patients who couldn't tolerate the GI side effects quickly stopped the orlistat and didn't lose much weight. My patients who remained on orlistat quickly found that they could eat more low-fat carbs without suffering from diarrhea, which resulted in a disappointing weight-loss plateau. The use of orlistat didn't reduce hunger.

Orlistat is not approved by the FDA to be taken safely during pregnancy, and strict compliance with adequate birth control for female patients is necessary. Adequate birth control must be discussed with the female patient's gynecologic provider before being prescribed orlistat, or before taking the over-the-counter form of orlistat. Orlistat should be stopped immediately if there is ever any suspicion of pregnancy and the patient should contact their gynecologic provider as soon as possible for advice.

Bupropion

The medication bupropion (Wellbutrin) has been associated with modest weight loss in studies. It is approved by the FDA for the treatment of "major depressive disorder" (Wellbutrin SR Package Insert, 2019) and "as an aid to smoking cessation treatment" (Zyban Package Insert, 2019). It is not approved by the FDA for weight loss and any use of bupropion for weight loss is off-label use. In discussing the use of bupropion for weight loss and weight maintenance, I want to be clear that what I am discussing is based on my personal experience with prescribing bupropion, on the FDA-approved package insert, and on the guidelines of the OMA. My discussion of how I might prescribe bupropion to my patients is meant to be advice only and is not meant to replace or supplant the FDA-approved package insert, the OMA guidelines, and the advice of patient's prescribing providers.

Bupropion comes in a sustained-release (SR) form and an extended-release (XL) form. I prescribe both forms in my office for weight loss. Bupropion SR comes in 100 mg, 150 mg, and 200 mg tablets. Bupropion SR is started at 150 mg once a day in the morning for three days and then is increased to 150 mg twice a day, usually once in the morning, soon after arising, and once again about eight hours later. Dosing of bupropion SR too late in the evening can cause insomnia in some patients. If needed, after 30 days of taking the bupropion SR 150 mg twice a day, the dose can be increased to bupropion SR 200 mg twice a day. Bupropion XL comes in a 150 mg and a 300 mg tablet and is started at 150 mg in the morning. After a month, if needed, the dose can be increased to 300 mg a day in the morning. The most commonly prescribed dose of bupropion for weight loss in my practice is 300 mg a day. In a study published in 2012 on 327 patients who took bupropion for up to 48 weeks, the ITT-LOCF weight loss results were 5.4% on the bupropion SR 300 mg per day dose and 6.9% on the bupropion SR 400 mg per day dose. The patients in this study were asked to reduce their caloric intake by 600 calories per day, to consume a liquid-meal replacement of 220 calories for breakfast and lunch, and to increase their expended energy through exercise by 1,000 calories per week. Seven percent of the patients on bupropion SR 300 mg per day withdrew due to side effects and 9% of the patients on bupropion SR 400 mg per day withdrew due side effects. The side effects that led to most of the withdrawals from the study were anxiety, insomnia, and palpitations (Anderson J. , 2002).

Bupropion also comes in a non-extended-release form called Wellbutrin that is available in 75 mg and a 100 mg tablets. The non-extended-release tablets are given twice a day in lower doses and three times a day in higher doses, up to a maximum daily dose of 450 mg/day. I don't prescribe the non-extended-release form of bupropion in my weight-loss practice.

Bupropion is in its own medication class and is called an aminoketone. Its mechanism of action in reducing appetite is unknown. While I only use bupropion SR and XL in my weight-loss practice, I have no reason to believe that plain bupropion wouldn't work just as well as the bupropion SR and XL at the same number of total milligrams per day.

Bupropion is contraindicated in patients with a seizure disorder; with current or prior bulimia or anorexia nervosa; that have recently and suddenly stopped alcohol, benzodiazepines, barbiturates, and seizure drugs; that have used linezolid or a monoamine oxidase inhibitor (MAOI) in the last 14 days; or that are hypersensitive to bupropion. Warnings in the package insert include neuropsychologic symptoms of depression, mania, psychosis, hallucinations, paranoia, delusions, homicidal ideation, aggression, hostility, anxiety, panic, and suicidal ideation. Also, seizures, elevated blood pressure, and angle-closure glaucoma have occurred in patients taking bupropion. The more common side effects that can occur while taking bupropion are headache, dry mouth, nausea, insomnia, dizziness, abdominal pain, tremor, sweating, and rash. There are a number of drugs that bupropion interacts with. See the full package inserts for the different forms of bupropion for a full listing of the contraindications, warnings, side effects, and drug interactions.

My experience in my clinic with bupropion as a single agent for weight loss is limited by the fact that I have rarely used bupropion as a single agent for weight loss. I have prescribed it many times for depression, sometimes as the first medication, but most often a second medication to other anti-depressants. I have prescribed it for smoking cessation, but this is in the face of stopping smoking, which causes weight gain. In the few patients that I have given it to first line for depression, I have not observed weight loss. However, these patients weren't seeing me monthly for a year, like in all of the medication-assisted weight-loss studies that I have presented above, and they weren't given a calorie-reduced diet and exercise instructions that were then reinforced at each monthly visit. Again, in my experience, it is not possible to get the results obtained in the studies I have presented above by giving patients weight-loss medications and then seeing them back in six months.

The final decision to prescribe bupropion off-label to a patient is the responsibility of the prescribing medical provider and should be made carefully after the medical provider considers the contents of the package insert and the patient's medical history.

The FDA has classified bupropion SR as a pregnancy category B medication, meaning there is no evidence of risk to humans. However, this classification is based on animal studies and small observational studies in humans. In the package insert, the FDA suggests that the prescriber should carefully consider the risk benefit ratio of prescribing bupropion during pregnancy against the risk of not prescribing bupropion during pregnancy. This makes sense in a woman that is taking bupropion for depression during pregnancy, since it would be dangerous to the fetus if the mother stopped the bupropion and the depression worsened. But it doesn't make sense to me in a woman that is taking bupropion for weight loss and is considering pregnancy. My advice is that bupropion should not be used for weight loss during pregnancy and that strict compliance with adequate birth control is necessary. Adequate birth control must be discussed with the female patient's medical or gynecologic provider before starting bupropion for weight loss. Bupropion that is being used for weight loss should be stopped immediately if there is ever any suspicion of pregnancy and the patient should contact their gynecologic provider as soon as possible for advice.

Canagliflozin

The diabetes medication canagliflozin (Invokana) has been shown to improve weight loss in studies as compared to placebo. Canagliflozin is approved by the FDA for the treatment of type 2 diabetes and for the prevention of the diabetic complications of cardiovascular disease and diabetic kidney disease. It is not approved by the FDA for weight loss. In discussing the use of canagliflozin for weight loss and weight maintenance, I want to be clear that what I am discussing is based on my personal experience with prescribing canagliflozin, on the FDA-approved package insert, and on the guidelines of the OMA. My discussion of how I might prescribe canagliflozin to my patients is meant to be advice only and is not meant to replace or supplant the FDA-approved package insert, the OMA guidelines, and the advice of patient's prescribing providers.

Canagliflozin comes in a 100 mg and a 300 mg tablet. It is started at 100 mg once a day before the first meal of the day. After one month, the dose can be increased to 300 mg once a day. In a study published in 2014 on canagliflozin for weight loss on 376 non-diabetic patients for 12 weeks, patients on canagliflozin 100 mg once a day lost 2.9% of their body weight and patients on canagliflozin 300 mg once a day lost 2.7% of their body weight. The patients were still losing weight at the end of the study and were expected to continue losing weight. The dropout rate due to side effects from canagliflozin was 3% and was due to genital yeast infections, nausea, and hypoglycemia (Bays, 2014). The finding that there was greater weight loss on the canagliflozin 100 mg once a day than on the 300 mg once a day was somewhat unexpected due to a previous study in patients with type 2 diabetes showing greater loss of weight for the 300 mg of canagliflozin at 3.4% (Rosenstock, 2012). In a 2018 12-month study of 201 type 2 diabetics, many of which were already on medications that caused weight gain, adding canagliflozin resulted in a 4.1% weight loss, suggesting that use of canagliflozin for 12 months in a weight-loss study of non-diabetics would result in at least a 4% weight loss (Carral, 2018). Based on the results of the studies above, I have listed 4% as the expected weight loss with canagliflozin in 12 months. Further studies are needed to better establish the 12-month weight-loss potential of canagliflozin in non-diabetics.

Canagliflozin is in the medication class of sodium-glucose co-transporter 2 (SGLT-2) inhibitors. Canagliflozin works by blocking the reabsorption of filtered glucose in the kidney, causing a loss of approximately 100 grams of glucose per day in the urine. Normally, a healthy human without diabetes loses almost no calories of glucose in the urine each day. The 100 grams of glucose that is lost in the urine per day is 400 calories lost per day. This loss of calories results in weight loss, if the patient doesn't increase their intake of food to compensate for the loss of calories from glucose being lost in the urine.

Canagliflozin is contraindicated in patients who have severe kidney impairment and in patients who have had a previous hypersensitivity reaction to canagliflozin. The package insert warns that in diabetic patients canagliflozin can cause lower limb amputations, low blood volume, low blood pressure, ketoacidosis, kidney injury if the patient is dehydrated, kidney infections, low blood sugar, gangrene of the skin of the genital area, and bone fractures. It is not known if these side effects will occur in non-diabetic patients taking canagliflozin. Common side effects of canagliflozin include genital yeast infections, urinary tract infections, and increased urination (Invokana Package Insert, 2019).

I have not used canagliflozin in my office for weight loss yet. Its present high cost limits my ability to use it for weight loss. I do plan on using it for weight loss in the future, after it goes generic and its price drops, for patients who have failed other medications, or that would like to lose a little additional weight after finding themselves at a weight-loss plateau. Canagliflozin does not reduce hunger or fatigue while dieting.

Canagliflozin is not approved by the FDA to be taken safely during pregnancy, and strict compliance with adequate birth control for female patients is necessary. Adequate birth control must be discussed with the female patient's gynecologic provider before being prescribed canagliflozin. Canagliflozin should be stopped immediately if there is ever any suspicion of pregnancy and the patient should contact their gynecologic provider as soon as possible for advice.

Of note, shorter studies of other medications in the same SGLT-2 drug class as canagliflozin have shown similar amounts of weight loss. These other SGLT-2 medications are empagliflozin (Jardiance), dapagliflozin (Farxiga), and ertugliflozin (Steglatro). Since weight loss is similar with all four of these SGLT-2 medications in studies, only the first to market (canagliflozin) will be listed in the figure above.

Zonisamide

Zonisamide (Zonegran) is a seizure drug that has been found to cause weight loss. Zonisamide is approved by the FDA for the treatment of seizures in patients down to two years of age and for migraine prevention in patients age 12 and older. It's not approved by the FDA for weight loss. In discussing the use of zonisamide for weight loss and weight maintenance, I want to be clear that what I am discussing is based on my personal experience with prescribing zonisamide, on the FDA-approved package insert, and on the guidelines of the OMA. My discussion of how I might prescribe zonisamide to my patients is meant to be advice only and is not meant to replace or supplant the FDA-approved package insert, the OMA guidelines, and the advice of patient's prescribing providers.

Zonisamide comes as 25 mg and 100 mg capsules. For weight loss, zonisamide is given at 400 mg once a day before bedtime. In a one-year study of 225 non-diabetic patients that was published in 2012, patients who took zonisamide 400 mg once a day lost 6.8% of their body weight in 12 months. Patients in the study were told to reduce calorie intake by 500 calories per day and to exercise. The patients returned to the research clinics once a month for the duration of the study. Diet and exercise were encouraged at each visit. About 6% of patients taking zonisamide dropped out of the study due to the side effects of headache, sleepiness, memory impairment, depression, and muscle weakness.

Zonisamide is in the medication class of seizure medications. It is not known how zonisamide works to reduce appetite or promote weight loss.

There are no contraindications to the use of zonisamide in the package insert. Zonisamide should be prescribed with close monitoring in patients who are already on another seizure drug that is similar to zonisamide, such as topiramate. Warnings include rare but serious skin reactions, hypersensitivity reactions, bone marrow damage, and heat-stroke like symptoms. Serious and more common side effects are suicidal behavior and suicidal ideation, seizures in seizure patients who stop the drug abruptly, excessive acidity of the blood (metabolic acidosis), birth defects, and neuropsychiatric symptoms of depression, psychosis, mental slowness, decreased ability to concentrate, sleepiness, and fatigue. Common side effects noted in the package insert are sleepiness, dizziness, difficult walking, agitation, short-term memory loss and mental confusion, nausea, double vision, altered taste, diarrhea, constipation, dry mouth, and headache. Nausea developed in 13.3% of patients on zonisamide at 400 mg once a day while 10.7% developed memory impairment and 18.7% developed headaches. See the package insert for zonisamide for a complete list of contraindications, warnings, side effects, and drug interactions (Zonegran Package Insert, 2016).

For side effects that are more than mild, including any rash, the zonisamide should be stopped immediately and the patient should immediately call their medical provider or go to an urgent care/ER. Once a patient has been taking zonisamide for more than a few weeks, some medical providers feel it should not be stopped suddenly. Patients should discuss in advance with their medical provider how to stop the zonisamide, should stopping it become necessary.

I have not used zonisamide for weight loss in my weight-loss clinic. I don't plan on using it in the near future due to its higher rate of side effects than other weight-loss medications, its smaller degree of weight loss than other medications, and because I am much more familiar with the seizure drug topiramate for weight loss.

The final decision to prescribe zonisamide off-label to a patient is the responsibility of the prescribing medical provider and should be made carefully after the medical provider considers the contents of the package insert and the patient's medical history.

Zonisamide is known to cause birth defects in humans and strict compliance with highly effective birth control for female patients is necessary. Highly effective birth control must be discussed with the female patient's primary care or gynecologic provider before starting zonisamide. In my weight loss practice, patients are required to be on a birth-control method that has a yearly pregnancy rate of less than 1% to be prescribed zonisamide. Hormonal methods of birth control are the only methods of birth control that have yearly pregnancy rates of less than 1%. Zonisamide should be stopped immediately if there is ever any suspicion of pregnancy and the patient should contact their gynecologic provider as soon as possible for advice.

Metformin

Metformin (Glucophage) has been used off-label by some medical providers for weight loss, even though the weight loss with metformin in studies has been small. Metformin is approved by the FDA for the treatment of type 2 diabetes in adults and children down to age ten. It is not approved by the FDA for weight loss. In discussing the use of metformin for weight loss and weight maintenance, I want to be clear that what I am discussing is based on my personal experience with prescribing metformin, on the FDA-approved package insert, and on the guidelines of the OMA. My discussion of how I might prescribe metformin to my patients is meant to be advice only and is not meant to replace or supplant the FDA-approved package insert, the OMA guidelines, and the advice of patient's prescribing providers.

Metformin comes in 500 mg, 850 mg, and 1,000 mg tablets that are not extended release and 500 mg and 750 mg tablets that are extended release. When used off-label for the treatment of obesity, metformin is usually prescribed at up to 1,000 mg given twice a day with meals. A slow taper from 500 mg once a day to the target dose of 2,000 mg a day should be carried out over three weeks. In a study published in 2012, 3,234 patients with impaired glucose tolerance, or pre-diabetes, were given metformin at an average dose of 1,700 mg per day. The subjects were encouraged to exercise 150 minutes per week and to reduce calorie intake in an effort to lose 5%-10% of their body weight. After one year, patients lost 2.7% of their body weight on the metformin. Gastrointestinal symptoms on the metformin were common at 28% in this study (DPP, 2012). In the study listed in the package insert for metformin, the discontinuation rate for metformin was 12% for diarrhea. Diarrhea was the most common side effect noted in the study on the package insert and occurred in 53% of patients (Glucophage Package Insert, 2018).

The contraindications to the use of metformin listed in the package insert are an eGFR (a measurement of kidney filtration) below 30, past hypersensitivity to metformin, and metabolic acidosis. There is a black box warning for a very rare side effect of metformin called lactic acidosis, which can cause death. Symptoms of lactic acidosis are not feeling good, muscle pain, difficulty breathing, sleepiness, and abdominal pain. Metformin must be stopped immediately if lactic acidosis is suspected, and the patient transported to an emergency room. Other warnings in the package insert are for vitamin B12 deficiency, which should be checked on a lab test every two to three years in patients taking metformin long term, and low blood sugar when metformin is added to insulin, or vice versa. The common side effects of metformin are diarrhea, nausea, vomiting, increased passage of bowel gas, indigestion, lack of physical energy, stomach pain, and headache. See the package insert for metformin for a complete list of contraindications, warnings, side effects, and drug interactions (Glucophage Package Insert, 2018).

Metformin is in its own medication class and is a biguanide. It is not known how metformin works to reduce weight.

I have not used metformin in my office for weight loss yet. Its high rate of GI side effects and low efficacy limits my ability to use it for weight loss. I do plan on using it for weight loss in the future for patients who haven't succeeded with other medications, or who would like to lose a little additional weight after finding themselves at a weight-loss plateau. Metformin does not reduce hunger or fatigue while dieting.

The FDA has classified metformin as a pregnancy category B medication, meaning that there is no evidence of risk to humans. However, this classification is based on animal studies and small observational studies in humans. In my opinion, that is not enough evidence to support the use of metformin during pregnancy for weight loss alone. Metformin is not approved by the FDA to be taken safely during pregnancy for weight loss, and strict compliance with adequate birth control for female patients is necessary. Adequate birth control must be discussed with the female patient's gynecologic provider before being prescribed metformin for weight loss. Metformin prescribed for weight loss should be stopped immediately if there is ever any suspicion of pregnancy and the patient should contact their gynecologic provider as soon as possible for advice.

Plenity

Plenity (cellulose and citric acid) is indicated by the FDA to aid in weight management in overweight and obese adults with a BMI of 25 to 40. In discussing the use of Plenity for weight loss and weight maintenance, I want to be clear that what I am discussing is based on the FDA-approved package insert. My discussion of how I might prescribe Plenity to my patients is meant to be advice only and is not meant to replace or supplant the FDA-approved package insert, OMA guidelines and the advice of patient's prescribing providers.

Plenity comes in 0.75 gram capsules and is prescribed as three capsules taken 20 to 30 minutes before both lunch and dinner with 16 ounces of water. If dosing before a meal is missed, Plenity can still be taken during or immediately after the meal. In the GLOW study published in 2018, 430 patients were randomized to take either Plenity or placebo. The subjects were encouraged to exercise 30 minutes per day and to reduce calorie intake by 300 calories per day below their calculated energy requirement. After 6 months, subjects on Plenity lost 6.4% of their body weight and subjection on placebo lost 4.4% of their body weight. Plenity was well tolerated with 3.6% of patient discontinuing the study due to side effects. The discontinuation rate for the placebo group due to side effects was 3.3%. In both the Plenity and placebo group, the most common side effects were gastrointestinal (Greenway, 2018) (Plenity Package Insert, 2019).

The contraindications to the use of Plenity listed in the package insert are pregnancy and a history of allergic reaction to cellulose, citric acid, sodium stearyl fumarate, gelatin or titanium oxide. Since the impact of Plenity on absorption of medications is not well known, then once a day medications should be taken in the morning or at bedtime. If medications need to be taken with meals, then this should be discussed with the dieter's medical provider before starting Plenity. The most common side effects of Plenity are mild to moderate abdominal distension, abdominal pain, bloating, bowel movement irregularity, constipation, diarrhea, acid reflux, difficulty swallowing, increased burping, increased bowel gas and vomiting. Up to 43% of users of Plenity have gastrointestinal side effects. See the package insert for Plenity for a complete list of contraindications, warnings, side effects, and drug interactions (Plenity Package Insert, 2019)

Plenity is in its own medication class. Plenity is non-systemic, meaning that it is not absorbed into the body. Each Plenity capsule contains thousands of superabsorbent hydrogel particles made of cellulose and citric acid that can absorb up to 100 times their weight in water. Once hydrated, the particles occupy about a fourth of the average stomach volume. When a person consumes food, the particles mix with the food and increase the sensation of fullness sooner. The particles break down in the colon and release the water that they absorbed in the stomach. The water is then absorbed in the colon. The Plenity particles are eliminated through normal bowl movements.

I have not used Plenity in my office for weight loss yet. It is only available through a national mail order pharmacy as of the writing of this book, which is a challenge for many patients. It is also more expensive than most other weight-loss medications that I have discussed above. I believe that Plenity will not help to reduce caloric intake for patients that are following a diet plan of eating six small meals per day, since I believe Plenity will not help a person to feel full when they are only eating small, measured meals. I do plan on using Plenity for weight loss in the future for patients who haven't succeeded with other medications, or who would like to lose a little additional weight after finding themselves at a weight-loss plateau. Plenity does not reduce hunger or fatigue while dieting.

The FDA has not given Plenity a pregnancy or breast feeding category that I am aware of. Therefore, Plenity should not be taken when trying to get pregnant, when pregnant, or when breast feeding, and strict compliance with adequate birth control for female patients is necessary. Adequate birth control must be discussed with the female patient's gynecologic provider before being prescribed Plenity for weight loss. Plenity should be stopped immediately if there is ever any suspicion of pregnancy and the patient should contact their gynecologic provider as soon as possible for advice.

Combination Weight-Loss Medications

Combining the above single-agent medications to achieve greater weight loss than with any single-agent weight-loss medication alone is intriguing. Medical providers have a long history of using two, three, four, and even five medications with different mechanisms of action to achieve better control of diabetes, hypertension, psychiatric disorders, asthma, and high cholesterol. The potential advantages of combining weight-loss medications are to:

1. Achieve greater weight loss.

2. Keep medications side effects lower by adding lower doses of two different weight-loss medications together.

3. Achieve better appetite control by affecting more than one pathway in the brain.

However, there are potential downsides to combining medications for weight loss:

4. The more agents that you add to treat a disease, the less effective each new agent is in changing the desired endpoint, which in this case, is weight loss.

5. Cost is increased.

6. Side effects can be increased, mostly by increasing the total number of unrelated side effects, but occasionally by additively worsening a single common side effect, such as nausea.

Those of us that have practiced weight-loss medicine for a long time have often used off-label medication combinations to enhance our patient's weight loss. Phentermine and fenfluramine (fen-phen) were used successfully in combination in the 1990s until fenfluramine was withdrawn from the market for heart valve damage. Phentermine was all we had for a while until it was discovered in the 2000s that phentermine and topiramate, when used together, were about as efficacious as fen-phen. Other weight-loss medical providers starting using the combination of bupropion and naltrexone in the 2000s with moderate success. Since then, multiple other off-label combinations have been used by weight-loss providers, some of which I will discuss below. As I present the medication combinations below, I will not repeat the information I have already provided above on the single-agent weight-loss medications, including how I use them in my practice, and their contraindications, warnings and side effects.

Combination Weight-Loss Medication Comparison	Bupropion + Naltrexone	Phentermine + Topiramate	Phentermine + Canagliflozin	Phentermine + Liraglutide	Phentermine + Topiramate + Liraglutide
Percent weight loss in 12 months (ITT-LOCF)	6	13	8[1]	Unk[2]	Unk[2]
Average weight loss in 12 months for a 250-pound person (pounds)	15	33	20	Unk[2]	Unk[2]
Average cost per month	$48	$34	$599	$1,311	$1,311
Drop-out rate due to side effects	30%	35%	4%	Unk[2]	Unk[2]
Helps to reduce hunger while dieting	Yes	Yes	Yes	Yes	Yes
Helps to reduce fatigue while dieting	No	Yes	Yes	Yes	Yes

Figure 9 - Combination Weight-Loss Medication Comparison

[1] *Result is from a six-month trial; the subjects in the trial were still losing weight when the trial was stopped and would have lost more in a longer study.*
[2] *Study results are inadequate, and results are unknown.*

All of the combinations of single-agent weight-loss medications listed above in Figure 9 are off-label and the decision to prescribe them off-label remains the decision of each weight-loss medical provider. The percent weight loss in 12 months is listed as ITT-LOCF results, unless otherwise specified. The average weight loss for a 250-pound person is calculated by multiplying the percent weight loss in 12 months by 250 pounds. The average cost per month is from various sources on the internet as of January 2020 and is at best an estimation of cost. I listed the cost of the similar-dose generic components of the two brand-name combination products, Qsymia (phentermine-topiramate) and Contrave (bupropion-naltrexone), instead of the more expensive cost of these brand name products. Not all possible combinations of the single-agent weight-loss medications are listed, due to a lack of study results and to my lack of experience with other combinations. In addition, it is possible to use three and even four of the single-agent weight-loss medications together in an attempt to achieve additional weight loss. However, these combinations have not been studied to see if adding additional medications will result in additional meaningful weight loss, and these combinations might result in excessive side effects from the total of the individual side effects of each medication.

Bupropion + Naltrexone

The combination of bupropion and naltrexone is approved by the FDA as the prescription medication Contrave. Contrave is approved by the FDA for "chronic weight management" in adults with an initial body mass index (BMI) of 30 or greater and in adults with a BMI of 27 or greater in the presence of at least one comorbidity (another existing medical condition) of obesity. Contrave comes as an extended release tablet of 8 mg of naltrexone and 90 mg of bupropion. The dose of Contrave starts at once a day in the morning for the first week and then is tapered upward over three weeks by one tablet per week to the usual dose of two tablets twice a day, or a total of 32 mg of naltrexone per day and 360 mg of bupropion per day. Please see the Contrave package insert for complete prescribing information on Contrave (Contrave Package Insert, 2014).

In two 56-week studies on a total of 3,238 non-diabetics that were published in 2010 and 2013, the patients on Contrave lost an average of 6.3% of their body weight. These results were reported as ITT-LOCF results. Subjects in these studies were instructed to reduce their caloric intake by 500 calories per day and to exercise. The dropout rate for the 2013 study was 24.3%

and the subjects reported nausea and headache as the two main reasons for stopping the study. The average rate of the most frequent side effect of nausea in the two studies was 29.5% (Greenway, 2010) (Apovian, 2013).

Naltrexone (Revia) is approved by the FDA for the treatment of alcohol or narcotic dependence. Naltrexone comes as a 50 mg tablet that is scored. Its medication class is an opioid antagonist. In studies as a single agent, naltrexone does not cause weight loss.

Naltrexone is contraindicated in patients that are taking opioids, are taking methadone or bupropion for the treatment of opioid addiction, are withdrawing from opioids, or are hypersensitive to naltrexone. Naltrexone has been shown to cause elevation of liver enzymes in high-dose studies in drug and alcohol addicts at five times the 50 mg dose of naltrexone. There is no report of liver enzyme elevation at the 50 mg dose of naltrexone. The side effects of nausea, headache, dizziness, anxiety, fatigue, insomnia, abdominal cramps, restlessness, bone pain, joint pain, muscle aches, and a runny nose have been seen with the use of naltrexone. Naltrexone should be used with caution in patients with renal impairment or liver impairment. Naltrexone should not be used for weight loss during pregnancy or breast feeding. For a complete list of warnings and side effects for naltrexone, see the package insert for naltrexone (Revia Package Insert, 2013).

It is not known how the combination of bupropion and naltrexone causes weight loss. The combination of bupropion and naltrexone has been used for weight loss as two separate medications for about two decades and was in use by medical providers for weight loss before the combination product Contrave was released.

In my weight-loss practice and in appropriate patients, I start bupropion XL 150 mg tablets once a day, as discussed under the single-agent weight-loss medication section above. If needed after a month, I increase the dose of bupropion XL to 300 mg once a day. At the same time that I start the bupropion XL, I start my patients on a half of a 50 mg tablet of naltrexone in the morning. If needed after a month, I increase the dose of naltrexone to 50 mg once a day in the morning. The maximum dose that I prescribe for weight loss for bupropion is 400 mg a day and the maximum dose of naltrexone that I prescribe for weight loss is 50 mg a day. Since these doses are not the doses used in the FDA-approved medication Contrave and since the individual medications bupropion and naltrexone are not FDA approved for weight loss, then the way that I use these medications in my weight-loss clinic is off-label.

Phentermine + Topiramate

The medication Qsymia, a combination of phentermine and topiramate, is approved by the FDA for "chronic weight management" in patients with a BMI of 30 or greater, or with a BMI of 27 or greater with one obesity-related comorbidity. Qsymia is a Schedule IV drug under the Controlled Substances Act. Qsymia comes in capsules in four different strengths of phentermine and extended release topiramate: 3.75 mg/23 mg, 7.5 mg/46 mg, 11.25 mg/69 mg, and 15 mg/92 mg. Qsymia is taken in the morning. Patients start Qsymia by taking the 3.75 mg/23 mg tablet for 14 days, then the dose is increased to the 7.5 mg/46 mg tablet. If the patient has not lost at least 3% of their body weight after 12 weeks on that dose, then the patient either should stop the medication completely, or increase the Qsymia to the 11.25 mg/69 mg tablet for 14 days and then increase again to the highest dose of 15 mg/92 mg. If the patient has not lost at least 5% of their body weight by 12 weeks on the highest tolerated dose, then the Qsymia should be stopped gradually by taking the dose they are on every other day for at least a week before stopping altogether. Please see the Qsymia package insert for complete prescribing instructions (Qsymia Package Insert, 2012).

In two 56-week studies with a total of 3,754 subjects that were reported in 2012, the patients on the highest dose of Qsymia lost an average of 10.4% of their body weight, reported as ITT-LOCF results. The patients in the study were instructed to reduce their calorie intake by 500 calories per day. The dropout rate for the highest dose of Qsymia was 17.4% and was due to blurred vision, headache, irritability, dizziness, tingling, insomnia, depression, and anxiety. The most common side effects of Qsymia, which occurred at least 2% more often than placebo, were tingling at 19.9%, nausea at 19.1%, and constipation at 16.1%. The side effects (that were greater than placebo) were most often dose related. See the package insert for Qsymia for a complete listing of contraindications, warnings and side effects (Qsymia Package Insert, 2012).

Please see the single-agent sections above for the way phentermine and topiramate work to reduce weight. Phentermine and topiramate were used by weight-loss providers as separate medications for more than a decade before Qsymia was approved by the FDA.

In my weight-loss practice and in appropriate patients, I start phentermine at one-half of a 37.5 mg tablet once a day in the morning for the first week and then I have the patient increase to the full 37.5 mg tablet once a day, as long as they are doing well, and their blood pressure is normal on the lower dose. I also have them start topiramate 25 mg tablets as an upward taper. The topiramate taper I use is one tablet at bedtime for a week, then two tablets at bedtime for a week, then three tablets at bedtime for a week, then four tablets at bedtime. I see the patient back in one month. If they are tolerating the dose of both medications, then I continue the phentermine at 37.5 mg once a day in the morning and the topiramate as a 100 mg tablet at bedtime. Since these doses of phentermine and topiramate are different than those in Qsymia, since phentermine is not indicated by the FDA for more than two weeks for weight loss, and since topiramate is not approved for weight loss, then my use of phentermine and topiramate in my office is off-label.

Phentermine + Canagliflozin

The combination of phentermine and canagliflozin (Invokana) is not FDA approved to be used together and the prescribing of this combination for weight loss is off-label. While I have not used this combination of medications in my weight-loss practice due to its high cost, I have used canagliflozin for some of my diabetic patients in my medical practice and have seen modest weight loss in a few of them.

In a 26-week study on 335 non-diabetic patients that was published in 2017, the patients that were given 300 mg of canagliflozin once a day and 15 mg of phentermine once a day lost 7.5% of their body weight. The subjects in the study were still losing weight at the end of the study and would have lost additional weight if the study had gone on for longer. The dropout rate for side effects was 3.6%, which was smaller than the dropout rate for the phentermine alone and the canagliflozin alone. The patients in the study were instructed to reduce calorie intake by 600 calories per day and to exercise for 150 minutes per week. The patients were seen monthly while on the study, with the diet and exercise instructions reinforced at each visit. There were no side effects that were different than expected from the individual medications that were used in the trial.

Canagliflozin is an expensive diabetic medication that results in modest weight loss by itself and some additional weight loss in this short trial when used with a half dose of phentermine. Although there is a coupon card that can lower the cost of canagliflozin to $0 in commercially insured diabetic patients, I doubt that the coupon card will work for non-diabetics that want to use the canagliflozin for weight loss. In my opinion, this drug combination deserves additional study at a higher dose of phentermine and for a full 12 months to determine the true efficacy of this combination.

Phentermine + Liraglutide

The use of phentermine and liraglutide together for weight loss is not approved by the FDA and medical providers that choose to prescribe it are doing so off-label. Please see the information above on each single-agent medication in this combination. Due to the high cost of liraglutide, even with a coupon card, and to the limited insurance coverage of liraglutide, I have not used this combination in my weight-loss clinic.

The medications phentermine and liraglutide have been studied together for weight loss in obese mice and produced a 9.2% weight loss in 12 weeks (Simonds, 2019). In another study, 45 human patients who had already been on liraglutide for a year and had lost 12.6% of their body weight were then given phentermine 15 mg once a day along with the liraglutide for 12 additional weeks. No additional weight was lost, but the combination of the two medications was well tolerated (Tronieri, 2019). There is inadequate evidence at this time to determine how much weight patients will lose on this combination over a one-year time period and what the dropout rate will be.

Phentermine + Topiramate + Liraglutide

This triple combination is not approved by the FDA and is off-label. In an observational report from 2018 on three diabetic patients who were treated with Qsymia (phentermine-topiramate) and liraglutide, the average weight loss was 15% at the one-year mark (Baloch, 2018). This is completer data, however, since none of the three participants stopped taking the two medications during the year. ITT results from a larger study would be smaller due to a 40%-50% dropout rate, which is typical for most large weight-loss trials. There is inadequate evidence at this time to determine how much weight patients will lose on this combination over one year and what the dropout rate will be.

Medical-Provider-Directed Very Low-Calorie Diets (VLCDs)

A very low-calorie diet (VLCD) is the most effective diet that is currently available. Participants in VLCDs lose more than twice as much in six months as all other diets that have been studied (Goday, 2016). Patients at our clinic lose about 54 pounds in six months on our VLCD, which is about twice the average weight loss we see for our patients to which are given two weight-loss medications and a standard low-calorie diet for six months. Dieters who are compliant on VLCDs feel little physical hunger, and this effect is durable for as long as the VLCD lasts. VLCDs are very safe but need to be closely monitored and supervised by a medical provider that is experienced in VLCDs. VLCDs have been around since the 1970s. The challenges of VLCDs are higher cost, frequent clinic visits, limited food choices, and the public's perceived lack of efficacy due to rapid weight regain after the VLCD.

A VLCD is classically defined as any diet where the dieter consumes less than 800 calories per day. This one-size-fits-all definition doesn't work well for many of my patients; so I use an alternate definition that was first proposed in 1989, that defined a VLCD is any diet where the dieter consumes 50% or less of their resting metabolic rate (RMR) (Atkinson, 1989). RMR is pretty much the number of calories that a person would spend if they were to remain completely still lying in bed for 24 hours. RMR varies with size, gender, and age. For a smaller woman, her RMR might be about 1,600 calories per day, while for a larger man it might be 2,000 calories per day. Therefore, per the alternate definition that I use, a VLCD for the smaller woman would be 800 calories per day or less and for the larger man it would be 1,000 calories per day or less. In addition, research has indicated that VLCDs of 400, 600, and 800 calories per day all result in the same weight loss (Ohno, 1989) (Foster, 1992). This is presumed to be due to an increase in fatigue on the lower calorie VLCDs resulting in decreased non-exercise and exercise activity. This leads to decreased daily energy expenditure by an amount that is equal to the decrease in calories consumed, resulting in no additional weight lost during an 800-calorie VLCD.

In my practice, for women five-feet tall and under, we prescribe a VLCD consisting of 700 calories per day; for women from 5'0" to 5'7", 800 calories per day; for women over 5'7" and for men under 5'7", 900 calories per day; and for men over 5'7", 1,000 calories per day. If our patients get excessively tired while on our VLCD, we add an additional 100 calories per day of protein.

The amount of carbohydrate I recommend on my VLCDs varies from 60-90 grams per day, depending again on the patient's sex and height. This is higher than early VLCDs, which were mostly, or completely, protein, but were very low in total calories per day. The very low, or absent, intake of carbohydrate in the early VLCDs was based on the theory that inducing ketosis was the mechanism by which VLCDs decreased appetite. Ketosis is the result of the body turning to stored fat to provide energy for the brain when there is an inadequate supply of carbohydrate in the diet. However, subsequent research has indicated that VLCDs with mildly higher levels of carbohydrate that don't produce ketosis have comparable levels of hunger reduction when compared to VLCDs that have little or no carbohydrate (Rosen, 1985).

A common question that is asked by patients who are considering a VLCD is whether they will be given weight-loss medication while on the VLCD to help with what they believe will be intense and worsening hunger with more and more weight loss. In my weight-loss clinic, I do prescribe at least phentermine to all appropriate patients who do a VLCD in my office.

I do this to help my VLCD patients through the fatigue that is common during the first two to three weeks on a VLCD, which gives them the opportunity to use and be comfortable with weight-loss medications that will be critical to help prevent weight regain during weight maintenance. In my experience, patients who have not used a weight-loss medication during a LVCD are much less likely to use a weight-loss medication during weight maintenance. The critical need for weight-loss medication to assist with weight maintenance will be discussed in Chapter 11.

A VLCD is hard because it is hard to give up the American diet that we are so addicted to, and to eat just shakes, soups, and bars that are purchased from the VLCD provider. It's hard to not eat the same food that your family is eating. It's hard to go to restaurants and have a protein bar while everyone around you is eating the foods you love. It's hard not to chew your food. And it's hard to be on the VLCD for long enough to lose 50, 100, or even 200 pounds. For those in my practice that have lost 200 pounds, it has taken up to a year on a VLCD to do it.

On the other hand, a VLCD is like a breath of fresh breath of air because it is so nice to diet without physical hunger. Most of us that are missing the loss-of-savor signal have been hungry 24/7 for most of our lives. Most of us that are not Muse Satiety Type 1s have dieted over and over again and have fought the increasing hunger that comes with each pound lost to the point that we say we are so hungry that we could eat the paint off the walls. But, when you're on a VLCD, you don't feel that hunger. Sure, you miss eating mentally, but you don't feel that gnawing pain of hunger in the pit of your stomach that you get when you diet on more than 800 calories per day. It is not known how a VLCD causes you to feel no hunger. The lack of hunger lasts, without fading, for as long as you're on the VLCD without cheating. It's so nice to be free of the hunger that many of my patient say, as they near the end of their VLCD, that they are afraid to go back to a regular diet because of the hunger they will again feel. An important point to make is that when a person on a VLCD cheats and eats just 200 calories more per day, then the hunger comes roaring back and it stays for one to two days, even if the person immediately reduces their intake back to the calories per day that they were supposed to be eating.

Typically, the food on a VLCD is comprised of nutritionally complete shakes, along with soups and protein bars. The dieter obtains all the food for the diet from the supervising medical provider for the length of the VLCD. Many patients wonder why they can't just do the VLCD on a diet of healthy protein with low-carbohydrate vegetables at 800 to 1,000 calories per day. This is a good question. In controlled circumstances in nutritional research centers, it doesn't matter what food is consumed to make up the 800 to 1,000 calories on the VLCD. The weight loss is the same and the level of reduction of hunger while dieting is the same. However, in the real world of dieter's own homes, a VLCD based on healthy protein, such as fish, chicken, and shrimp, and low-carbohydrate vegetables, such as broccoli, cauliflower, and zucchini, goes well for about six weeks, in my experience. The patients do lose about 10 pounds of fat and five to 10 pounds of water weight the first six weeks, just like they would on a VLCD done with the supplements from the medical provider's office. However, even though they are not physically hungry on a VCLD, they are mentally hungry, so, after a while, they start nibbling on the leftovers calling to them from their refrigerators. Or they start adding condiments, such as cheese, steak sauce, or shrimp cocktail, to their small servings of food. They start adding olives, chopped apples, salad dressing, croutons, and cheese to salads. As the VLCD goes on, they stop measuring exact portions and start guessing at portion sizes instead. As soon as they start eating 200 extra calories per day over what they have been prescribed by their VLCD provider, they become hungry. Due to the increase in hunger, they begin adding even more food to their daily intake. Their weight-loss plateaus, and they give up. I've let people try to do a VLCD in the past while eating their own food, but it has not worked in my clinic for more than six weeks. I've tried doing a VLCD myself with food from my home, but I have failed as well. I don't recommend trying to do a VLCD with food from the dieter's pantry at home.

A VLCD requires the following additional ingredients to be successful:

1. Strict journaling. Strict journaling of every calorie consumed each day improves weight loss by 50% in research studies (Hollis J. , 2008).

2. Attendance at a weekly support group. Support group attendance improves weight loss by 20% in research studies (Sacks F. , 2009).

3. Weekly follow-up visits with the diet counselor. This is especially important during the first month when the dieter is getting accustomed to being on a VLCD.

4. Monthly follow-up visits with the medical provider supervising the VLCD. This is important both for encouragement while on the VLCD, to have questions answered about the VLCD, and for medical safety.

5. A mandatory limited palate of food at each meal. Patients on a VLCD only get one item per meal at each of the four or five meals per day. These meals are mostly nutritionally balanced shakes, along with an optional single serving of soup, and/or one protein bar.

Most of patients on a VLCD do well for the first month, or so, but then they get busy, become lax on the journaling, and start coming to the support groups only every other week. The patients who stop carefully following the VLCD always plateau. A VLCD is an amazing opportunity to lose a lot more weight than any other diet on this planet. Those who chose to do a VLCD should follow the VLCD exactly as prescribed and not waste the opportunity.

There are a number of vendors of the supplements that are used for commercial VLCDs, including Medifast, Optifast, Bariatrix Nutrition, HealthWise, and Robard. Some of these vendors require the medical provider to exclusively sell only their supplements to their customers, while the rest permit medical providers to buy supplements from any company that they would like. Some of these vendors sell their supplements directly to consumers, but most sell them only to medical providers of VLCDs. Some of these vendors have their own franchised weight-loss clinics, such as Medifast, but most don't.

Humans tolerate consuming a very-low carbohydrate diet well. For centuries, the Inuit consumed a low-carbohydrate diet of fish and the flesh of marine animals for about half of each year. In a VLCD analysis report by a group of European experts published in 2002, it was stated that millions of patients had participated in VLCDs with no known deaths related to a VLCD (Saris W. , 2002).

However, there are a number of possible side effects related to being on a VLCD. Some of these side effects can be serious and can be prevented with the help of an experienced medical provider. For safety reasons, VLCDs should not be done by individuals on their own. The VLCD side effects are listed below:

1. Low sodium – VLCDs are inherently low in sodium. The daily sodium intake on a VLCD can vary from 800 to 1,500 mg of sodium per day, depending on the VLCD supplements that are consumed. This is a very low intake of sodium, and, in time, it can cause low blood pressure, fatigue, light-headedness, and even fainting. Low sodium is prevented on a VLCD by the dieter consuming one bouillon cube per day. Bouillon cubes contain about 900 mg of sodium. Those who don't like bouillon can substitute a quarter teaspoon of salt for a bouillon cube. A fourth of a teaspoon of salt contains about 600 mg of sodium. Even with the intake of additional sodium in the bouillon cube, patients on our VLCD still are not exceeding 2,300 mg of sodium per day, which is the recommended upper limit of daily consumption of sodium (USDA, n.d.). Consuming extra salt has concerned some of our VLCD patients, at least until we have explained that they were still on a low-sodium diet in spite of the extra sodium.

2. Low potassium – A person on a VLCD consumes much less potassium than the amount of potassium they consume on their usual diet. This can lead to low blood levels of potassium, which can cause muscle cramps, muscle weakness, palpitations, and rarely serious heart arrhythmias. While on a VLCD through our office, all patients are required to take 20 milliequivalents of prescription potassium per day to prevent low potassium. Since the 20-milliequivalent tablets of potassium are quite large, we give our patients 10-milliequivalent tablets of potassium and have them take two tablets a day. A potassium blood level is checked after the first week on a VLCD,

and then monthly until the end of the VLCD. The patients on our VLCDs are given potassium citrate, instead of the cheaper potassium chloride, because the citrate form of potassium reduces kidney stone risk, as discussed below.

3. Gallbladder attacks – Any diet that is low in fat and that causes rapid weight loss can cause gallstone attacks. Gallstone attacks are costly, cause individuals to take time off work, and can have serious side effects. The risk of developing non-symptomatic gallstones during a VLCD is as high as 25% in one study, with up to 5% of patients on a VLCD having a symptomatic gallstone attack while on a VLCD (Broomfield, 1988). Use of the medication ursodiol has been shown to reduce the risk of gallstone attacks in patients on a VLCD (Broomfield, 1988) (Liddle, 1989). For our patients on our VLCDs that haven't had their gallbladder removed, we prescribe ursodiol 250 mg or 300 mg once a day. It has been years since we have seen a gallstone attack in one of our VLCD patients. The only side effect of ursodiol is diarrhea. However, since a VLCD is constipating, the ursodiol helps to treat the constipation. This will be discussed further below. Of note, once patients have achieved their desired weight, the ursodiol is stopped, since there isn't an increased risk for gallstones during weight maintenance, and since ursodiol doesn't help with weight loss or weight maintenance.

4. Kidney stones – Patients participating in a VLCD have a slightly higher risk of developing kidney stones (Kielb, 2000). Substituting potassium citrate for the potassium chloride that is usually given for potassium supplementation in a VLCD significantly reduces the risk of developing kidney stones in patients on a VLCD (Muscogiuri, 2019) (Guirguis-Blake, 2014). In my practice, patients on a VLCD are given potassium citrate 10 milliequivalent tablets and are asked to take two tablets a day. The potassium is stopped after the VLCD is completed, since there isn't an increased risk of kidney stones during weight maintenance and since potassium citrate doesn't help with weight maintenance.

5. Gout attacks – Patients participating in a VLCD are at a slightly higher risk for developing gout attacks at a rate of about one out of every 100 participants (Palgi, 1985). I have seen one patient with gout during a VLCD in the last 10 years of doing VLCDs for more than 500 patients. Patients with a history of gout should confer with their VLCD provider before starting a VLCD, and adequate fluid intake should be maintained during the VLCD. The patient should notify their VLCD provider as soon as possible if they develop unexplained warmth, pain, and swelling in any joint during the VLCD. The VLCD provider can then make a proper diagnosis and begin treatment.

6. Low blood pressure – Symptomatic low blood pressure can occur during a VLCD and can lead to a feeling of light-headedness as well as fainting spells. Occasionally, injuries can occur if a person faints while standing. Blood pressure drops during a VLCD due to a decreased intake of fluids as well as a very low intake of sodium. Both occurrences result in a drop in blood volume and an accompanying drop in blood pressure. Low blood pressure can be prevented by drinking eight 8-ounce glasses of liquids per day and by consuming one bouillon cube per day while on a VLCD. Low blood pressure can especially be a problem for individuals who start a VCLD while on blood-pressure medication for high blood pressure and for other illnesses. Patients taking blood-pressure medication at the start of a VLCD should notify their VLCD provider. The VLCD provider will then determine if a dose adjustment of the patient's blood-pressure medication(s) is needed both before starting the VLCD and during the VLCD.

7. Low blood sugar – Symptomatic low blood sugar can sometimes occur during a VLCD in a person with a history of hypoglycemia, or low blood sugar. During an episode of low blood sugar, a person can experience shakiness, sweating, light-headedness, palpitations, and mental slowness. The treatment for hypoglycemia is to consume a small amount of something that contains glucose. The symptoms

resolve moments after eating a glucose-containing snack, and this can confirm for the patient that the most likely cause of their symptoms was hypoglycemia. For non-dieters, episodes of hypoglycemia can mostly be avoided by reducing carbohydrate consumption at meals and by consuming a small protein-based snack two hours after each meal. Patients who experience episodes of hypoglycemia while on a VLCD, especially if hypoglycemia is not common for the patient, should notify their VLCD provider.

Hypoglycemia can also happen in diabetics that are on insulin or are on diabetic medications that stimulate the pancreas to produce extra insulin. A type 2 diabetic patient who is on these medications should carefully plan what changes need to be made with their diabetic medications with an experienced VLCD provider before they start a VLCD. Type 1 diabetics are not allowed to do a VLCD. In my practice, type 2 diabetics that are on insulin will need to reduce the dose of the insulin by about a third before starting the VLCD. This applies to both short- and long-acting insulin. Also, in my practice, the dose of medications that increase secretion of insulin from the pancreas are also reduced by about 50% at the start of the VLCD. My staff then calls the patient every few days for the first week to ask for the patient's current dose of diabetic medication(s), morning blood sugars, and for the presence or absence of episodes of symptomatic hypoglycemia. The VLCD providers in our office can then make changes to the patient's diabetic medication as needed. The goal is to keep fasting morning blood sugars between 140 and 160 while on the VLCD to avoid hypoglycemic episodes. As a diabetic loses weight rapidly on the VLCD, the need for insulin, or for drugs that stimulate the release of insulin, decreases quickly, and frequent downward adjustments are needed. Again, only experienced VLCD providers should treat type 2 diabetics that are on insulin, or on drugs that stimulate the release of insulin, with a VLCD.

8. Constipation – Due to the low volume of residue from the small amounts of food that are consumed on a VLCD as well as the

decreased intake of fluids that occur in patients who don't drink the recommended amount of fluid while on a VLCD, constipation can be a common side effect. For patients who are given ursodiol to prevent gallstone attacks, the diarrhea from the ursodiol counteracts the constipation from the VLCD and most VLCD patients on ursodiol don't experience constipation. For those who don't need the ursodiol because they don't have a gallbladder, or those who choose not to take it, and then develop constipation, over-the-counter medications will be needed to control the constipation. These medications include MiraLAX, Colace, and Dulcolax. If the constipation persists after using these medications, the VLCD provider should be contacted for further advice.

9. Fatigue – Fatigue can occur in the first few weeks of a VLCD, which is likely due to the marked drop in carbohydrate intake that occurs when an individual stops a high-carbohydrate American diet and then starts a VLCD. If the fatigue is more than mild, the patient's VLCD provider should be contacted for advice. Use of the stimulant-weight-loss drug phentermine early in the VLCD can help patients with fatigue. At the same time, the VLCD participant should be patient, since the vast majority of VLCD patients feel a rebound in energy by the third week on the VLCD. Many feel even more energy than they did before they started the VLCD.

10. Mental food craving – While the science behind a VLCD allows the VLCD participant to diet without feeling physical hunger for as long as the dieter remains compliant on the VLCD, a VLCD doesn't prevent the mental craving for favorite foods, or the craving for chewing solid food. Weight-loss medications, and especially phentermine, can help to reduce the mental craving. The mental craving also improves with time, at least to a degree. Particularly difficult is the occasional complaint of an intense need to chew solid food that is not satisfied by the shakes, soups, and bars which comprise the diet on the VCLD. The need to chew something usually fades after the third week, but when it is an ongoing concern, chewing sugar-free

gum can help, although chewing more than one piece every two to three hours can result in gas and diarrhea from the sugar alcohols that are used as sweeteners in sugar-free gum. It is tempting for VLCD providers to let patients who are desperate to chew something to chew on celery or beef jerky. However, introducing these foods can promote cheating on the VLCD.

11. Social pressure to eat with friends and family – The longer that a patient is on a VLCD, the more difficult it is for family and friends that don't get to eat socially with the patient. These mostly well-meaning family members and friends may put pressure on the VLCD participant to return to eating regular food with them. The anxiety caused by this social pressure to eat with family and friends can undermine a VLCD patient's commitment to remain faithful to the VLCD. I strongly recommend to all my new VLCD patients to avoid as much as possible going out to restaurants during the VLCD, and especially during the first month. During the first weeks of the VLCD, when fatigue is significant and food craving is intense, it is nearly impossible to sit in a favorite restaurant with family and friends and not give in and have a bite. And cheating on diets never stops at one bite. I also recommend that VLCD patients who must prepare dinnertime food for their family should not sit at the dinner table with them for the same reason. As a VLCD goes beyond the first month, some patients find that they can sit at dinner with family and friends, and then just eat a protein bar with water or a diet drink. However, this often backfires for my VLCD patients and many start cheating on dinnertime food.

I strongly encourage my VLCD patients to avoid eating meals with people who are critical of the VLCD diet, even if it is family members. I have experienced this negative talk firsthand when I was on a VLCD. One of my family members once told me, when I was on a VLCD, that they wouldn't go out socially with my wife and I until I was willing to eat regular food at dinner with them. They weren't being mean about it. They were just not comfortable eating dinner in front of me while I wasn't eating anything. Other family members have told me that VLCD is unhealthy and that I needed to eat vegetables while dieting, or I will get sick.

12. Doubt – As boredom with the limited food choices on the VLCD increases, as social pressure to eat with friends and family mounts, and as the fatigue that VLCD participants have in the first few weeks drags on, it is natural for VLCD participants to start to doubt whether they can continue the VLCD. My first advice is always to hang in there; it gets easier by the third week. That is, unless the VLCD participant is cheating by eating more than their allotted daily calorie limit. In that case, they remain famished throughout their attempt at the VLCD and almost always plateau and/or quit before the first few months have passed.

Like most difficult tasks that humans tackle, a VLCD is easier if it is taken day by day, in small mental pieces. The dieter should tell themselves, "I can make it through one day on the VLCD." Then, on the next day, the dieter should tell themselves that they can make it through another day. Take it one day at a time. Another way to stay committed to a VCLD, when doubt rears its ugly and destructive head, is to remind yourself of all the negative consequences of being obese that led you to start the VLCD in the first place. This might include weight-related knee pain with walking, shortness of breath with climbing stairs, fear of getting fired, and fear of health consequences, such as type 2 diabetes, sleep apnea, stroke, and heart attack. Some of my patients have taped lists of all the health and social problems that their weight has been causing them through-out their house. Others have placed a picture of themselves at their heaviest on the fridge door.

Again, when doubt threatens to end your commitment to a VLCD, be positive, focus on the benefits of the rapid weight loss that will occur on the VLCD, and stay away from people who try to undermine your commitment.

13. Hair loss – Thinning of hair is a common and frustrating consequence of any diet and tends to be more pronounced with the more weight that it is lost. Excess hair loss appears to also occur in diets that are low in protein. The loss of hair related to dieting is not permanent and the hair that has been lost will completely regrow by six to twelve months after the diet has ended, if the dieter is otherwise healthy and depending on how long a person's hair is.

The natural life cycle of a human hair is two to six years. The varying length of the life cycle of a human hair is due mostly to differing genetics from person to person. The active growth part of the life cycle of a human hair is called the anagen phase. Normally, 85% to 90% of hair follicles are in the anagen phase. In the last one to four months of the hair's life cycle, the hair follicle goes into a dormant phase, or telogen phase, during which the hair stops growing and then falls out. Within about two weeks of the hair falling out, new hair begins growing.

During a diet, the body conserves protein for essential body functions and furnishes less protein to the hair follicles for hair growth. More than the usual number of hair follicles move into the telogen phase and the growth of new hairs can be delayed. In one study, 35% of VLCD patients consuming 420 calories per day reported mild hair loss (Ryttig, 1997). I have personally not seen that frequent of hair loss with my VLCD participants at the levels of calorie intake that I prescribe. In my VLCD patients who complete a six-month VLCD, hair loss occurs in less than 25% and is mild. Many don't lose any discernable hair. A small number of our patients have reported hair loss weeks after the VLCD has ended. My theory on how this happened is that up to 25% of these patients' follicles went into telogen phase during their VLCD, but that the hair didn't fall out of the follicle. After the patients completed the VLCD and their calorie intake increased, new hairs began to grow in those follicles, pushing the still attached hairs out of the follicles.

This made it appear that their hair was falling out even though they had stopped the VLCD.

All of our patients who have lost hair during or after one of our VLCDs have regrown all of their hair. We believe that the reason that our VLCD patients don't lose as much hair as is discussed in the literature is because our VLCD diets provide adequate protein.

14. Bad breath – Bad breath, or halitosis, occurs frequently in patients who are on a VLCD. The exact cause for this is not well understood but is at least in part due to the mild ketosis that VLCD participants experience, as well as the dry mouth that can occur during a VLCD. The dry mouth on the VLCD occurs because the dieter drinks less fluids because they are eating less. The dry mouth is also in part due to phentermine that many of our patients take during their VLCD. The solution is to drink more water and to use diet gum, diet candy, and diet mints; although the dieter shouldn't use more than one mint, candy, or piece of gum every few hours, due to the gas and diarrhea that can be caused by excess consumption of the sugar alcohols that are used as sweeteners in the sugar-free mints, gum and candy.

While our patients are on a VLCD, they are seen weekly by trained diet counselors, such as registered nurses or medical assistants. These weekly visits are comprised of a 10- to 15-minute group class on various topics related to weight loss and weight maintenance, and a 10-minute private diet consultation with the diet counselor. During the consultation, the diet counselor reviews the patient's journal of their food intake, reviews compliance on the prescribed prescription and over-the-counter medications, and discusses challenges and side effects that might be occurring. Questions are answered.

Once a patient is compliant and comfortable on the VLCD and weight is being lost steadily month by month, the next big question for patients is how long they should remain in the VLCD. This answer is different for every patient and is based on many factors, including cost, time commitment, desired body image, and how long the drive to eat socially can be denied. We allow our VLCD patients to stay on a VLCD for up to one year. This one-year time limit is based on our experience with VLCDs and not on scientific studies. This time limit does not indicate that we believe that VLCDs that last longer than a year a harmful in any way. Many VLCD patients find that they easily reached their initial weight loss goal, but that they still have an unacceptable amount of fat on their abdomens and thighs. It is perfectly safe for them to continue the VLCD for a few more months until they reach a weight at which they are happy with their body shape, although losing weight lower than ideal body weight is never acceptable. In addition, for patients over 40-years old, I encourage them to stop losing weight at five to 10 pounds over their ideal weight, since patients over 40 look older if they lose too much fat in their faces (Guyuron, 2009). Since patients have a lower body water content due to being on a very low sodium diet, our VLCD patients are encouraged to lose to five pounds below their desired weight, since they will gain five pounds of water weight when they stop the VLCD and begin eating a weight-maintenance diet.

Ending a VLCD and starting weight maintenance is a stressful time for the VLCD participants in our clinic. A number of our patients have lost more than a 100 pounds on our VLCD and some have lost more than 200 pounds, all without feeling physical hunger. However, each of our patients know from experience just how hungry they will be when they start weight maintenance on a higher intake of calories per day. This hunger is due largely to the high levels of ghrelin that are present by the end of a successful VLCD. Some have asked if they can stay on the VLCD forever, so they wouldn't ever have to feel hungry again. Of course, the answer is no, they couldn't stay on a VLCD forever. In our clinic, we transition our VLCD patients, over the span of a month, to a maintenance diet of shakes, soups, and bars four to five times during the day and one protein-and-vegetable-based meal with their family and/or friends in the evening—all totaling about 1,600 calories per day. They continue the appetite suppressing medications that they have been using during the VLCD long term, to suppress the massive surge of hunger that occurs at the end of a successful VLCD. Exercise at 500 minutes per week of brisk walking is strongly encouraged. The principles of successful weight maintenance will be discussed further later in this book.

Weight maintenance after a VLCD is difficult for almost all VLCD participants. The more weight that a dieter loses correlates with how fast they will gain it back after the diet, and since a VLCD produces rapid and significant weight loss, then rapid and significant weight regain is an undesired but common occurrence after a VLCD. The weight regain, in my observation, is generally faster in Muse Satiety Type 5s than in Muse Satiety Type 4s and is faster in Muse Type 4s than in Muse Type 3s. The use of appetite suppressants after a VLCD, along with aggressive efforts at following the principles of weight maintenance, help a lot. But inevitably, after six to 12 months, some weight is regained. In our clinic, we strongly encourage our VLCD participants to return to repeat in VLCD at any time that they have gained back more than 20 pounds. We allow them to redo the VLCD at a lower cost.

There is a temptation by well-meaning medical providers to have patients do a VLCD every other month, believing that the patients will better tolerate the VLCD that way and will be able to restart the VLCD each month without difficulty. After treating more than 500 patients with a VLCD, I can tell you that the answer is resoundingly don't do it. Starting a VLCD is hard for almost all patients, and restarting is just as hard. Once you're on a VLCD, staying on it is pretty easy, as long as you don't cheat. In my experience, most patients who mess up and cheat on a VLCD have a hard time restarting. Also, in my experience, many patients who go on a vacation during a VLCD and then try to get back on the VLCD after the vacation have a hard time restarting. A medical-provider-supervised VLCD is safe enough and easy enough to stay on that patients should stay on a VLCD until they reach their weight-loss goals, whether it be 50 or 200 pounds.

A VLCD results in over twice as much weight lost over every other diet, including prescription-appetite-suppressant-based diets. VLCDs are just as effective as weight-loss surgery. A common statement that I hear from patients who have more than 50 pounds to lose is that they are going to do a less effective diet for a while, and then if it doesn't work, they will do a VLCD. What almost always follows is that patients do the other diet, lose 10 to 20 pounds, and then never return to do the VLCD. They end up with a disappointing amount of weight lost, instead of losing all the weight that they wanted to through a VLCD. If you're on the fence on whether to do a VLCD, a prescription-based-appetite-suppressant diet, or any other diet, then just do the VLCD. You'll be glad you did.

WEIGHT LOSS IN CHILDREN AND TEENS

Before finishing this chapter, I would like to briefly address weight loss in children and teenagers. I do treat both age groups for weight loss. If we can keep our children and teens thinner, they will be significantly less likely to be obese as adults (Lifshitz, 2008). Many of the principles taught in this chapter and in the rest of this book apply to teens as well, although there aren't as many medications that can be used for weight loss in teens. Weight loss for children 12-and-under is different than for teens and will be discussed below. Obesity in children and teens is defined as having a BMI that is at the 95th percentile or greater.

Depending on maturity and motivation, teens who are obese that are taught the proper principles and tools that lead to weight loss can decide on their own that they need to lose weight and succeed. Teens that are obese that have stopped growing, or are still growing but are severely obese, should be started on a diet. Teens that are mildly to moderately obese and have not stopped growing should probably be considered for a reduction of calorie intake to prevent weight gain while the teen grows taller, instead of being placed on a diet that causes weight loss. Regardless, teens and their caregivers should consult with pediatric weight-loss specialists to determine the appropriateness of dieting for the teens and to receive counseling on activity and dietary goals. Medications to assist with weight loss can be discussed at that time with the medical provider.

Due to the independent nature of teens, many will resist suggestions that they lose weight. The same resources that are effective for adults in helping them to get ready to lose weight in "Chapter 15 – Breaking down the Barriers that Keep You from Trying to Lose Weight" can help teens. Teens that decide to start a diet are high risk for stopping their diet due to their limited ability to see how sacrificing pleasure today can bring greater pleasure in the future. For example, after a month on a diet, when a teen's friends call for the teen to go to the local fast-food joint to hang out, the teen will probably immediately place the value of going out with friends to the fast-food joint higher than staying on their diet. For this reason, teens have a short diet-attention span. All you can do when a teen cheats on their diet is to encourage them to get back on their diet, since they can't be forced to diet when they don't want to. If you try to force a resistant teen to diet, it might work somewhat while they are at home, but they will then overfeed themselves at friend's houses, church, and sporting and school activities. They will also use their also own money to purchase food outside the home.

Children 12-and-under are much less independent and are more willing to diet when their caregiver tells them to do so. However, children 12-and-under, and especially children 10-and-under, do not have the ability to consistently choose to resist eating highly palatable food if it is readily available to them in their homes. If parents want an obese child to lose weight, then the food environment in the home that was the major contributor to the child's obesity must change, and not just for the obese child, but for the whole family. Food at meals must be changed to single-serving plates of food that are appropriate in size. The only drinks allowed must be calorie free, besides white milk. No snacks can be available in the whole house that the child will try to find and consume between meals. The child's inactive time needs to decrease, and the child's active time needs to increase. If the family goes on a diet with the child, and especially if the mother goes on a diet with the child, then child is more likely to lose weight (Andriani, 2015). Before placing your 12-and-under child on a diet, I strongly recommend consulting with a specialist trained in pediatric obesity to discuss if and what kind of a diet is appropriate for your child.

As I complete the chapter, I want to stress that a diet ends on the last day of the diet. The diet either resulted in meaningful weight loss or it didn't. If a person gains the weight back after ending the diet, it doesn't mean that the diet failed. It means that the dieter's efforts at weight maintenance failed. Weight maintenance is a vastly different animal than weight loss and it is significantly more difficult than weight loss. If not done correctly, weight maintenance most often fails. The only predictor of weight regain after a successful diet is the amount of weight that was lost on the diet and not how it was lost (Wing R., 2005). Those who have lost more weight typically gain the weight back faster, but over a longer period of time. Those who have lost less weight typically gain back the weight slower, but over a shorter period of time. Gaining the weight back after a diet doesn't mean that the individual should go looking for another diet, in hopes that the next diet will finally help with weight maintenance after the weight is lost again. I can't tell you how often I've seen dieters in my office lose 100-plus pounds and then not follow the correct principles of weight maintenance, resulting in gaining back all the weight they have lost. I have found out later that they have tried another diet program and that they have only lost 10 or 20 pounds. Why didn't they come back to me and repeat the diet in my office that resulted in the 100-plus pounds of weight loss? It's because dieters who gain it all back after a diet can't separate in their minds the successful weight loss from the failed weight maintenance. Dieters who have regained the weight they lost should lose weight again with the most effective diet that they have done before, or that they can find. Once they have lost the weight again, they must simply try harder to comply with the correct principles of weight maintenance that will be discussed in Chapter 11.

In summary, the best diet for weight loss is the diet that affords the most weight lost at the smallest cost per pound lost, while promoting heart health and maintaining safety. I have shown in this chapter that all diets work, although some result in more weight loss than others. Certainly, different people will find different diets to be the best for them. For me, as a member of Muse Satiety Type 5, the VLCD works best. I have done a VLCD of varying lengths at least 20 different times in the last 10 years. No other diet works as well as a VLCD for me. In my experience, patients who have 50 pounds or more to lose and are members of Muse Satiety Types 4 and 5 have the highest chance of losing that 50 pounds through a VLCD. If a VLCD just isn't something that the dieter who needs to lose 50 pounds or more can wrap their mind around, then the next best diet is a medication-assisted diet using two medications along with a 1,000-calorie-per-day diet. For overweight patients with less than 50 pounds to lose, I recommend a medication-assisted diet using two medications, along with a 1,000-calorie-per-day diet.

CHAPTER 11

I LOST IT, SO HOW DO I KEEP IT OFF?

MAINTAINING WEIGHT LOSS after a diet is much more difficult than losing weight. Weight loss requires a person to maintain a daily calorie deficit for a long enough period to lose a desired amount of weight. It is difficult but doable. Almost all overweight individuals have successfully dieted at least once in their life. Other the other hand, it is nearly impossible for individuals to maintain weight after a diet, since it requires eating the exact number of calories that they have burned each day, no more and no less, day after day, for the rest of their lives, in the face of the high ghrelin and low metabolism that occur with dieting. Since dieters are members of Muse Satiety Types 2 to 5, they lack one or more satiety signals that they need to be able to know and feel when to stop eating. It is difficult to find studies of the rate of success for the general public in maintaining weight after a diet. A general estimate from low-quality research is 80% of individuals who lose weight will gain back most of what they have lost in one to three years (Wing R. , 2005). The risk of regaining weight after dieting for members of Muse Satiety Types 2 to 5 has not been studied. From my clinical experience, for individuals who are Muse Satiety Type 2s, I estimate the risk of regaining all of the weight lost from a diet is greater than 50% over a one to three-year period after dieting. For Muse Satiety Type 3s, I estimate the same risk to be greater than 70%, and for members of Muse Satiety Types 4 and 5, I estimate the same risk to be 90% to 100%. Many members of Muse Satiety Types 3 and 4 have a lifetime cumulative weight loss ranging between 100 to more than 800 pounds. For Muse Satiety Type 5s, the fluctuations up and down in weight can be so large as they diet, and can occur so frequently throughout their lives, that many have repeatedly lost and regained between 500 and 2,000 pounds in their lifetimes.

As you may remember, I am a Muse Satiety Type 5. As a Muse Satiety Type 5, I have lost and gained back more than 1,500 pounds in my lifetime. Gratefully, I now know there are tools that have been proven to work to prevent weight regain after a diet. With the use of these tools, which I will discuss below, members of Muse Satiety Types 2 to 5 can reduce the amount of weight they regain after a diet by 50% to 75%. In fact, some of the dieters in my weight-loss practice are successfully maintaining their weight with no weight regain, year after year. It's not easy for them, but they are doing it. I personally have not done as well as these successful weight maintainers, but I have been able to reduce the amount of weight I regain per year after dieting from as much as 50 pounds a year down to 10 to 20 pounds a year. For me that has been a great accomplishment!

I have heard many say that if weight maintenance after a diet doesn't keep a person from regaining the weight they have lost, then it wasn't worth doing the diet in the first place. This is just not true. Even though I hate dieting repeatedly, I enjoy the health benefits and social benefits of being thinner, even if it is only for six to twelve months out of every two to three years. The years of being thin delay the onset of knee and hip arthritis, delay the onset of type 2 diabetes, lower blood pressure and cholesterol, and prevent single-car accidents related to sleep apnea—just to name a few benefits. Just the improvement in social success for the short years of being thinner make the effort at dieting worthwhile. I'm quite certain that other dieters feel the same way I do. Because of this, we're not going to stop trying to lose weight every time we gain it back. If weight regain is inevitable for each of us after our diets, then we are grateful for any help to lengthen out the time in between our diets. For me, if I can increase the time between my 30- to

50-pound diets from six months, like it was in my early adulthood, to the present 18-month average between major diets, then I am ecstatic.

Repeated cycles of weight loss, followed each time by weight gain, have been derogatorily labeled as yo-yo dieting, or more scientifically, weight cycling. For years, overweight individuals have been told that weight cycling increases death, increases body fat, and permanently lowers metabolic rate. Because of this, overweight individuals have been told that it is better to stay heavy than to repeatedly lose and then regain weight. Gratefully, this myth has been refuted in recent years (Stevens VL, 2012).

As I have discussed in a previous chapter, a serious mistake made by many dieters is to assume that the method they used to lose weight was a failure if they gained back all the weight. As a result, dieters are often unwilling to return and will instead try a diet that worked best for them before. They move on to other less effective diets, hoping in the back of their minds that they will one day find a diet that will help them lose weight and then never gain it back. They don't realize it, but what they are really forever searching for and never finding is the diet that will turn them into members of Muse Satiety Type 1. As I have explained above, that is just not possible. You are either born with the three satiety signals or not.

The exact definition of successful weight maintenance is difficult to pin down. Many weight-loss programs consider weight maintenance to be a success if their dieters keep off at least 10 pounds of the weight they lost on the diet for two years after the end of the diet. Some diets use a percentage of the total body weight lost that was then maintained as a measure of success, with maintenance of a 5% weight loss by two years being considered successful weight maintenance. For example, that would be like a 200-pound person losing and keeping off at least 10 pounds of their weight loss for two years. It is true that a 10-pound weight loss that is maintained long term does have small but significant health benefits. However, gaining back all but 10 pounds after a diet would be disappointing for all my patients. We want better weight maintenance results than that. In my practice, the goal for all of my weight-loss patients with at least 30 pounds to lose is to lose at least that 30 pounds, or more if needed, and then to gain back no more than 10 pounds in the next five years. Now that's real weight maintenance. And the successes that I have had with my patients prove that it can be done.

I want to be sure that it is understood that the statements "rapid weight loss ruins your metabolism" and "slow weight loss is better weight loss because you are less likely to gain the weight back" are false. The best that I can determine is that these are just erroneous statements started by someone to explain why overweight individuals can't keep the weight off after a diet. As to the first statement, studies have shown that peoples' basal metabolic rates don't change in between and after repeated dieting (Das, 2003) (Das, 2007). The average person's basal metabolic rate drops about 200 calories per day by the end of an average diet and doesn't return to its pre-diet level until all the weight that was lost is regained. However, the metabolic rate does return to its pre-diet level after the dieter gains back all the weight they have lost. As to the second statement, in my experience, slow weight loss just results in very little weight lost. People tolerate diets only so long. Diets make you feel hungry, tired, and deprived. A study has indicated that dieters who have lost weight quickly are no more likely to regain their weight than those who lose weight slowly (Toubro, 1997). The best diet is one that gets as much weight as possible off of you as fast as can be done safely. The more weight lost, the longer it takes to gain it back (Anderson J. , 2001).

In the worldwide medical literature, there are no studies that I have been able to find that have successfully taken a group of dieters who have lost weight on a diet and then have kept the majority of them from gaining back most of the weight that they lost. Sure, there are individuals scattered here and there that have successfully lost weight and have kept it off. There are even studies where up to 34% of the participants have been able to maintain their weight loss after a diet for as long as 10 years (Apolzan, 2019). That is great for the 34% of successful weight maintainers, but 66% of the participants were not able to maintain their weight loss. That is just not acceptable. It must be pointed out, we don't know what percent of each Muse Satiety Type there were in these studies. For all we know, the 34% that kept the weight off in these studies were members of Muse Satiety Types 2 and 3, since most Muse Satiety Type 2s and 3s do maintain weight more successfully than members of Muse Satiety Types 4 to 5.

There are three proven ways to maintain weight lost after a successful diet. They are prescription medication, exercise, and calorie counting.

Prescription Medication for Weight Maintenance

The first landmark study to show that weight can be successfully maintained by the use of medication after a diet was done in 1992 (Weintraub, 1992). In this study, 121 obese patients lost an average of 32 pounds on phentermine in the first 33 weeks of the study. They then continued with phentermine for three additional years. The patients regained an average of one pound per year. This was, and still is, astounding. At the end of the three-year maintenance period, the patients were taken off the phentermine. Over the next 20 weeks, almost all of the patients gained back almost all of the weight they had originally lost. While unfortunate, this fits with what I have already presented, that high ghrelin and low metabolism after a diet result in 80% of patients gaining back most of the weight they have lost from a diet within two to three years. This study gave us the first proof that the long-term use of a weight-loss medication can provide most patients with the ability to maintain weight loss long term, if they keep taking the medication.

I was intrigued immediately by the news that my patients and I could take phentermine off-label for maintenance for long periods of time and not gain back the weight we have lost over and over again. However, changing the mindset of most of my patients concerning the use of medication long term for weight maintenance has been difficult. So many of my patients still believe what they have been told by dietitians, other medical providers, and diet books, that if you can just learn to eat right, then you will never again gain back the weight lost from a diet. At the end of their various diets, my patients who are members of Muse Satiety Types 2 to 5 have often said to me, "I feel so good that I will never gain the weight back. I don't need phentermine for weight maintenance," "I refuse to take a drug long term for weight maintenance; if I can't keep it off by diet and exercise, then so be it," or "I'll just exercise, and I won't need phentermine." Sadly, they have almost all gained back the weight they lost within six to 24 months of stopping phentermine. I have had patients on phentermine in my practice for more than 20 years as of writing this book. Their weight remains stable for as long as they take the phentermine. If they stop taking it because they can't get back to my clinic for a refill, then almost always their weight starts to rise.

It takes more than one study to establish medical fact. Gratefully, there are more studies that prove the long-term use of phentermine helps patients to successfully maintain weight. In 2011, 10,500 patients from three separate weight-loss clinics were given phentermine for five years. There was no placebo group in this study. The patients in this study lost an average of 20 pounds in the first six months on phentermine. After five years of continuous phentermine use, the average weight regain was two pounds. There were no deaths, serious side effects, or addictive behaviors that were attributable to the phentermine (Rader, About 2014). Again, this is astounding. It's like the holy grail of weight maintenance has finally been found.

I have discussed the use of the combination of phentermine and topiramate for weight loss in Chapter 10. Patients who had lost 13% of their body weight on phentermine and topiramate at the end of one year were then continued on the same dose of phentermine and topiramate and only gained back three pounds by the end of the second year (Garvey, 2012). There were no deaths, serious side effects, or addictive behavior that were attributable to the phentermine component in the combination.

Taken together, these three studies have demonstrated that the medication phentermine, when taken alone for weight maintenance, is quite effective and safe. It is important to remember that the medication phentermine is only approved by the FDA in obese patients for "a few weeks." Any use of phentermine for longer than a few weeks for weight loss and weight maintenance is off-label use. Finally, I must stress that phentermine is not a miracle pill that allows a person to maintain weight while eating poorly and not exercising. The three studies above all included a recommendation to diet and exercise while taking the phentermine and involved regular follow-ups with the prescribing weight-loss medical providers.

The medication liraglutide has been studied for weight maintenance as well. In a study done on 2,254 patients that was reported in 2017, subjects that received liraglutide lost about 8% of their body weight, or about 18 pounds, in about one year. Those who continued to the end of the three-year study only gained back four pounds. Subjects on placebo lost 2.6% of their body weight, or about eight pounds, in about one year. Those placebo patients who continued to the end of the three-year study gained back two pounds (Roux, 2017).

Metformin was studied for its ability to promote weight maintenance. In a study of 994 patients who had successfully lost 3% of their body weight while taking metformin, or about seven pounds, the average weight regained after 10 years was about two pounds. The placebo group in this study lost one pound and had gained back two pounds by the tenth year (Apolzan, 2019).

I have discussed topiramate for weight loss in Chapter 10. In a study published in 2004, 293 patients first lost about 22 pounds on a low-calorie diet and then were either given low-dose topiramate, high-dose topiramate, or placebo for up to 14 months. The patients on both low-dose and high-dose topiramate lost about 15 additional pounds over placebo by 32 weeks and then gained back about four pounds by the end of 14 months. There were no serious side effects in this small trial (Astrup, 2004). Topiramate has not been approved by the FDA as a single agent for weight loss or weight maintenance, although it is part of the FDA-approved combination-medication Qsymia that was already discussed in the previous chapter. Like phentermine, the use of topiramate alone for weight loss and weight maintenance is off-label use.

Phentermine, liraglutide, metformin, and topiramate are more effective than diet alone for weight maintenance after a diet. None of these medications have been compared head-to-head in clinically significant studies as of writing this book. As discussed above, none of these medications are completely effective in preventing weight regain after a diet. But, without question, they can slow down and sometimes even stop the discouraging cycle of weight loss with a diet followed by weight regain.

For patients who are members of Muse Satiety Types 2 to 5 that have ever been more than 30 to 50 pounds overweight, have lost that weight, and are struggling to keep from gaining it back, I plead with you to carefully think about the information that I have presented. Ask your medical provider to consider prescribing one of these medications to you long term to help you to slow down the weight regain that so often occurs after a diet. And don't get overconfident one, two, or three years later and decide that you no longer need the medication for weight maintenance, and that you can do it on your own. Like most successful weight maintainers on medications, it won't go well for you off the medications. Last of all, if you choose to ignore what I am recommending and try to maintain weight without medication, be vigilant to weigh often so that you can monitor for the first 10 pounds of weight regain. Then, don't delay and return to your medical provider and get back on medication for weight maintenance.

For the medical providers, I plead with you to stop telling your patients that once they have lost weight that they should stop the weight-loss medications that they used to lose weight. For members of Muse Satiety Types 2 to 5, it almost never goes well. The side effects of the single-agent medications that I have presented above, whether used alone or in combination, are most often mild, if they occur at all. In my experience, patients who have successfully taken these medications for more than six months while dieting, with minimal or no side effects, rarely develop significant side effects later. Of course, be aware of the side effects and safety information in the package insert for each of these medications before prescribing them to your patients. Also, before prescribing these medications, be aware of your local and state laws governing the prescribing of long-term weight maintenance medications.

Exercise for Weight Maintenance

Researchers have conducted a number of studies to determine how much exercise per day is needed to maintain weight after a diet. One of the first landmark studies to establish the amount of exercise needed to maintain weight after a diet was published in 1995 (Ewbank, 1995). In this study, subjects initially lost an average of 62 pounds on a VLCD. At the end of the diet, they were instructed to exercise and eat right to maintain their weight loss. The subjects were interviewed by the researchers two years later. The patients who had exercised enough to burn more than 2,000 extra calories per week had only gained back 13% of the weight they had lost. It would have taken a 140-pound person walking four miles per hour, 71 minutes per day, seven days a week, to burn at least those 2,000 calories per week. Those in the study that exercised enough to burn more than 1,500 extra calories per week gained back 24% of the weight they had lost. Those who exercised less than 1,500 extra calories per week gained back about 75% of the weight they had lost. Walking was the chosen source of exercise for 65% of the study participants.

A second study that further validated exercise as a weight maintenance tool was published in 1997 (Schoeller, 1997). In this trial, 32 women who had lost between 31 and 70 pounds on a diet were then asked to exercise mildly, moderately, or not at all, to prevent weight regain. Careful monitoring of the women's diets and exercise for the next year indicated that it required 80 minutes per day, seven days per week, of moderate exercise to maintain weight after a diet. Lesser amounts of exercise per day were less effective.

Jakicic found in 2008 that it requires between 60-90 minutes per day, six days a week, of at least brisk walking to maintain weight after a diet (Jakicic, 2008).

These studies establish the fact that it takes a lot of exercise, approximately 80 minutes per day, seven days per week, or 500 minutes per week, to prevent weight regain after a diet for members of Muse Satiety Types 2 to 5. The amount of exercise required to maintain weight after a diet is difficult to wrap one's mind around, because it is more exercise than most of us can conceive of finding the time for. In addition, many of us would not be able to tolerate that much exercise per day due to orthopedic problems, such as knee and back pain. On the other hand, I have seen exercise work to maintain weight after a diet for a small number of my patients. These successful patients have been able to maintain weight for six to 24 months by exercising more than an hour per day, seven days a week. However, ultimately, something happened to each of them that led them to either stop exercising, or to sharply reduce their minutes of exercise per day. The reasons that this occurred have varied from patient to patient, but included injuries, the need to work two jobs, cold weather, the lack or loss of an exercise partner, vacations, and the need to care for sick family members. Once these patients stopped their daily exercise, they regained weight rapidly, just like they would have if they had stopped a long-term medication for weight maintenance.

Moderate intensity exercise at 80 minutes per day, seven days a week, works just as well in maintaining weight after a diet as do the weight-loss medications I have presented above. Exercising less than 80 minutes per day is not as effective in preventing weight regain after a diet. However, not being able to find the time to exercise 80 minutes per day to prevent weight regain is not an excuse to throw up your hands in frustration and all avoid exercise. Exercising 60 minutes per day, seven days a week, is moderately effective in promoting weight maintenance after a diet. And while exercise 30 minutes per day, five days a week, doesn't work at all for weight maintenance, this amount of exercise has other health benefits, including reducing heart disease, depression, blood pressure, and cholesterol. All adults should be exercising a minimum of 30 minutes a day, five days a week, if they are first cleared to do so by their medical provider. Weightlifting and strength training help to build muscle and trim waistlines, but do not help prevent weight regain after a diet.

Calorie Counting for Weight Maintenance

Counting calories to achieve weight maintenance after a diet is effective but is difficult to adhere to for most. The biggest problem with counting calories for weight maintenance is that the vast majority of humans underestimate how many calories they consume per day by more than 30%. That translates into a person saying they are eating 1,500 calories per day, but they are really consuming 2,000 calories per day. Why do most humans underestimate how many calories they consume per day? There are many reasons, including not knowing how many calories there are in the foods they are eating, not measuring the portion sizes of foods that are being consumed, not counting little bites and sips of this and that throughout the day in the total calories per day, and just plain forgetting something they ate.

There are a few studies that show that counting calories can help with weight maintenance. In the Diabetes Prevention Program study, 37% of dieters maintained a 7% loss of weight for about three years by calorie counting (DPP, 2012). Also, 36% of the members of the National Weight Control Registry have maintained weight after a diet for as long as 10 years by counting calories (Wing R. , 2005)

Medications, exercise, and calorie counting work to help dieters to succeed at weight maintenance after a diet. Many successful weight maintainers use two or three of these methods at the same time to increase their success at weight maintenance. Besides these three methods of weight maintenance, there are no other proven ways to successfully maintain weight after a diet. There is no berry-based diet from the far East that will magically keep us all thin. None of the myriad of commercial diets and book diets have accurate and dependable information on long-term weight maintenance after their diet programs.

National Weight Control Registry

I'd like to shift gears a little and present the largest and most successful long-term registry of successful weight maintainers. It is called the National Weight Control Registry (Hill J. , 1994). The National Weight Control Registry (NWCR) was established in 1994 by Drs. James Hill and Rena Wing (Hill J. , 2005) (Wing R. , 2005). To be a member of the registry, an individual must have lost 30 pounds or more and then must have kept it off for at least a year. More than 10,000 individuals have become members of the NWCR since its initiation. The average weight loss for members of the registry is 66 pounds and they have kept it off for an average of 5.5 years (The National Weight Control Registry, 2020). It is important to recognize that registering with the NWCR has been voluntary and the observations of the behaviors of this group cannot completely represent the behavior of all overweight individuals. However, the findings from the registry have strongly suggested that there is a common method of long-term weight maintenance that can work for a large group of individuals. If those of us that struggle with maintaining weight want to succeed with weight maintenance, then we need to be doing what the members of the NWCR are doing.

The NWCR is not a diet program or diet study, and the members of the NWCR have not been sent information on how to lose weight and maintain weight. Instead, the members participate in yearly follow-up questionnaires to examine the behavioral and psychological characteristics of successful weight maintainers, as well as the strategies that the members of the registry are using to successfully maintain weight (Hill J. , 1994).

In my estimation, the NWCR is mostly made up of members of Muse Satiety Types 3 to 5, since members of Muse Satiety Types 1 and 2 only occasionally gain enough weight that they could meet the requirement of having lost at least 30 pounds to join the registry. Since the average weight lost for members of the registry is 66 pounds, it is even more likely that most of the members of the NWCR are from Muse Satiety Types 3 to 5.

The demographics of the members of the NWCR as of 2020 were as follows:

1. 80% were female (The National Weight Control Registry, 2020).

2. The average age for the women was 45; for men, the average age was 49 (The National Weight Control Registry, 2020).

3. 55% of members of the NWCR reported that they lost weight through one of the many commercial weight-loss programs, a medical provider, or nutritionist (The National Weight Control Registry, 2020).

4. 45% reported that they lost their weight completely on their own (The National Weight Control Registry, 2020).

5. 89% lost the weight through diet combined with exercise (Wing R. , 2005).

6. 10% lost the weight with diet alone. (The members of the NWCR used a number of different weight-loss methods to lose their excess weight (Wing R. , 2005). There wasn't one weight-loss method that was significantly more successful than the others.)

7. 1% lost the weight by exercise alone (Wing R. , 2005). As discussed elsewhere in this book, exercise alone doesn't cause weight loss, so we can probably assume that these exercisers ate lower-calorie foods while they were exercising but didn't consider that to be a diet.

8. 15% of the members of the NWCR lost their weight quickly. Others took up to 14 years to lose their weight (The National Weight Control Registry, 2020).

9. The amount of weight lost by the individuals in the NWCR ranged from 30 to 300 pounds (The National Weight Control Registry, 2020).

10. The duration of the successful weight maintenance ranged from one year to 66 years (The National Weight Control Registry, 2020).

I will now discuss the successful behaviors that this group has been doing to maintain weight. About 5% of them, or about 500 members of the registry, are taking phentermine long term (Klem, 1997). They have found medical providers that are willing to prescribe phentermine long term for weight maintenance. What do you think the other 95% of the members of the NWCR are doing? From what I have explained above, if they aren't taking phentermine, then the only other thing that works well is exercise. Sure enough, 90% of the members of the registry are exercising an average of 60 minutes per day, seven days a week, or 420 minutes per week. The majority (76%) are walking briskly as their form of exercise. Other forms of exercise that they are doing are resistance training (20%), cycling (20%), and aerobics (18%) (Wing R. , 2005).

The members of the NWCR are quite consistent in their dietary behaviors:

1. 78% eat breakfast every day (Wing R. , 2005).

2. Almost all members continue long term on a low-calorie diet. Even more specifically, they do this by limiting the intake of certain foods (92%), limiting the quantity of food eaten (49%), limiting fat intake (38%), counting calories (36%), and counting fat grams (30%) (Wing R. , 2005). They almost certainly have the low-calorie and low-fat meals at restaurants and they most likely skip the fries with their sandwiches. In the NWCR, there isn't a difference in long-term success at weight maintenance, whether a person consumes a high-protein diet or a high-carbohydrate diet (Sacks F. , 2009). It's the calories that count.

3. More than 90% of the members of the NWCR eat the same number of calories on the weekends and on holidays as they do during the

week (Wing R. , 2005). They don't overeat at restaurants, at parties, or on cruises.

4. Approximately 80% weigh their food at least once every four days to keep their food portions from slowly trending upward in size. This can be done easily by consuming a calorie-measured meal for at least one meal a day, such as a protein bar, protein shake, string cheese, frozen diet meal, etc.

5. 75% weigh themselves at least once a week and 44% weigh themselves every day (Wing R. , 2005).

6. The members of the NWCR consume five to six small, pre-measured, and protein-based meals throughout the day (Wing R. , 2005).

I want to drill down a little deeper into some of these dietary behaviors. Ninety-two percent of the members of the NWCR limit the intake certain foods in their diet. While I don't have access to the exact foods that the members of the NWCR are limiting in their diets, I have no doubt that they are limiting foods that they can't resist. Foods that they can't resist are foods that they are addicted to. A food that a person is addicted to is a food is a person looks at on a serving plate or bowl and says to themselves, "I really shouldn't eat that," and then comes up for air 20-30 minutes later and the food is either mostly gone or completely gone. The types of food that individuals are addicted to vary widely from individual to individual, based on upbringing, taste preferences, and current food environment. Some prefer salty foods over sweet foods. Some prefer Italian food over Mexican food. And the triggers that induce the overuse of addictive foods also vary widely from individual, and include worry, anxiety, sadness, depression, anger, fatigue, and poor self-image.

The only solution to addictive foods is to remove them completely and permanently from a person's diet for the rest of their life. It sounds harsh, but it is no different for food addictions than it is for addictions to anything else in life. No, a person isn't addicted to all foods. Once a person has stopped any type of addictive behavior and are in recovery, then returning to experience that addictive behavior again just once will invariably result on a rekindling of the addictive behavior. That is why I stopped eating ice cream, my favorite food, 20 years ago as of writing this book, and I don't dare take even a little bite. I was eating up to a half-gallon per day by myself 20 years ago and I would return to eating a half-gallon a day if I started eating ice cream again. I will be addressing the topic of food addiction and strategies to overcome food addiction more in a later chapter.

As to weighing at least weekly, if not daily, during weight maintenance, I have discovered in helping my patients with weight maintenance that this is truly a crucial component of weight maintenance. For members of Muse Satiety Types 2 to 5, it is normal and expected to have days and weeks where they gain weight. Even members of Muse Satiety Type 1 gain a little weight on a cruise for a week, because they eat right up to their nausea at almost every meal. Members of Muse Satiety Type 1 return home from the cruise and without thinking about it, forget a few breakfasts, subconsciously eat less on their plate for a few meals, and are back their pre-cruise weight within a week or so. For members of Muse Satiety Types 2 to 5, they will have to consciously recognize that they have gained weight on the cruise and then consciously go on a one to two-week diet after the cruise to get the weight back off. They will have to do the same thing for every other event that increases food intake or decreases activity, repeatedly, totaling hundreds of diets, for the rest of their lives. To differentiate these repeated little diets from the more drastic yo-yo dieting, I call these little repeated diets serial dieting. Events that cause an increase in weight for members of Muse Satiety Types 2 to 5 are vacations, deaths in the family, working two or more jobs, injury, sick family members that need continuous care, and stress. Of course, members of Muse Satiety Types 2 to 5 need to try to be consistent with their weight maintenance diets and exercise rules during these difficult times of life. But even then, there will be times when their weight creeps up. There should be no guilt over these weight increases, just recognition that it's time to do another five- or 10-pound diet. It's not hard to lose five to 10 pounds with a two- to four-week diet. It is much harder when a person neglects to recognize little episodes of weight gain, here and there, until they add up to a 20- or 30-pound weight gain. I encourage my weight-maintenance patients to weigh every day, so they can catch the little weight gains occur, and to catch them before they make your pants or dresses too tight to wear. If a person gains five pounds every two months and then loses five pounds every two months, then they will weigh the same after two years. But, if they gain five pounds every two months and don't lose five pounds every two months, they will weigh 60 pounds more at the end of two years. Again, whatever you do, don't beat yourself up over these little episodes of weight gain. Just get to work and lose it back off each time. If you go to a theme park for a week, just plan on going right on a seven-day diet when you return home, because you're going to need it.

Members of the NWCR eat multiple small meals throughout the day to prevent weight regain. They eat 5.2 small meals a day but do eat out 3.5 times per week on average. It would seem to me that they are eating about 4.2 small meals a day and then eating a meal with family or friends once a day. Why do they continue eating about four small meals a day during weight maintenance? First, they have discovered that if they under eat throughout the day and then inevitably overeat at dinner, despite their best efforts not to do so, they will come out neutral for the day. Second, 78% of the members of the NWCR still say they are on a diet. They are consuming the frequent small meals during the day to try to lose more weight.

These small meals can be a protein bar, protein shake, or something made from grocery food, such as a few thin slices of turkey on a rice cake, Greek yogurt, one string cheese, a small serving of cottage cheese, etc. The guidelines for the small protein-based meals from grocery food are to keep the protein content at about 15 grams, the carbohydrate content at no more than 18 grams, and the total calories at 150-200. Of note, this must be where the members of the NWCR weigh their food frequently, as they endeavor to keep these frequent small meals to about 150 calories each.

The idea of eating only one regular meal a day of the foods that I love, instead of three, was a hard one for me to accept. However, after observing the successful weight maintainers in my practice, I realized that all of them were replacing two regular meals a day with protein bars or shakes just like I had told them to do. I was struggling with weight maintenance because I wasn't following my own advice. I finally started replacing breakfast and lunch with protein bars or shakes and eating just one meal a day with my family in the evening. It became so much easier to maintain weight! For a person who burns about 2,000 calories per day, which is the average for most of us non-construction workers, replacing breakfast and lunch with four small protein meals throughout the day adds up to 600 calories, leaving 1,400 calories to be eaten for dinner to then be weight neutral for the day. Most of us in Muse Satiety Types 3 to 5 will try not to overeat for dinner, but we probably will, like we always have. Even if we end up eating a whole plate of food, which we shouldn't, we will still end up at about 1,400 calories for dinner and 2,000 calories for the day. We will not have gained weight for the day. If that same pattern can be consistently followed day after day, then we will successfully maintain weight.

One last commonality that is shared amongst the members of the NWCR that needs to be discussed is consistency in effort. Sixty percent of the members of the NWCR reported that they followed the same dietary rules discussed above on weekends and on holidays. They also reported consistency in weight-loss efforts. Those members of the NWCR that reported an increase in fat in the diet or a decrease in average minutes exercised per day for the previous year reported an increase in weight for the same year. Members of Muse Satiety Types 2 to 5 are never cured of the disease of obesity, no matter how long they have successfully maintained their weight. The missing signals of fullness, loss of savor, and nausea with overeating can't be learned, and it is hard to overcome the effects of high ghrelin and low metabolism after a diet.

It is important to recognize that few to none of the members of the NWCR are maintaining the weight that they have lost while being sedentary. The only exception might be those who take phentermine long term for weight maintenance. Saying this another way, members of Muse Satiety Types 2 to 5 have little to no chance of ever maintaining the weight they have lost from a diet if they are not exercising or are not taking a medication like phentermine. I should repeat this three times to get this into people's heads, but hopefully that is not necessary. Exercise, exercise, and exercise. It appears that it doesn't have to be consecutive minutes, but I would be cautious with breaking the 60 minutes per day into too many small of periods. I believe that part of the reason that exercise works is that getting the heart rate above 100 and keeping it there for at least 20 minutes activates the sympathetic nervous system and the activation of that system promotes appetite suppression for up to an hour afterward. Lacking any study to guide my advice, I will play it safe and recommend not breaking up the exercise into any more than two 30-minute periods of exercise per day.

How well have the thousands of patients that I have seen in my practice done with weight maintenance? Some have done very well for years and others have disappeared from the day they finished their diet and I have never seen them again. I don't have aggregate data to share from my own practice on my patients' success with long-term weight maintenance. I would like to share the weight-loss graphs of a few of my patients to demonstrate some of the different patterns that I see in patients who have continued to come to me for long-term weight maintenance after initially losing weight in my office.

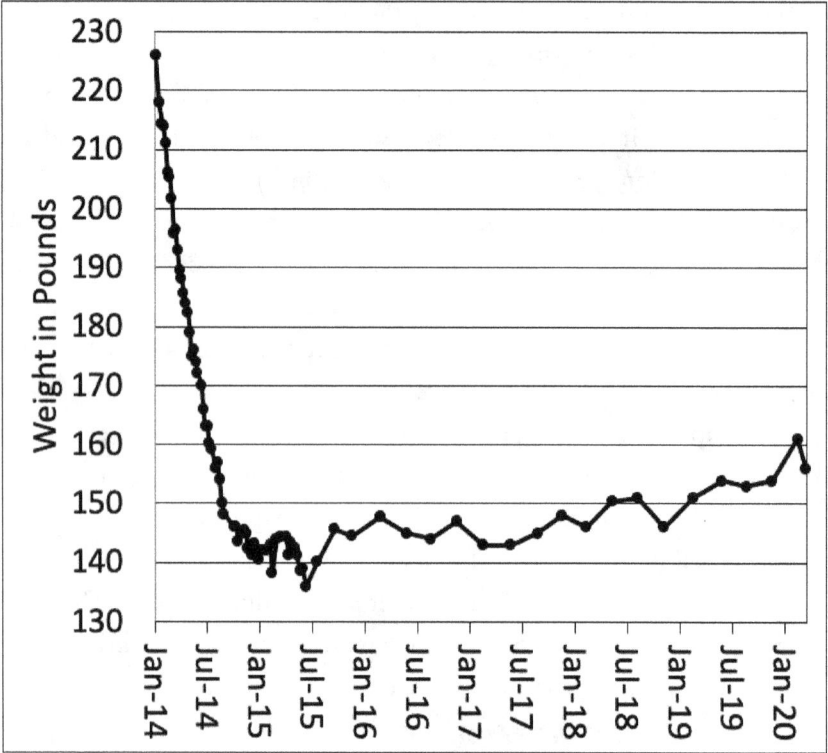

Figure 10 - Patient 1 Weight-Loss Graph

Patient 1 lost 90 pounds with a VLCD in my office from January 2014 to June 2015, as can be seen in Figure 10. The patient is a Muse Satiety Type 5. The patient has been in weight maintenance since that time. The patient has been consistently taking phentermine and has been consistently exercising daily for 60 minutes. Although the stress of COVID-19 in the first quarter of 2020 caused a little rise in the patient's weight, the patient is working on losing 10 pounds to get back to where she wants to be. Patient 1 is a shining example of how I envision weight maintenance should go for everyone. However, since human behavior is not homogeneous, then not everyone will be as successful as patient 1.

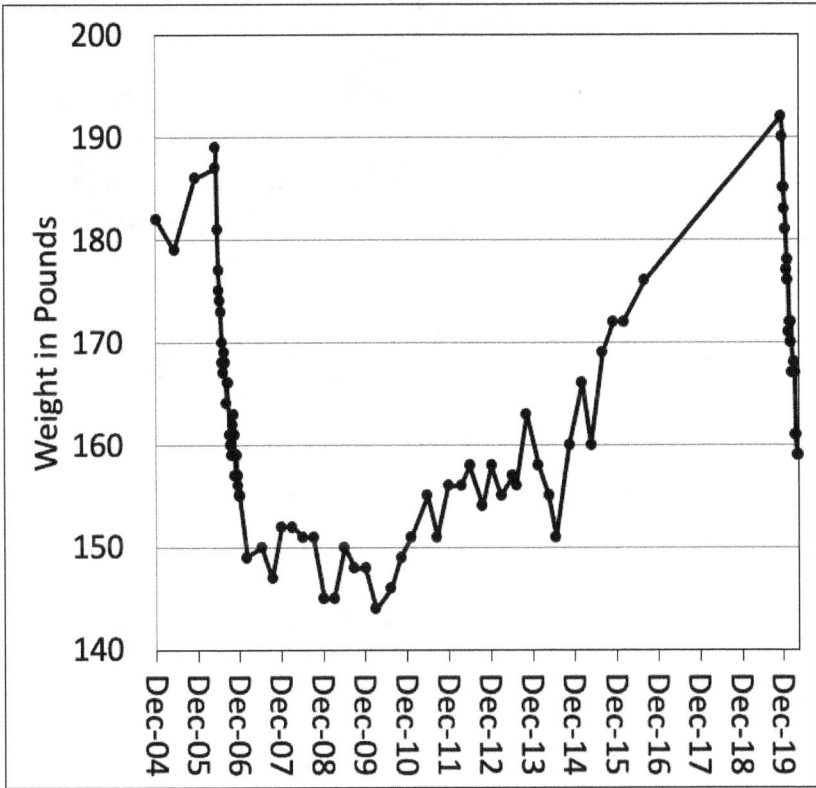

Figure 11 - Patient 2 Weight-Loss Graph

Patient 2 lost 40 pounds with a VLCD in my office between May 2006 and February 2007 as can be seen in Figure 11. Patient 2 is a Muse Satiety Type 3. After the successful weight loss, patient 2 started weight maintenance and did well with phentermine and daily exercise until near the end of 2015 when the patient's mother fell ill. The patient had to care for their ailing mother while working full time to make ends meet. This caused an immense amount of stress for the patient, and their compliance with their maintenance program suffered. As the patient's mother worsened, the patient stopped coming to our office in 2015 for more than three years, during which time the patient regained all the weight they had originally lost plus a little more. The patient's mother died in 2019, and the patient returned in November 2019 to again lose the weight they had lost via our VLCD. Weight maintenance is much harder than weight loss. Patient 2 did very well at maintenance for eight years, at least until severe family stress occurred and derailed their successful efforts at weight maintenance. I'm proud of this patient for returning and losing the weight again, now that their stress level is significantly less.

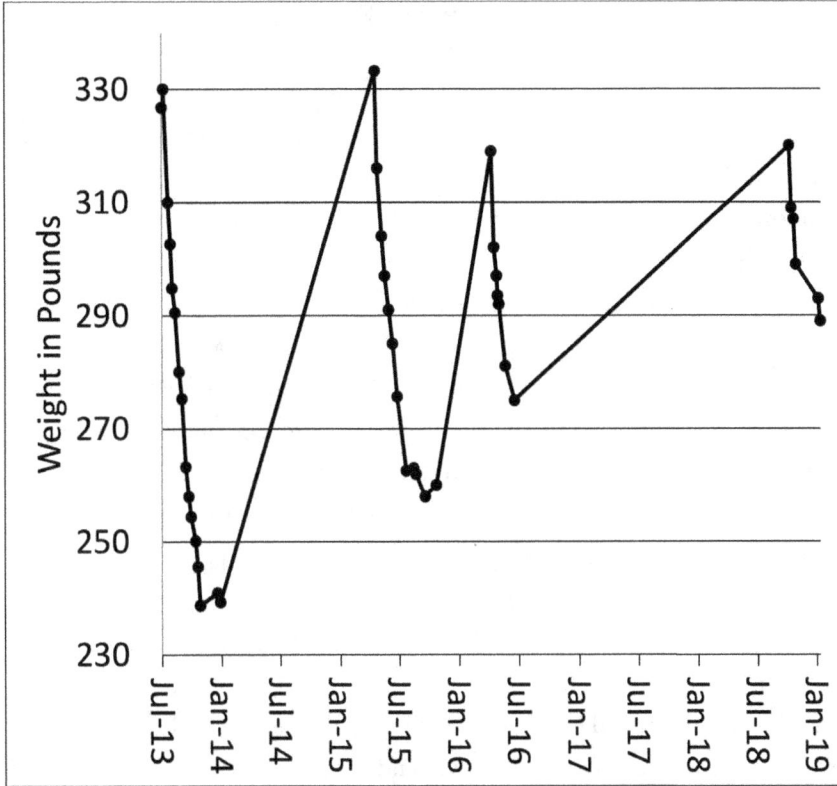

Figure 12 - Patient 3 Weight-Loss Graph

Patient 3 lost 91 pounds on a VLCD in my office from July 2013 to November 2013, as can be seen in Figure 12. The patient is a Muse Satiety Type 5. Despite teaching the patient how to be successful at weight maintenance, the patient disappeared for more than a year. During the patient's time away from our office, the patient regained all the weight they had lost. The patient restarted a VLCD in May 2015 and lost 75 pounds in the next five months. Again, despite our teaching and encouragement, the patient disappeared for six months and gained back 61 pounds. The patient again did a VLCD starting in May 2016 and lost 44 pounds. The patient again disappeared for two years and regained all the weight they had lost. The patient started another VLCD through our office in November 2018 and lost 31 pounds. The patient has not been back since.

Patient 3's experience of on-and-off-again efforts at weight maintenance is, unfortunately, a common occurrence in my office. I am convinced that my patients know and remember what I have taught them about weight maintenance. If these patients are anything like me, then life gets in the way of weight maintenance and the rules of weight maintenance go out the window. I can't be unhappy with patients like patient 3, since I am just like them. The good things that can be said about patient 3 is that the patient keeps coming back to try again, and that it was healthier for the patient to be thinner for half of the last seven years than never at all.

Weight maintenance is within the grasp of all frustrated members of Muse Satiety Types 2 to 5. The principles of weight maintenance discussed above, if followed consistently, will result in members of Muse Satiety Types 2 to 5 never again seeing themselves regain all the weight they have lost from a diet. Many of my patients have gained back less than 10 pounds of what they lost years ago by following these principles. That is not saying that they haven't had periods where they became lax in following the principles of weight maintenance. The successful weight maintainers in my practice have had to do mini-diets over and over again when they have gained a little weight and even have had to do bigger diets over and over again when they have really overdone it. With weight maintenance, our motto must be, "Never give up, never surrender" (1999, Jason Nesmith, *Galaxy Quest*). It's okay to lose a few battles against weight regain when you're still going to win the war.

CHAPTER 12

FOOD CRAVING - ANOTHER LAYER OF COMPLEXITY ON TOP OF AN ALREADY COMPLICATED DISEASE

FOOD CRAVING, OR the almost irresistible desire to eat a person's favorite foods, is the third disease causing obesity. Food craving is also called food addiction. It follows closely on the heels of the other two causes of obesity: Muse's Satietopathy (Chapter 2) and maximum weight memory (Chapter 7). Right from the beginning of this chapter, I want to set straight the mistaken concept that obesity is just an addiction to food. I hope that the previous chapters have made it clear that obesity is much more complex than just a food addiction. However, food craving affects many people. About 80% of people in the US report one or more food addictions. Most humans, given one of their favorite foods, will overeat it, even though they know they shouldn't. Despite knowing that they shouldn't, most people repeatedly overeat their favorite and addictive foods for most of their lives, even though they know that it will cause them to gain weight. That is what addiction is, per the online Merriam-Webster Dictionary, "a persistent compulsive use of a substance known by the user to be harmful."

Food craving affects individuals of all Muse Satiety Types, as far as I can tell. Food craving is genetically and environmentally based. Different individuals find more or less pleasure with the consumption of different foods. Some find ice cream irresistible. Others can't resist candy. For some, chocolate reigns supreme. There are even others that eschew these and instead find delight in salty foods, such as crackers, pretzels, and nuts. Some are addicted to only a few foods and others to a larger number of foods. Although I don't have a study to prove it, I have asked hundreds of patients if they have more than 10 foods that they repeatedly find to be irresistible, and the answer thus far has always been "no."

I've heard some patients say, at my first meeting with them, that they are addicted to everything. That is not true. There are some foods that very few, if any, people are addicted to, such as whole raw apples, baked potatoes without toppings, raw broccoli, or raw cauliflower. It is difficult to eat two raw apples, two baked potatoes without toppings, or two cups of raw broccoli or cauliflower in the same hour. The same applies to most fruits and vegetables that are high in fiber and that aren't flavor enhanced with butter, salt, sugar, and fat. The fiber in these fruits and vegetables prevents overconsumption. Cooking does break down the fiber in fruits and vegetables, which then allows for overconsumption. A person can eat a lot more cooked broccoli and cauliflower, especially with added butter and salt, than they can eat raw broccoli and cauliflower.

The presence of food craving is harmful to humans because it increases the amount of weight gained per year by members of each Muse Satiety Type. A Muse Satiety Type 1 that doesn't control their food addictions might gain 20 pounds over their lifetime, instead of zero to 10 pounds. A Muse Satiety Type 5 can gain hundreds of pounds more during their lifetime due to failure to control their food cravings as compared to another Muse Satiety Type 5 that doesn't experience food craving.

Addictive eating in individuals who crave one or more foods can be triggered by boredom, loneliness, stress, frustration, anxiety, depression, anger, fatigue, sleepiness, feelings of helplessness and hopelessness, social situations where eating is tradition or expected, grief over the illness, injury, or loss of a loved one, grief over the loss of a cherished possession or position, and sadness and depression over personal illness or injury. In addition to these emotional, social, and situational triggers, environments that offer easy access to addictive foods are a big trigger for repeated episodes of addictive eating. Finally, a common trigger for addictive eating is eating for the sheer pleasure of eating. The human brain is wired to enjoy pleasure. Even though the above triggers are sometimes factors in triggering addictive eating, most of us just eat more than we should for the fun of eating.

Once an addictive food has been experienced enough times by the brain that the brain's pleasure center finds that food irresistible, then addictive behavior with that food will be very hard to resist for the rest of a person's life. Just like most smokers can't return to dabbling with smoking years after quitting, and most alcoholics in recovery can't return to an occasional drink years after quitting, most food addicts can't return to their addictive foods for the rest of their lives.

Once a food addiction is in remission, three things can happen that make most humans more likely to relapse and return to their use of an addictive food. First, the loathing and disgust that led people to stop their addictive behavior with food fades over time. Second, the brain's memory of the pleasure of the addictive foods fades only a little over time. Third, most humans are overconfident in their belief that they will never return to their addictive eating behaviors again. These three things set humans up to easily fall back into food addictions. The solution to the first pitfall is to keep the loathing and disgust for food addiction alive by continually reminding one's self of the physical and social misery caused by the obesity that resulted from the food addiction. Some put signs and posters on their mirrors and refrigerators to remind them of the misery they once experienced when they didn't control their food addictions. The solution to the second pitfall is to remind one's self that addiction to certain foods is no different than addiction to any other substance. Once you are in remission, you can never go back to your addictive substance again, because it will beat you almost every time. The solution to the third pitfall is to never be overconfident when it comes to trying to eat favorite foods. Once an addict, always an addict. It really isn't fair, but there is nothing that can remove the addiction from the brain. The only solution is to abstain from addictive foods for life.

A common complaint coming from those who suffer from food addictions is that with almost every other addiction, you can stop the addictive substances and avoid the environment that has that substance in it completely, whereas with food, you still must eat every day. The answer is simple. You're not addicted to most foods. You must stop each of the foods that you are addicted to and never consume them again. Since most people don't have more than 10 foods that they are addicted to, they can still eat the other foods that they are not addicted to. If they identify the foods they are addicted to and stop consuming them, only to find that their brain discovers a few more foods to crave, then those additional foods must join the list of foods that should be avoided for life.

Like other addictions, food addictions are complex, and the underlying triggers can often require professional counseling and therapy. Medication can often help to treat the triggers for food addictions; these medications were discussed Chapter 10.

Food addiction affects most members of all the Muse Satiety Types. Food addictions have a number of triggers, many of which may require ongoing therapy with medication and counseling to address them. The mainstay of treatment for food addiction is to strive for 100% avoidance of addictive foods. Carefully planned, continually revised, and strictly followed food rules are needed to prevent relapse.

CHAPTER 13
FOOD RULES

AVOIDING THE TRIGGERS for food craving must become a compulsive and intensely involving process. You must establish an extensive set of rules for what you can and can't eat in different environments and in the face of different triggers. You must then stick to those rules rigorously. In the case where your adherence to those rules fails and you fall off the wagon, you must have a plan to get back in recovery. You must continually be on the watch for new addictive behaviors with new foods, new environments, and new triggers.

I want to make it clear that no two individuals will have the same food cravings, food environments, and food triggers, so no two people will have the same rules for their specific food addictions. It took years for me to realize this. I read other author's books on how to keep from gaining weight over time, and as I read their books, I became frustrated because what worked for the authors and their cravings just didn't pertain to me. Now, I realize that those authors were sharing the specific food rules they had instituted in their lives based on their food cravings, environments, and triggers. The principles underlying those author's needs to have food rules are what applies to everyone with food craving.

I will now share some of my many food rules that I try to follow religiously. When I don't follow them, I overeat my addictive foods and gain weight. It is an ongoing process to overcome food craving and to get it completely under control. If I can say at end of the month that I used my addictive foods less often and to a lesser degree than the previous month, then that month was successful in respect to food addiction. Of course, the goal must always be in sight, and that is completely abstaining from my addictive foods.

I've heard patient's say, "I just can't live without my soft drinks," "I have to have my dessert each evening," and "I plan my whole day around my snacks; I can't do without them." That's no different than what my patients say when I tell them to quit smoking or stop drinking. These are all just addictions, and anyone can stop them and remain in recovery.

My most addictive foods, listed in order from most addictive to less addictive are cookies-and-cream ice cream, cookie-dough ice cream, plain M&Ms, regular Skittles, red licorice, Costco poppy seed muffins, white bread with butter and honey, movie popcorn with butter, cashews, and peanuts. Those are the snack foods that I will consistently choose over any others and that I will consistently overeat, even though I know I shouldn't. This list of my 10 addictive foods doesn't include many foods that I have overeaten on different occasions in the past. That list is more than 100 items long. However, most of the foods I have overeaten on different occasions are not foods that I consistently crave and consistently choose over all other foods. I do have to have food rules for these less addictive foods as well.

You will probably notice right away that there are many foods that others are addicted to that are not on my list, and vice versa. We humans are all so different. Keep that in mind as I share some of my food rules concerning the foods that I crave. Your food rules won't be the same as mine because your food triggers, environment, and food cravings are different than mine. These rules can be a guiding or starting point in helping you to determine your own.

Some of my food rules:

1. No sugar (refined sugar, high-fructose corn sugar, fruit juice, and sugar soda). This makes sense for me since the first seven items on my list are full of sugar. I haven't had a single bite of most of them

since about the year 2000. When one of my daughters was 16, she asked me what my favorite food was. My response was, without hesitation, ice cream. She replied, "But, Dad, I've never seen you eat it." I allow a few exceptions to this rule of mine of no sugar, and unfortunately, those exceptions can occasionally result in overeating. My exceptions to this rule are:

a. I can have honey and jam on bread sometimes. If I am honest with myself, I know I can't eat bread, especially white bread, with honey or jam because any time that I have tried to start eating bread again, within days I had been eating four to six slices per day.

b. I can have Jell-O, but I don't like it much and only eat it rarely. Since I'm from Utah, and since Utah is the Jell-O capital of the US, then Jell-O is served occasionally at family gatherings.

c. I can have a single muffin for breakfast when I am traveling, and I can't find anything else to eat. I only travel a dozen times per year, and I can only have one muffin per day.

d. I can eat whole fruits, although I have to watch out for seedless grapes, since I have overeaten them a number of times in the past. I never drink fruit juice or fruit smoothies.

e. I can eat sugar in main and side dishes. I am very aware that there is a lot of sugar in ketchup, barbeque sauce, and sweet-and-sour sauce. And yes, I am more prone to overeat when there is a lot of sugar in the main and side dishes.

2. I never purchase peanuts and cashews. Exceptions to this are that I can buy snack-size bags of peanuts and cashews to help myself stay awake on long drives, and I can have nuts in main and side dishes. I try hard to buy only as much as is called for in the recipe since I will eat the unused nuts, despite trying not to.

3. I don't purchase Costco poppy seed muffins. When someone else buys them and brings them home or to social events, I try not to start eating them, because I always overeat them.

What is the underlying commonality in the above rules? If you're addicted to a food, you must withdraw from eating it and never return to eating it again.

CHAPTER 14

DIET MYTHS SET STRAIGHT

WEIGHT LOSS AND weight maintenance are hard. So hard, in fact, that virtually everyone from Muse Satiety Types 2 to 5 that loses weight will then gain back the weight they have worked so hard to lose. Members of Muse Satiety Types 2 and 3 gain it back in two to three years, members of Muse Satiety Type 4 in one to two years, while members of Muse Satiety Type 5 gain it back in as little as six months. Dietitians, personal trainers, medical providers, vitamin hucksters, and next-door neighbors have claimed to have the answers to this dilemma for years, but what they have recommended has not helped the vast majority of overweight people to lose weight and to keep that weight off. Many well-meaning individuals have tried to wrap their minds around this problem and have come up with their best guesses for why people are obese and what works for successful weight loss and maintenance. Frequently, their answers range from not being completely correct to being plain wrong.

Overweight individuals often state that they don't know why they gain weight because they don't eat any more than anyone else. Thin medical providers in the industry have tried to come up with some explanation for why they are thin, and others are overweight. I have heard thin medical providers say in lectures:

1. "There has to be something more than just calories going on here, because I overeat and don't gain weight and my obese patients overeat and gain weight."

2. "The body has a set point and when people lose weight, their body does everything it can do to prevent them from going below the set point."

3. "The obese have no chance at weight maintenance, since after weight loss their metabolism is so low that they have no choice but to gain back all of the weight they have lost."

In the sections below, I will discuss some of the various diet misunderstandings and the facts behind the fiction:

1. Everyone has a set point for what their body thinks it should weigh and you can't lose weight below that set point.

Many individuals believe that once that they lose so much weight, that no matter what they do, they will not lose any more because that is what their body wants them to weigh. This is not true.

The three main enemies of diets are hunger, fatigue, and boredom. Plateaus during diets occur when a dieter has allowed their calorie intake to subtly increase to where their calorie intake equals their calories burned per day. Calories consumed per day increases as a dieter gets overconfident in their ability to eyeball their food and then guess how many calories they are eating. They stop measuring and often stop recording their food intake. Without measuring, a cup becomes a cup and a half, and four ounces becomes eight ounces. Also, the dieter's calories burned per day are lowered by a drop in their resting metabolism of 200 to 500 calories per day and a drop in their levels of non-exercise activity and exercise activity. It is common for dieters to become more and more tired as they lose more and more weight. This fatigue then causes the dieter to decrease both their non-exercise physical activity and physical activity, leading to an additional significant drop in calories burned per day.

By maintaining a 600-calorie difference per day between calories burned and consumed, a dieter can lose about six pounds per month. If the dieter then adds back 300 calories of food per day, which is still less than what they were eating before the diet started, has a decrease in metabolic rate of 200 calories per day, and decreases their overall activity by 100 calories per day, the 600-calorie deficit has been erased and they will stop losing weight. Since dieters can't really perceive the small increase in the amount of food that they are eating per day and in the small drop in their activity level, they are confused and state that even though they are eating the same and exercising like always, they are no longer losing weight. They erroneously believe this to mean that their body has reached a plateau and is keeping them from losing any further weight.

Many members of Muse Satiety Type 1 have maintained their weight within the same five pounds for many years. This has occurred because almost subconsciously their brains have signaled them to stop eating at the proper point in their meals consistently throughout their lives, even with varying activity levels. Members of Muse Satiety Types 2 to 5 have less than effective, or absent, satiety signals and tend to get in a rut of eating about the same portion of food at every meal, with no significant change in intake in spite of changes in activity level, which results in weight gain over time. However, it is true that the very overweight can reach a point where the higher number of calories that they burn by moving their heavier bodies around can equal their excessive calorie intake, at which point the very overweight can remain at a fairly stable weight. However, if something happens to decrease their activity level, such as a broken leg, a change in job, or a need to work two or more shifts a day at a sit-down job, or if something happens to increase calorie intake, such as retiring and entertaining for work more, they will start to gain weight. Weight loss has always been mostly about calories consumed minus calories burned.

What can a person do if they reach a diet plateau? In the case of the person above, they can recommit to carefully counting calories and keeping their intake at 600 calories less than when they started their diet. They can also increase daily exercise and daily non-exercise activity by 300 calories per day. Together, these efforts will restore the 600-calorie-per-day deficit and they will resume losing six pounds per month.

Individuals don't have a weight set point beyond which they can't lose weight. A weight plateau can be overcome by the dieter reducing calorie intake and by increasing activity.

2. Colon cleanses cause weight loss.

This is an easy one. Colon cleansing has been around for centuries. It was quite popular in the early 20th century but fell out of favor as its purported benefits were never proven. There has been a resurgence of interest in colon cleansing in recent decades. Colon cleansing can be accomplished using oral or rectal herbal and pharmaceutical products, or by flushing out the colon contents via the rectum by a colon-cleansing practitioner. While flushing stool out of the colon causes a temporary loss of weight, there are no studies that have proven that colon cleanses cause permanent weight loss. All a colon cleanse does is remove stool from the colon which is then replaced within 24 hours of returning to a normal diet. The theories that toxins from the retained stool in the colon cause fatigue, weight gain, infertility, etc., are not based on fact. In addition, colon cleanses can be dangerous and even deadly (Mishori, 2011).

To lose weight a person needs to reduce the amount of fat stored in the fat cells in their body by having the body burn the fat for energy. Colon cleanses don't cause you to burn fat. Colon cleanses don't cause long-term weight loss, and I don't recommend colon cleanses to patients who want to lose weight.

3. Drinking water promotes long-term weight loss.

This myth has been around as long as I have been practicing weight-loss medicine. It is recommended all over the internet and is even recommended by medical providers. It does seem like such a safe thing to do, to drink more water. However, it doesn't work for long-term weight loss.

A number of studies have shown that water consumed within an hour before a meal reduces the amount of food eaten at that meal, but only in seniors age 55 and older. However, the amount of the reduction in calorie intake has been small, only 50 to 75 calories (Daniels, 2010). The researchers didn't know to control the study so that there was an even distribution of Muse Satiety Types in each group, so that could have confounded the study results. As far as I can tell, none of the studies followed subjects for the next four hours to see if the members of Muse Satiety Types 2 to 5 went home, became hungry again after their stomachs emptied, and then consumed additional food. There is no evidence in these studies that drinking water at the previous meal prevents snacking in the four to five hours until the next meal. As previously mentioned, I am a member of Muse Satiety Type 5. My wife is a member of Muse Satiety Type 1. We have been married since 1984. During all that time, I have consistently consumed three to four times as much water as my wife at restaurants and have still finished my plate of food and started eating her food. Being a member of Muse Satiety Type 5 is so frustrating for me!

Drinking water does cause the body to expend a tiny number of calories, according to research done in Germany in 2003. The research study showed that 40% of the energy burned from drinking 1.5 liters of water per day was used to warm the water from cold to body temperature. The other 60% was burned by activation of the sympathetic nervous system, to facilitate the absorption, utilization, and excretion of the water. Added together, the total energy burned by the ingestion of 1.5 liters of cold water in one day was 48 calories (Boschmann, 2003). That would amount to a little less than half a pound lost per month or five pounds lost in a year. That is pretty underwhelming. It's especially underwhelming when an overweight individual who has been gaining 10 pounds a year since their last diet then tries to lose weight by drinking water. They will still gain five pounds a year, assuming that they are 100% compliant with the water drinking, seven days a week, 365 days a year. Other studies have shown that water is the only beverage that works to reduce intake of calories at the subsequent meal. Calorie intake is increased when any other caloric beverage is consumed before a meal (Daniels, 2010).

There is no evidence that long-term water drinking before meals reduces long-term weight gain or promotes weight loss (Daniels, 2010). I don't recommend water drinking before meals as a way to lose weight to my patients.

4. Eating slowly promotes weight loss.

After learning about members of Muse Satiety Types 2 to 5 in previous chapters, it should be easy to understand that eating slower doesn't cause a member of Muse Satiety Types 2 to 5 to lose their savor for food. If members of Muse Satiety Types 2 and 3 eat more slowly, it is possible that they might stop eating a little earlier at a meal, but they will then return to eat more of the meal later. Eating more slowly doesn't cause members of Muse Satiety Types 4 and 5 to feel full before their stomach is filled to its maximum capacity. I have asked hundreds of members of Muse Satiety Types 4 and 5 if eating more slowly has helped them lose weight and the answer has been no every time.

Research in this area is limited and the research that has been done is often interpreted incorrectly by editorialists. A small study in 2009 showed that the hormones that increase satiety rose to higher levels in men who ate a meal over 30 minutes versus eating the same meal over five minutes (Kokkinos, 2009). Measures of satiety were done right after the five- and 30-minute meals. This study has led to a number of editorial comments at different websites stating that this study proves that eating slower causes weight loss. However, a 1991 University of Pennsylvania study showed that the effect of eating slower is short lived and that after 10 months there is no difference in weight loss between fast and slow eaters (Rolls, 1991). Another study from 2007 showed that slower eating lowered calorie intake by men by 10%, but slower eating didn't decrease calorie intake for women (Martin C. , 2007).

The glaring problem with these studies is assuming that all patients have the same satiety signals, and that overweight people defeat their satiety signals by eating faster. I propose instead that the average speed of eating in the first minutes of a meal is the same for most hungry individuals, whether skinny or overweight. The rate of eating at a meal, in my opinion, is largely determined by ghrelin levels at the beginning of a meal (levels are the same for the skinny and obese) as long as it has been about the same time since the last substantial meal. I also propose that a second determinate of speed of eating is the palatability of the food in the meal, which is not the same for all foods for all people. Lastly, I do agree that speed of eating at meals is partly a learned habit and that to some degree it can be unlearned.

Another way to state this is that members of Muse Satiety Types 1, 2, and 3 start to slow down and then stop only part way through their plate of food, due to the counter-regulatory effects of the satiety hormones that block the hunger stimulated by ghrelin and induce fullness. If asked in a study, members of Muse Satiety Types 1, 2, and 3 would self-classify themselves as normal to slower eaters. Members of Muse Satiety Types 4 and 5 feel no signal to stop in the middle of the plate, so their ghrelin-induced hunger continues unabated, and they eat the rest of the food on their plate at the same rate that they started. If asked in a study, they would self-classify themselves as medium to fast eaters. A well-done retrospective-analysis study has demonstrated that more overweight individuals eat faster than thinner individuals, but of the weaknesses that the authors noted in their study, missing was the fact that the overweight individuals are more likely to be members of Muse Satiety Types 4 and 5, who do consider themselves to be faster eaters. The researchers did report that individuals who self-reported that their eating speed was fast at the beginning of the study, and then reported normal or slow eating speeds at the end of the study did consume less food than when they had self-reported that they were eating faster (Hurst, 2018).

I do advise my patients, when they ask me, that eating slower might help members of Muse Satiety Types 2 and 3 to lose a little extra weight on a diet and to maintain weight more successfully at the end of a diet. However, in my experience, eating slower doesn't help members of Muse Satiety Types 4 and 5 to lose weight or maintain weight after a diet.

5. Overweight people absorb more calories from their food than thin people.

We have all heard this one many times throughout our lives. It is a mostly incorrect assumption arrived at by both thin people and overweight people as they attempt to understand what causes obesity. I have often heard overweight individuals lament that they don't know why they are heavy because "they don't eat any more than anyone else." Even the relatives of many overweight individuals have stated to me that they haven't seen their over-weight relatives eat any more than anyone else. From their observations, it is understandable that people might draw the conclusion that overweight individuals must be absorbing more calories from their food.

It was proposed by researchers in the 2000s that differences in levels of some bacteria in overweight versus thin individuals caused the overweight individuals to absorb more calories from their food. The extra calories came from certain species of bacteria in the intestine breaking down indigestible carbohydrates into absorbable short-chain fats.

A study of special mice bred to have no bacteria in their small intestines showed that these mice absorbed 30% less calories from their food as com-pared to mice with a normal amount of bacteria in their small intestines. The special mice, therefore, remained thinner. However, studies in obese and thin mice that both had a normal amount of bacteria in their small intestines have indicated a smaller difference in energy absorption at around 10% more for the obese mice, but this has not been consistently found in all studies. When thin mice have the bacteria from obese humans transplanted into their small intestines, the mice gain weight. Studies in humans have shown that after obesity surgery in humans, the types of bacteria in the small intestine change to be more like the bacterial populations of thinner humans (Lean, 2018) (Al-Assal, 2018) (Li, 2011).

Research into the role of bacteria in the human small intestine causing excess absorption of calories from otherwise indigestible carbohydrates is difficult to apply to humans. This is because most of the research has been done in rodents, the results are not consistent from study to study, and we don't know if the differences in bacteria between thin and overweight humans are the cause of obesity, or just a result of being thin. The kind of diet that is proposed to improve the types of bacteria in the small intestine of over-weight people to those that are associated with being thin are similar to the heart-healthy foods that I recommend my patients consume while dieting. I recommend my patients lose weight while consuming small portions of foods from the American Heart Association's Mediterranean Diet, namely, non-starchy vegetables, whole grains, nuts, berries, highly unsaturated oils, fish and chicken, with very little sugar and fruit, and very little red meat.

6. Some people have such a low metabolism that they can't lose weight.

Low metabolism is blamed by so many for such a large portion of our problem with losing weight and maintaining weight. I would love to place a blimp over every major city in the world with giant letters emblazoned on the side of the blimps stating, "It's not your metabolism, it's your inactivity."

Our basal metabolic rate (BMR) accounts for 60%-70% of the energy we burn each day and is the amount of energy that it takes to breathe, think, beat your heart, move your food through your intestines, etc. BMR can also be thought of as the energy that would be burned if a person lay in bed all day long without moving. Basal metabolic rate does vary a little between individuals of the same body size, with males having BMRs about 200 calories higher per day more than females, and 20-year-olds having BMRs about 200 calories higher per day than 60-year-olds. Exercise, for most people, accounts for 0% to 10% of their daily calories burned per day. A person who burns about 10% of their energy per day via exercise is exercising vigorously for about 30 minutes a day. The remaining 20%-30% of the calories that we burn each day come from non-exercise activity. Non-exercise activity is all the little things we do all day that burn more energy than lying in bed and not moving a muscle. Many of those things seem minor, like walking around the office at work and taking out the trash at home. Over the 16 hours or so that we are awake each day, the hundreds of little things we do add up to the 20%-30% of the calories that we burn each day from non-exercise activity. Clearly, there are individuals who do little more than sit all day, and then there are others that are very active and are on the move all day long, either tapping their feet constantly, walking here and there, or working at a job that requires a lot of manual labor.

We can't increase our BMR much, but we can increase how many calories we burn per day by increasing non-exercise activity and exercise activity. We can walk or bike to places instead of driving, park farther away from our destinations, take a walk during lunch, take out the trash ourselves, weed the garden, and sweep the floor. Standing in meetings, while watching TV or streaming videos, and while talking to friends burns more calories than sitting. We can make time for more non-exercise activity and exercise in our busy lives.

When overweight patients of mine have continued to insist that their metabolism is lower than thin people, I have tried to help them understand by explaining the following three things. The first is that overweight individuals require a higher basal energy expenditure per day just to breathe against their heavier chest wall, pump blood through more and longer blood vessels, and to keep their larger bodies warm. Increased muscle is needed just to be able to complete non-exercise activity. Plus, overweight individuals burn a lot more energy walking from point A to point B, due to having carry around their extra weight. Overweight individuals burn more calories per day then thin individuals of the same sex, age, height, and body composition.

Second, I explain that if they really have a lower metabolism than other people, then that means they can walk a mile burning less calories than other people of the same sex, age, height, and body composition. Of course, I then tell them that the human body is efficient enough that they really can't walk a mile while burning less calories than another person of the same sex, age, height, and body composition, and that the real problem is they don't walk the mile. They have a low level of non-exercise and exercise activity.

Last, if they still are struggling to abandon their pre-set notion that they are overweight because they have a low metabolism, then I gently say to them that if they really have a lower metabolism than other people, and they are burning less calories per day than other people, then why are they eating more than they should? It doesn't matter if a member of Muse Satiety Type 1 burns a little or a lot of energy in a day, because they will still feel full and stop eating as soon as they have eaten enough to satisfy their calorie needs for the day.

I hope that this helps to dispel the myth that overweight individuals have a lower metabolism than other people. The truth is that members of Muse Satiety Types 2 to 5 are overweight because they innocently and impercep- tibly consume more food than members of Muse Satiety Type 1.

7. Some people have such a high metabolism that they can't gain weight.

The definition of the word *metabolism*, in laymen's terms, is different than the definition of the word *metabolism* when it is used by medical providers and researchers. This difference is, at least in part, the source of the confusion that leads to statements like this and other similar statements.

As I mentioned in the previous section of this chapter, basal metabolic rate (BMR) is the number of calories burned by individuals at complete rest and accounts for about 70% of the calories we burn per day. The rest of the calories that we burn per day is from non-exercise activity and exercise activity.

When someone tells me that they know someone that can eat whatever they want and never gain weight, then I ask them if they have ever followed that person around for a day, mimicking their every move. They would be exhausted, since the person they are describing must be an athlete, a construction worker, or is hyperactive. Manual laborers and athletes burn 1,000 to 2,000 extra calories per day over what sedentary individuals burn. Hyperactive individuals burn 400 to 800 calories more per day than other people just through their excessive movements. They gesture a lot and expansively, constantly fidget, and often turn left when they should be turning right so they must retrace their steps to complete their tasks. Manual laborers, athletes, and hyperactive individuals spend so much extra energy that they need to eat an extra meal per day, or even more, to keep from becoming emaciated.

The laymen's term *metabolism* is misleading and needs to be banished from our vocabulary. Instead, the words "low-activity level" or "high-activity level" should be substituted for "low metabolism" and "high metabolism". Then, the diet myth that we are discussing, that some people have such a high metabolism that they can't gain weight, would instead be stated that some people have such a high level of activity that they can't gain weight. That statement is not a myth. It is a factual statement of what would happen to any individual who burns a high number of calories per day.

8. Eating frequent small meals promotes weight loss.

This idea was originally proposed as a solution for successful weight loss that involved eating six small 150- to 200-calorie meals per day resulting in a consumption of about 1,000 calories per day. The suggestion of those promoting this diet was that the dieter wouldn't be as hungry by eating more often and would better comply with the diet. From a dieting standpoint, there is nothing wrong with this type of a diet and it does work, if the 150- to 200-calorie-per-small-meal restriction is maintained.

Somewhere along the way, after hearing the "frequent small meal" mantra from many sources for years, the general public began to believe that eating frequent small meals suppressed appetite enough that it caused weight loss. Patients have frequently come to me and asked why they are not losing weight since they are eating frequent small meals throughout the day. A few questions later and I find out that they are not measuring the calories being consumed in those "small" meals, nor are they counting the number of small meals per day. Research has proven that eating six small meals per day doesn't increase metabolism, doesn't burn fat, does cause more weight gain, and does cause more hunger versus eating three times a day (Ohkawara, 2013).

In contrast to the above, I want to be sure that the reader is aware of the success that participants in the National Weight Control Registry have had by eating four small 150-calorie meals throughout the day in place of breakfast and lunch and then having a larger meal in the evening with their family. This was discussed in Chapter 11 on weight maintenance.

For me, as a member of Muse Satiety Type 5, nothing could be more dangerous than being allowed to eat six meals a day. I can easily eat 1,000 calories per meal six times a day because nothing but pain when I reach my stomach's maximum capacity tells me to stop. Even then, I'm still hungry, even though I know that I can't physically eat any more. Such is the life of almost all Muse Satiety Type 5s. Muse Satiety Type 4s have the same problem with eating six small meals a day, because they too are lacking a full signal. Muse Satiety Types 2 and 3 can do better when eating six meals a day, because they have a full signal, but they must be sure not to snack between the six small meals.

I want to stress that it is not wrong to lose weight or maintain weight by eating four 150-200 calorie meals throughout the day and then a somewhat larger meal at dinner. For those dieting to lose weight, the daily intake of food should be around 1,000 calories per day. For those trying to maintain weight after a diet, the daily intake of food should be around 1,600 calories per day, depending on activity level and body size.

Eating frequent small meals does not promote weight loss any more than any other diet. Weight loss comes from maintaining a calorie deficit between calories consumed and calories burned. It doesn't matter how frequently or infrequently the calories are consumed.

9. **People had normal satiety signals when they were young but lost them because their caregivers made them eat all their food at mealtimes.**

I do hear this statement a lot from overweight people in their thirties or older. They tell me that they were thin until they were in their twenties, and then they started to gain weight. I also hear this statement from thin members of Muse Satiety Types 1 and 2 that are searching for a reason why people are overweight. With no knowledge of the Muse Satiety Types, they can only think that something went wrong with their family members, friends, and colleagues along the way from their thin childhood to being overweight as an adult. The only thing that they can think of is that the ability to gain excess weight as an adult must have come from the overweight individual's parents making them clean their plate when they were children, which then caused them to lose their satiety signals. What they don't understand is that overweight individuals have been missing one or more of the three satiety signals from birth. If you take children from Muse Satiety Type 1 and try to make them finish all of the food on their plates, they will just sit there and cry, because they know that if they do eat more, they will throw up, or at least feel like throwing up. On the other hand, children who are Muse Satiety Type 4s and 5s will finish all of their food and start eating everyone else's leftover food from off their plates as soon as they are old enough to get up on a chair and handle a spoon. Even mothers that have nursed or bottle-fed individuals who are later found to be members of Muse Satiety Types 4 and 5 will remark just how much and how often that their child would eat as an infant. Babies and toddlers from Muse Satiety Types 4 and 5 are hardly ever described by their parents as finicky eaters.

On the other hand, children from Muse Satiety Types 2 and 3 feel full at the exact point in their meals where they have eaten enough to satisfy their calorie needs. They will then ask their parents if they can be excused so they can return to doing whatever they were doing before the meal. When their fullness signal fades in 10 to 15 minutes, they are either too engrossed in what they are doing to return to the table to eat more, or if they do return to eat more, their mother has cleaned the food off the table and there is nothing for them to eat. Children 12 and under don't often raid the fridge and pantry in between meals without parental permission, so they just go back to whatever they were doing before they returned to the kitchen. Carrying this forward, youth 12 to 18 that are in Muse Satiety Types 2 and 3 that are often in sports, music lessons, cheerleading, school clubs, and school extracurricular activities are often too busy to wait for the full signal to fade at mealtimes. They leave their remaining food on their plate and depart in a rush to get to the next class or fun activity. Also, they are active enough throughout the day that they are burning extra calories, which helps to compensate for any overeating that they might do in between meals. They remain thin through grade school. In college, members of Muse Satiety Types 2 and 3 often live off campus on limited funds, study in the library where most people don't snack, and spend very little time in their living quarters around their fridge and personal food. They are always busy with school, part-time work, having fun with friends and dating, and often discard the rest of their food at meals, once they feel the satiety signal of fullness. They remain quite active, which helps to compensate for in-between-meal snacking. Then, when members of Muse Satiety Types 2 and 3 finally get out of school and start making money, they find that there is almost always extra food to eat at work and that they can buy whatever food they want to stock their fridge and pantry at home. Work and family responsibilities cut into exercise time. They start to gain weight. The satiety signals that they were missing from birth were always missing, but there wasn't a chance to eat more calories per day than they were burning until in their mid-20s.

If these same members of Muse Satiety Types 2 and 3 think back carefully to their childhood, they will remember days where they were stuck at home all day long and how they popped by the kitchen every 30-60 minutes for a few extra bites from their last meal, an unfinished dessert, or a snack from the pantry. Children from Muse Satiety Type 1 might head to the kitchen with them but won't ever snack on more than one bite of food in between meals. Otherwise, it would make them feel nauseated.

There are individuals who do temporarily become members of Muse Satiety Types 2 to 5 after starting out life as members of Muse Satiety Type 1. A person can temporarily move from Muse Satiety Type 1 to Muse Satiety Types 2 to 5 due to pregnancy. I have had a number of women who are members of Muse Satiety Type 1 tell me that they have gained 60 and 80 pounds above their ideal weight during a pregnancy, only to lose all the way back down to their pre-pregnancy weight within six months of the delivery. Another cause is due to the use of medications that tend to cause weight gain in almost everyone. An example of a medication that can causes some members of Muse Satiety Type 1 to become ravenous at mealtimes and also to snack excessively between meals is prednisone, a powerful anti-inflammatory steroid used for asthma, rheumatologic diseases, back and neck pain, allergic reactions, arthritis, and even strep throat. I have seen many patients gain 50 or more pounds while on prednisone and then lose it all after they stopped the prednisone.

Obesity is not caused by people being trained to overeat as children. Individuals are born with or without satiety signals that do or do not stop them from overeating.

10. The previously overweight can learn how to eat right and be thin forever.

Members of Muse Satiety Type 1 stop eating subconsciously in the middle of their first serving at mealtimes, day after day, for their whole lives. The presence or absence of the satiety signal of loss of savor that only Muse

Satiety Type 1s have is the double-yellow line in the road between members of Muse Satiety Type 1 and members of Muse Satiety Types 2 to 5. A lack of this signal is the main reason that two-thirds of the world's population is either overweight or obese. In my opinion, the origin of the myth above is based not on facts from studies, but on a well-meant, although erroneous, effort by members of Muse Satiety Type 1 to try to understand why others are overweight. Thinking that everyone feels the same satiety signals that they do, members of Muse Satiety Type 1 look at members of Muse Satiety Types 2 to 5 and could possibly think to themselves, "They eat past their feeling of fullness, they keep eating even though they are no longer hungry, and they keep eating even when it makes them nauseated. How can they?" What the members of Muse Satiety Type 1 don't understand is that members of the other Muse Satiety Types have never experienced all three satiety signals like they have.

Members of Muse Satiety Types 4 and 5 will never feel the almost subconscious satiety signal of fullness and will always eat past the exact point at each meal where they should have stopped. It is nearly impossible to model almost subconscious behavior consciously. It is true that members of Muse Satiety Types 2 to 5 can try to model the behavior of members of Muse Satiety Type 1, and depending on compliance, they will gain weight more slowly and will be able to last longer in between diets. However, almost all will still end up becoming overweight again.

The discussion of the components of a successful weight maintenance program is in Chapter 11. As you review Chapter 11, either in your mind or by rereading it, don't forget the most important component of weight maintenance is to either exercise for 80 minutes every day, take an appetite suppressant long term, or do both. Doing neither will result in almost guaranteed weight regain after a diet.

Some well-meaning individuals have stated that all that obese people need to do to keep from gaining weight is a "lifestyle change." I don't know if a lifetime of food deprivation and more exercise than a person wants to do, or has time for, can be adequately summed up by the politically correct term "lifestyle change." Members of Muse Satiety Type 1 don't have to suffer through food deprivation and frequent and lengthy exercise to stay thin.

Weight maintenance is like walking up a moving escalator the wrong way. If you want to get to your goal, the top of the escalator, you never get to rest. Every time you take a rest, you're gaining weight. Weight maintenance for members of Muse Satiety Types 2 to 5 can be achieved only through great and continuous effort. "Eating right" by itself has been proven to not work for weight maintenance for member of Muse Satiety Types 2 to 5.

11. Eating some foods make you lose more weight than others.

While it is true that digesting some foods requires the expenditure of more calories than other foods, the energy expended in digesting these foods is far smaller than the total calorie content of the foods. Protein, for example, requires 10% more energy to metabolize than carbohydrates, but that 10% difference will only result in 30 pounds lost on a diet of mainly protein instead of 27 pounds on a diet of mainly carbohydrate. That's not a big difference! I'm not saying that a low-carbohydrate diet is a bad thing to do. In fact, reducing carbohydrates is a great way to diet if it is done in a nutritionally sound manner.

It is also true that some individuals extract more energy from their food as it travels through the small intestine. I have already discussed this above under diet myth number 5. This effect is small compared to the total calories consumed and doesn't make a big enough difference in weight loss to matter much. It might matter more in weight maintenance, but research on humans in the area is limited and contradictory.

Eating certain foods over other foods doesn't make a significant difference in weight loss while dieting. The best regimen to consume while dieting is foods from the heart-healthy Mediterranean Diet.

12. Denying yourself snacks and desserts during diets makes you start binging on those same foods later, causing you to gain back all the weight you have lost.

The most common reason that I hear this myth is as an attempt to explain why dieting doesn't work. Others use it as a rationale for a diet during which a dieter doesn't deny themselves any of their favorite foods.

I haven't been able to find research to prove or disprove this statement. What we do know from experts in the field is that 60% to 80% of the US population suffers from at least one food craving, with some having up to 10 foods that they crave. For the purposes of this book, food craving and food addiction describe pretty much the same thing, that an individual has an intense desire for and repeated loss of control with the eating of one or more foods. Food cravings can worsen immediately after stopping the addictive foods but do fade over time.

With an understanding of the body's defense against starvation that was discussed in Chapter 2, we now have greater understanding of what happens at the end of a diet. At the end of a successful diet, ghrelin is high, resulting in the dieter feeling more hunger and craving more than they did before they began the diet. The more weight lost, the higher the ghrelin rises. Higher levels of ghrelin make the dieter eat more, snack more, and consume more of their favorite foods. The extra calorie intake rapidly results in the dieter regaining the weight they had lost. At that point, ghrelin returns to its pre-diet level and the excess hunger resolves.

I do know plenty of dieters who have permanently stopped eating certain foods which they haven't previously been able to stop overeating, in an effort to help with weight loss and weight maintenance. It is not wrong to deny the human body of pleasant activities that potentially result in negative consequence. Examples are stopping smoking, stopping driving faster than the speed limit, and stopping the use of illegal drugs. Many people successfully stop these and other pleasurable activities for years. Anyone that stops an addictive behavior will likely need to have another surrogate activity to take its place to help to mitigate the chance that a moment of intense psychological need will result in relapse.

Humans can stop participating in intensely pleasureful activities successfully and can remain in remission for years. This applies to giving up food cravings and addictions as well. Certainly, there will be at least a few relapses during the process of stopping addictive foods, but that doesn't mean the determined dieter can't ultimately triumph.

13. If you lose weight fast, then you will gain it back fast; and the more weight you lose on a diet, the more likely you are to gain it back.

To start with, about 80% of individuals gain back most, if not all, of the weight they have lost on a diet within one to three years (Kraschnewski, 2010) (Weiss, 2007). Weight maintenance is just plain hard. In the weight-loss industry, successful weight maintenance after a diet is most often defined as maintaining a weight loss of at least 5% of the pre-diet weight for one year. For a person who weighed 200 pounds before their diet, this would be maintaining a weight of 190 pounds or less for at least a year after starting the diet. Research has indicated that the factors that predict success at weight maintenance are an older age, an active lifestyle, and less than four hours a day of screen time (Anderson J. W., 1999) (Weiss, 2007). In addition, the more weight that a person loses on a diet, the greater the risk for weight regain in pounds (Weiss, 2007), but the greater the chance of not having gained it all back by one year (Nackers, 2010).

As to slow weight loss resulting in better weight maintenance than fast weight loss, research has shown that rapid weight loss over a three-month period versus slow weight loss over a nine-month period resulted in 30% more patients losing to the goal of 12.5% of their body weight in the rapid weight-loss group versus the slow weight-loss group. After about two and a half years, both groups gained most of the weight back with no significant difference between the groups (Purcell, 2014). This finding, that the rate of weight loss does not predict weight regain, was confirmed in a similar study in 2016 (Vink, 2016).

In summary, slow weight loss is not better than fast weight loss in preventing weight regain after a diet. Fast weight-loss results in more patients getting to their weight-loss goal than slow weight loss. The more a person loses, the less likely they are to gain it all back by the end of 18 months.

14. Eating at night makes a person fat.

The theory behind this myth is that if you eat calories late at night and you are not burning as many calories while you are asleep, then those calories are more likely to be stored as fat. This explanation is true but isn't why eating at night can cause weight gain. Studies have shown that when humans are placed in metabolic units, where every calorie consumed and burned is meticulously tracked, and are placed on a 1,000-calorie-per-day diet, it doesn't matter whether the 1,000 calories per day is eaten once a day, five times a day, or all at bedtime. The weight loss is the same. When calories are consumed at night before bed, the body isn't needing as many calories for muscle activity while in bed, so it stores some of the calories of food in the muscles and liver, and the rest is converted to fat for storage in fat cells. However, fat being stored in fat cells is not just a one-way street. As soon as the body wakes up the next morning and needs energy, at least some of that energy comes from fat. Sedentary individuals burn up about 10% of their calories at rest from their fat stores, while marathon runners burn up to 50% of their resting calories from their fat stores.

The real reason why eating late at night causes weight gain is that for most humans, a late-night meal is usually a fourth meal for the day, putting the person over their needed calorie intake for the day. The extra calories eaten late at night are dutifully stored as fat by the body, but unless the body burns off those extra calories stored as fat the next day, those fat calories will remain with the rest of the fat calories in the fat cells, and the person eating late at night will slowly but surely become overweight. In contrast, remember that Muse Satiety Type 1s that have had an adequate dinner earlier that evening might go with you to the fast-food joint or to the kitchen for a late-night snack, but once given the food, they won't eat more than a bite because they have lost their savor from eating dinner and they won't get their savor for food back until the next morning.

Eating at night does not cause weight gain, if an individual's daily calorie intake does not exceed their daily calories burned.

15. You don't have to count calories to lose weight.

This statement is true to a degree because some people do lose weight without counting calories. However, what is truer is that a person must take in less calories per day than they are burning in order to experience weight loss. Weight loss requires a calorie deficit. Many people struggle to maintain a daily calorie deficit as a diet goes along due to rising hunger and increasing fatigue. The first 5 to 10 pounds lost on a diet is fairly easy, whether the diet is calorie counted or not, but the next 5 to 10 pounds lost is much harder due to rising ghrelin and falling metabolism. The more weight loss desired from a diet, the more success is seen by dieters who count calories as opposed to those who do not count calories. Studies have shown that dieters who count calories while dieting lose about 50% more than individuals who don't count calories (Mockus, 2011) (Baker R. , 1993).

The purveyors of diets that don't require calorie counting use other ways of lowering total calories consumed per day. Some instruct their dieters to cut out almost all fat, hoping that their dieters will then keep their calorie intake of protein and carbohydrate to less than the calorie intake they had previously consumed before they started. Others instruct their dieters to cut out almost all carbohydrates, hoping that their dieters will then keep their calorie intake of protein and fat to less than the total calorie intake prior to starting. Some sell their dieters pre-prepared and pre-calorie-measured meals for the dieter to eat at prescribed times during the day. The hope is that the dieter will avoid eating food outside of the provided meals. Others alternate a much lower food intake one day and a mildly increased food intake on the next day, hoping that the average daily food intake will be less than calories burned over time. No matter how the different diets function, they all must cause an average daily calorie deficit, or the dieter will not lose weight. That is because the body is programed to try to keep us at the same weight. It does this by making us hungry at each meal, which starts us eating, and then makes us feel full at exactly the point in the meal where our calorie needs are met. If you stop eating before you have met your calorie needs, then you will still be hungry. It takes a lot of willpower to consistently stop eating at mealtimes when we are still hungry, and to not to snack between meals when we haven't eaten enough at the previous meal and are still hungry.

A consistent daily calorie deficit causes weight loss. This is best accomplished by calorie counting. Any method can be used for calorie counting while dieting, however, most of my patients are using one of the excellent free apps on their cellphones, such as "Lose It!" and "MyFitnessPal."

16. Eating carbohydrates makes you fat.

The thought behind this myth is that the body treats the calories from carbohydrates differently than calories from protein and preferentially converts them to storage fat. This is just not true. To test out what kind of misinformation is available on the internet on this topic, I typed "does eating carbohydrates make you fat" into the search bar and the results I got were split with about half of the search results saying that carbohydrates make you fat and the other half saying that carbohydrates don't make you fat. I then added "scholarly article" at the end of the initial search phrase, and the results I then got all reported the same thing: eating a diet high in carbohydrates doesn't cause any more weight gain than a diet that is low in carbohydrates (Sartorius, 2018) (Gaesser, 2007) (Ma, 2005).

When ingested carbohydrates are digested, converted to mostly glucose and fructose before entering the blood stream, insulin is released from the pancreas to stimulate the muscles and liver to take up the glucose and store it as glycogen. Once the muscles and liver are full of glycogen, insulin then stimulates the fat cells to take up the rest of the glucose to be stored as fat. While this sounds like a bad thing for the excess carbohydrate to be stored as fat, especially to those of us who are overweight, it is instead a normal and necessary process. The lay person tends to think that fat is a storage process that is a one-way street, with no easy way for the fat to leave the fat cells. However, the fat in fat cells easily leaves the fat cells to be used by the body for energy. In between meals and at rest, as much as 66% of the fuel being used by our bodies is coming from fat and the rest is from carbohydrates (Lowery, 2004). The longer a person exercises, the more that glycogen stores in the muscles and liver are depleted and the more that the fuel being used by the body for energy during exercise is coming from stored fat.

When protein is consumed, it is digested into amino acids that are then absorbed into the blood stream. The amino acids are used by the body to produce proteins found in muscles, tendons, collagens, enzymes, structural components, hormones, etc. The body has no way of storing excess amino acids and converts them to glucose. The body then uses the glucose from the excess amino acids in just the same fashion as the glucose from carbohydrates, as was discussed in the previous paragraph.

The theory that the glucose from ingested carbohydrates is preferentially stored as fat over the glucose from excess ingested protein has been proven to be false. The most accurate studies on this topic are controlled-feeding studies. These studies are performed in metabolic rooms where changes in energy intake and expenditure are very accurately measured. The study subjects remain in these rooms for the duration of the study, which can be as long as six months. One researcher analyzed the results of 32 controlled-feeding trials on a total of 563 patients where the dietary carbohydrate intake varied from 1% to 83% and dietary fat intake varied from 4% to 84%. Protein intake was kept the same, at about 17%, and total calorie intake was maintained at the same level throughout the studies. Across all of these studies, there was a slight weight loss in the high-carbohydrate diets that would have amounted to three pounds lost in three months over the high-fat diets (Hall, 2017). In another controlled-feeding trial on 15 subjects for 13 weeks, total calorie and protein intake were kept the same for the duration of the study. Wide variations in carbohydrate versus fat intake didn't result any difference in body weight (Hirsch, 1998). Finally, a study was performed on 16 men, nine lean and seven obese, in a controlled-feeding trial. The men were fed a high-carb diet that supplied 150% of their daily calorie needs for 14 days and were then switched to a high-fat diet that supplied 150% of their daily calorie needs for 14 days. There were no differences in change in body weight and lean mass during the high-carb and high-fat parts of the study. There was a slightly greater increase in fat mass during the high-fat part of the study. There was no difference in the change of body weight and lean mass between the lean and obese men (Horton, 1995).

Before you grab your doughnut and chocolate milk, it is important to understand that not all carbohydrates are the same. Some are significantly healthier than others. Examples of healthy foods containing carbohydrates are non-starchy vegetables, whole grains, and dried berries. Examples of less healthy foods containing carbohydrates are candies, cakes, cookies, sugar-sweetened drinks, and ice cream. The main reasons that these less healthy foods are not good for us is that they result in overconsumption of calories and weight gain due to their being highly palatable, calorie dense, lacking in fiber that promotes satiety, and containing too much fructose, which can lead to fatty liver and diabetes. Since heart disease affects about half of our population later in life, it is important to note that these less healthy foods are not a part of proven heart-healthy diets, such as the Mediterranean Diet (Martínez-González, 2019).

Carbohydrate ingestion is no more likely to cause weight gain than protein ingestion. It is the overconsumption of all three energy sources—carbohydrate, protein, and fat—that results in weight gain and not preferentially carbohydrate consumption. Both dieters and weight maintainers should consume the heart-healthy diet espoused by the Mediterranean Diet.

17. People who overeat are just addicted to food.

Food addiction, also known by the more scientific term *food craving*, is a reality for many people, both thin and overweight. It is the third disease causing obesity. I have discussed in more detail in Chapter 12 that food addiction is not the only cause of the obesity epidemic. Food addiction affects members of all Muse Satiety Types. It is not known whether it affects the members of each Muse Satiety Type with an equal frequency or not.

In the United States, per one researcher, 60% to 80% of individuals are addicted to between one and five foods (Pelchat, 1997). I have found that some people can be addicted to up to 10 foods. Food addiction can be defined as repeated consumption of highly palatable foods despite negative consequences. The consumption of these foods is most often in response to triggers that don't include hunger and is not related to the timing of the most recent meal. These are foods about which an individual might say out loud or silently to themselves, "I can't have that food around because I overeat it every time." These are the foods that a person goes looking for in between meals, in the fridge or pantry, and if they are not found, the person shuts the door of the fridge or pantry in frustration. The person is not addicted to anything else in the fridge or pantry. Addictive foods are often different from person to person and from males to females. Younger persons have more food addictions than older persons (Pelchat, 1997). Food addictions appear to be related to both genetic predispositions and to environmental factors. Food addictions can be lessened to a degree through behavioral modification (Hill A. , 2007).

Is it true that food addiction is the only contributor to the obesity epidemic? No. Is food addiction part of the problem? Yes. Food craving is one of the three disease that I have proposed are causing our epidemic of obesity.

18. Starvation diets permanently lower your metabolism, making you gain more weight than if you had never dieted.

This is just another myth that is not based on science. It is true that human metabolism drops about 200 calories per day soon after starting a diet, which can be felt by the dieter as they notice more fatigue, dry skin, constipation, cold intolerance, and hair loss. The amount of drop in metabolism during and after a diet varies by the amount of weight lost, sex, age, and body frame. A study indicated that, depending on the amount of weight lost, some dieter's metabolism drops by as much as 500 calories per day by the end of a diet (Fothergill, 2016). From the same study, we also know that dieter's metabolism remain consistently low for as long six years after the end of their diet and don't rise at all, even though the dieters gain weight over time. Does this mean that their metabolism is permanently lower for the rest of their lives? No. As soon as they gain all the weight they have lost back, which occurs commonly, then their metabolism returns to what it was before they started losing weight in the first place.

Why does the body lower metabolism during and after a diet? One thought is that it is an adaptive behavior from when humans lived off the land with little ability to save food beyond one growing season. During years of famine, the human body lowered its metabolism when food was scarce to help the human to survive. Whatever the cause for this state of lowered metabolism after weight loss, it makes weight maintenance a formidable challenge.

Dieting does not permanently lower a person's metabolism. Dieting repeatedly doesn't cause a person to be heavier than if they had never dieted at all.

19. Losing muscle during weight loss is bad.

A person's body does not store extra muscle beyond what is needed to accomplish its daily physical tasks. If a person increases their activity level, then the body increases muscle to more efficiently allow the person to accomplish their desired level of activity. If a person becomes inactive, then the body decreases muscle to a level that is necessary for the new level of activity.

If a person on a diet is not exercising, then they will lose some muscle due to their total weight decreasing during the diet. Their trunk and leg muscles will lose muscle mass proportionally to the amount of weight lost, since the muscles don't have as much weight to move around. A protein-calorie deficient diet is a diet that supplies less than the US recommended daily allowance (RDA) of protein for adults, which is about 55 grams per day for a 5'9" tall man and 45 grams per day for a 5'4" tall woman. If a dieter consumes less than their RDA of protein per day, then they will lose additional muscle mass because the body will have to use protein from their muscles to make glucose to feed their red cells. Excess muscle lost in this fashion should be avoided by sticking with diets that supply at least 55 grams of healthy protein per day for males and 45 grams of healthy protein per day for females. People who exercise during weight loss lose more fat and less muscle than people who lose weight without exercising, even though the amount of weight lost is similar (Layman, 2003). Regardless of how much muscle is lost during weight loss, a person can still increase their muscle mass after their diet by exercise to where the individual would like it to be.

There is no permanent harm to body muscles from diet-related muscle loss.

20. Skipping breakfast makes you gain weight.

We have been told for more than 100 years that breakfast is the most important meal of the day. Eating breakfast has been associated in studies with improved academic performance in children and adolescents (Adolphus, 2013). However, eating breakfast appears to cause a small amount of weight gain in a summary study of 13 studies that was published in 2019 (Sievert, 2019). In this study, called a meta-analysis, the individuals who ate breakfast weighed one pound more and consumed 260 calories more per day than those who skipped breakfast. The authors did state that the quality of the data from the 13 studies used in their meta-analysis was low and that their findings should be interpreted with caution.

So, what is the correct answer? Does eating breakfast cause weight gain or weight loss? These are my thoughts, keeping the Muse Satiety Types in mind. Whether a Muse Satiety Type 1 eats breakfast and two more meals in a day or skips breakfast and only eats two meals a day, they will stop at exactly their calorie needs at each meal and won't gain or lose weight. Members of Muse Satiety Types 4 and 5 will always take at least one extra bite of food they are served at any meal and will tend to gain weight over time. The more plates of food that they are served per day, the more extra bites they will take per day.

On the other hand, 78% of the 10,000-plus members of the National Weight Control Registry (NWCR) who are successfully maintaining weight after a diet report eating breakfast every day (Wing R. , 2005). However, the frequent small meals eaten by members of the NWCR are small 150-calorie meals as part of their effort to eat four small, evenly spaced meals throughout the day leading up to a small dinner in the evening. The members of the NCWR are not eating breakfast from a standard plate of American breakfast food.

A number of patients have asked me over the years if it was okay that they were not eating breakfast, since they had heard that it was unhealthy to skip breakfast. My patients who have asked this have all told me that they just aren't hungry in the mornings and some have said that they would get nauseated if they ate before noon. What I have told them in the past is what I'll tell you now. If you're not hungry in the morning and you feel perfectly fine, then don't eat breakfast. If you're not hungry in the morning and you skip breakfast, but then you feel mentally slow an hour or two later, then pull out a healthy 150-calorie snack and take a bite or two. If that picks you up, then great. If not, you should check with your medical provider to see if they can help you. If you are hungry in the morning, then have a small heart-healthy breakfast.

Skipping breakfast doesn't cause weight gain for Muse Satiety Type 1s. As for members of Muse Satiety Types 2 to 5 that are struggling with their weight, the answer is less clear, but if breakfast is eaten, it should be small and should consist of mostly healthy protein.

21. Overweight people just need to push away from the table.

People don't say this very often anymore, or at least I hope not. It is completely untrue. Saying it just informs others that you don't really understand the problem of obesity.

As I mentioned in Chapter 2, members of Muse Satiety Type 1 stop eating mostly subconsciously via an intact signaling system that has been present since birth. I also discussed how it is nearly impossible to train members of Muse Satiety Types 2 to 5 to consciously mirror the mostly subconscious behavior of members of Muse Satiety Type 1 when it comes to stopping eating right at the proper calorie. Lacking some or all these subconscious signals, members of Muse Satiety Types 2 to 5 end up overeating at virtually every meal and then gaining weight over time.

Telling overweight members of Muse Satiety Types 2 to 5 to just to push away from the table really means that you are probably a member of Muse Satiety Type 1 and that you just can't figure out why overweight people don't stop like you do. If you still don't understand, then read Chapter 2 again.

22. Yo-yo dieting is dangerous.

I haven't been able to figure out exactly how this widespread myth was born. It could have been hatched out of a psychological need of overweight people to find an excuse for not having to restart the difficult and tiresome task of another diet once again. Then again, it could have had origin in the frustration that members of Muse Satiety Type 1 have with the seemingly valueless efforts of overweight members of Muse Satiety Types 2 to 5 to lose weight, only to gain it back again.

The truth is that repeatedly losing weight and gaining the weight back again is not harmful to the human body. In a 20-year study of 45,000 women that was published in 2009, researchers reported that individuals who repeatedly gained and lost 20 pounds or more, and individuals whose weight didn't fluctuate, didn't have a difference in overall death rate. In addition, they didn't have a difference in rates of death from stroke and heart disease (Field A. E., 2009).

While repeatedly losing and then regaining weight may seem pointless to many, they don't understand the positive value related to even short time periods of weight loss. Without question, during a diet and during the time that a previously overweight person is thin, the pancreas is under less metabolic stress, lengthening the time to the development of diabetes for those who are at risk for diabetes. Sleep apnea is improved by 50% with a 20-pound weight loss and usually completely resolves with a 50-pound weight loss. Overweight individuals are at higher risk for knee replacement due to weight-related wear and tear on their knee joints. With even intermittent reduction of weight, overweight individuals significantly prolong the time until they need a knee replacement. Finally, psychologically, most overweight individuals would vastly prefer being thin for half of their lives rather than never being thin at all.

So, when your loved one, friend, or colleague is ready to start a new diet, don't talk trash to them. Just smile and wish them success.

23. Fat people have poor self-control.

As I have mentioned elsewhere, when a human being doesn't lose their savor in between substantial meals, like what happens with members of Muse Satiety Types 2 to 5, then it takes superhuman willpower to keep from eating when they remain hungry. Maybe this will make it easier to understand. When members of Muse Satiety Type 1 are hungry, they always go and get something eat. As they swallow their first bite and hungrily get ready to eat the second bite, what if they were suddenly struck by a jolt of energy of some kind and, as a result, were stuck with that same degree of hunger that is compelling them take their second next bite, forever. 24/7. 365 days a year. Just like the members of Muse Satiety Types 2 to 5. If you are a member of Muse Satiety Type 1, it makes you think, doesn't it? How would you know when you'd reached your calorie needs and you needed to stop eating your meal? Happily, there isn't really such a jolt of energy that turns Muse Satiety Type 1s into Muse Satiety Type 5s, so members of Muse Satiety Type 1 will continue to eat until they feel full and will then lose their savor for food until the next meal, just like always.

Members of Muse Satiety Types 2 to 5 have just as much willpower in other areas of their lives as members of Muse Satiety Type 1. No amount of willpower is enough to prevent weight gain for more than 90% of the members of Muse Satiety Types 4 and 5. Members of Muse Satiety Type 2 and 3 can sometimes do it by sheer willpower, but it is still tough. However, as the years go by, most members of Muse Satiety Types 2 and 3 succumb and gain weight.

24. All you have to do to lose weight is exercise.

This myth just won't die, even in the face of overwhelming evidence that exercise by itself doesn't cause weight loss. I will only briefly touch on this myth at this point in this book, since this topic is addressed more extensively in Chapter 17. I believe that this myth is enduring because of the observed financial success of commercial gyms across the country and because of their non-stop media ads. This myth is also enduring because of the astounding weight loss that viewers saw firsthand on *The Biggest Loser*. In 2019, 71.5 million Americans had a gym membership at a total cost of about $32 billion per year (Gym Market Research & Industry Stats 2019 , 2019). That is up from 22 million Americans that had a gym membership in 1993.

A 2010 study on 34,079 women for 13 years that examined the relationship between weight maintenance and minutes of exercise performed per week (Lee I.-M. , 2010) reported that no group of women lost weight, no matter how much exercise they did. On the other hand, the only group that maintained weight for the duration of the study were the women who were thin to start with and that exercised 420 minutes a week, or 60 minutes per day. In the NWCR of 10,000 individuals who have lost an average of 70 pounds and that have kept it off for an average of 5.7 years, only 1% report that they lost their weight by exercise alone. 89% of the women report that they lost weight by adding exercise to a fixed-calorie diet, while 10% report that they lost their weight by diet alone (Wing R. , 2020).

Why doesn't exercise cause weight loss? That is because the human machine is made to reliably and consistently consume the same number of calories it has burned in the last 24 hours. If not, skinny people who started an exercise program would become emaciated. Michael Phelps, the Olympic swimmer, has been reported to burn about 8,000 calories a day when he is training for the Olympics. The next day he eats about 8,000 calories of food. If he didn't, and only ate a still large 4,000 calories the next day, then he would lose more than one pound per day.

With this in mind, the real heroes of *The Biggest Loser* program were the unsung dietitians that kept the program participants on a lower-calorie diet. Otherwise, no matter how many calories that the personal trainers could get the participants to burn, if they weren't on a lower-calorie diet that was very closely monitored, then they would have eaten back what they had burned each and every day and would have lost next to nothing.

I know that the legions of personal trainers around the country bristle at the suggestion that exercise, including weightlifting, rarely, if ever, causes weight loss. It is because they have personally seen countless people in their weight-training programs lose weight. But the weight loss is only occurring in their clients that are following the fixed-calorie diets that these same trainers are giving them. Exercise versus diet studies, such as Sopko et al (1985), in which non-exercisers reduced their caloric intake by 500 calories per day and exercisers increased their exercise by 500 calories per day for the duration of the study, have demonstrated that equal amounts of weight are lost when equal amounts of calorie reduction by diet or calorie expenditure by exercise are present. But, in these studies, dietitians are present to be sure that the exercisers don't just go home and eat back the calories that they just burned, which is what almost all humans naturally do.

Please don't get me wrong on aerobic exercise and weight training. I am a big advocate of exercise, both during weight loss and especially during weight maintenance. Exercise has a host of benefits besides helping with weight maintenance. For those who use and can afford them, weight trainers are a great help to people. I would just encourage the weight trainers to be sure that their overweight clients are constantly reminded to maintain their caloric intake at a healthy fixed level while they are increasing their exercise.

Exercise doesn't cause weight loss. However, exercise is critical for weight maintenance and promotes good health. Everyone should try to exercise at least 30 minutes a day, five days a week. A medical provider should be consulted before starting an exercise program if there is any question of poor health that might be adversely affected by exercise.

25. Drinking sugar-free soda makes you fat.

Consuming sugar-free soda has not been proven to cause humans to gain weight. This has not stopped some from cherry picking the results of the occasional low-quality study that supports their point of view as proof that diet drinks cause people to gain weight. These inflammatory claims have then made it into the news media and, as a result, the public at large now believes that drinking sugar-free soda is a significant contributor to the worldwide obesity problem. As previously discussed in this book, the obesity problem in the world is due to a genetic absence of satiety signals, or Muse's Satie-topathy, maximum weight memory, food craving, and a calorie-rich food environment. Even if consuming sugar-free soda were ever proven to cause weight gain, then the amount that it would contribute to the total problem would be small.

In addressing this myth, it is important for the public to know that there are two main types of studies that are presented by the media. First are observational, or epidemiologic, studies, which are based on research on large databases to see if cause-and-effect patterns can be found. Examples of just a few of the databases studied are the Canadian healthcare database, the Kaiser health plan database, and the Dutch healthcare database. Observational dietary studies cannot establish cause and effect, and this is most often stated in the discussion section of observational dietary studies. This type of study is hampered by an inability to confirm what diet the subjects in the database were really consuming. These studies are biased due to reverse causality and residual confounding. Reverse causality is defined as a misidentification of the cause and effect, so that the effect is really the cause. An example would be to assume that consuming diet drinks causes obesity, but in reality, obese people are more likely to consume diet drinks to help control their weight, and that is why an observational trial can draw the wrong conclusion from its study of a database. Residual confounding is when the potential effect of a confounding variable in a study is not completely accounted for in the analysis of the data. An example would be studying a database to see if obese people have more cancer than thin people. However, the researcher of this study fails to adequately correct for the fact that a significant number of thin people are more likely to be thin because they smoke. The smoking will increase their cancer rates. This might erroneously lead the researcher to conclude that obese people don't have a higher rate of cancer than thin people, when in fact obese people do have more cancer than thin people. The vast majority of dietary studies are observational, like I have just discussed, so that we often hear of dietary studies that say that a certain food is good for you one month and then is bad for you the next month.

In contrast to observational studies, randomized controlled trials are less subject to bias and can prove cause and effect. However, randomized controlled trials are more expensive, don't always reflect the real world in their tightly controlled clinical environments, are smaller in size, and have shorter durations. Randomized controlled studies are the gold standard of studies, but only represent a small portion of the total number of studies that are published. The media doesn't tell their listeners that the study they are presenting is an observational trial or a randomized-controlled trial, which creates confusion.

I took the time to explain the above because in humans, the majority of observational trials have suggested that sugar-free-soda consumption is associated with weight gain (Azad, 2017) (Fowler, 2016), and the majority of randomized-controlled trials have shown that sugar-free-soda consumption is associated with weight loss (Miller, 2014) (Tate, 2012) (Ruyter, 2012). Since the randomized controlled trials are much more reliable, then the answer is that sugar-free-soda consumption does not cause weight gain. In fact, it helps contribute to weight loss.

Why has so much been written about these unreliable observational trials on sugar-free soda? Why has so little been written about the randomized controlled trials on sugar-free soda? I don't know for sure, but here are my thoughts. Organizations and companies that benefit from denigrating sugar-free-soda consumption are probably behind this. Often, the biased research is being supported by big money from these companies. I'll leave it to the reader to research this area further, since it is beyond the scope of this book. In my weight-loss practice, I don't ask my sugar-free-soda drinkers to stop their sugar-free-soda intake while on a diet. I do encourage moderation in the consumption of sugar-free sodas, as well as all other low-calorie drinks.

Sugar-free-soda consumption doesn't cause weight gain in humans. Although it can cause weight loss, the amount is small, and its use cannot be relied on to help a person lose a significant amount of weight.

26. Certain body types can't lose weight no matter what they do.

This is a common myth found on many of the body building/weight training web sites on the Internet. The body type these web sites associate with having a hard time losing weight is the Endomorph Body Type. According to these web sites, Endomorphs are genetically designed to be "larger" than other people and the best that they can do is work out so that they can be heavy, but still fit. These web sites suggest that there are two other body types: The Ectomorph Body Type whose members can't gain weight and struggle to bulk up, and the Mesomorph Body Type whose members bulk up more easily and lose weight more easily. In my opinion, overweight members of Muse Satiety Types 2 to 5 that are the same sex, body frame, weight, height, muscle mass, and activity level will lose pretty much the same amount of weight on an identical diet, no matter if they are Endomorphs, Ectomorphs, or Mesomorphs. I also propose that individuals with the genetic ability to build more muscle with exercise are evenly distributed across Muse Satiety Types 1 to 5.

27. A ketogenic diet causes more weight loss than a non-ketogenic diet.

Ketogenic diets have been around for 60 to 70 years and are defined as diets that are so low in carbohydrate consumption that the body must produce ketones to feed the brain. The brain can only derive energy from glucose from carbohydrates and ketones. Fat is not able to cross the blood-brain barrier and therefore can't be used by the brain for energy. When a human consumes less than 20 grams of carbohydrates per day, then the body begins to convert fat into ketones to cross the blood-brain barrier and feed the brain. It is widely believed amongst laypersons and medical professionals that a very low carbohydrate diet that causes ketosis to occur causes more weight loss than a diet that doesn't cause ketosis, even if the diets allow the same number of calories per day. This is theorized to occur by a number of mechanisms, including ketosis suppressing appetite, making ketones using extra energy, and calories being lost in the urine as ketones spill into the urine.

Just because the whole world believes something doesn't mean it's true. Human studies in metabolic units, which are the most accurate studies available, have shown that ketogenic diets don't cause any more body fat loss than non-ketogenic diets (Hall K. , 2016). I addressed this more in depth in Chapter 10.

The above diet myths are just a fraction of the many diet myths circling the world. I encourage dieters to use only scholarly articles as well as university and medical-specialty websites to evaluate dietary claims to determine for themselves if a claim is fact or myth.

CHAPTER 15

BREAKING DOWN THE BARRIERS THAT KEEP YOU FROM TRYING TO LOSE WEIGHT

IN MY WORK as an obesity specialist, I have been surprised to meet new weight-loss patients in their fourth, fifth, and sixth decades of their lives that have never really tried to lose weight. They have come to see me to start their first diet. Or, maybe, they have tried once to lose weight, but had lost a few pounds in the effort and had gained it back. Many had already been struggling with their weight by age 20 and most had been gaining weight steadily throughout their adult lives. The need to lose weight just hadn't been important enough to motivate them to get going with weight loss. I haven't noticed a difference in Muse Satiety Types for these individuals. Why hadn't they ever tried to diet before? What made them suddenly ready to diet? Hopefully, in answering these questions, I can elucidate some of the things that have been holding many people back from losing weight.

There is a science behind successfully changing human behavior, and understanding the steps required to change behavior can improve the chance of success in getting ready to lose weight. The steps to changing behavior are:

1. Recognize the need to change.

2. Formulate a plan for change.

3. Maintain a positive attitude about the need to change.

4. Initiate the plan for change.

5. Celebrate successes in changing your behavior.

6. Have a plan for setbacks.

7. Maintain the change.

Each of these steps can be directly applied to starting and succeeding at weight loss and successful weight maintenance. I will address each of these steps in the sections below.

1. Recognize the need to change.

Every person who is overweight already knows that they are overweight. They are frustrated by their weight, at least to some degree, and would like to lose their excess weight if they could. However, many other priorities loom larger in their lives that make the decision to lose weight comparatively less urgent, and possibly the need to lose weight is so far down their list of priorities that weight loss is not even considered an option. The key to recognizing the need to change a behavior is to elevate the importance of changing that behavior to the highest level possible in their personal list of priorities, so the individual's brain will assign not only a knowledge of importance to the behavior change of weight loss, but an emotional urgency to the behavioral change of weight loss.

Love is a strong emotion for humans and is a strong motivator to action. Fear is another strong emotion. Hate is a powerful emotion as well. These three emotions are strong enough that they motivate us to almost immediate action. The emotional urgency that a person needs to have attached to the need to lose weight would be well served by using the emotions of love, fear, and hate as motivators to action. You have to love weight loss for all the good that it will do for you. You have to fear your current weight for the health risks it might bring and for the risks of loss of social opportunity that it could cause. You need to hate your obesity because of the health problems it is already causing you and for the loss of social opportunities you have already suffered.

What can you do to augment the emotions needed to make weight loss a higher priority in your mind? Make a written list of all the health and social benefits that would come with weight loss. Think carefully because there are many. Some of the benefits from losing weight from my personal list are less knee and back pain, being able to bend over to do something without getting really short of breath, being able to lie flat on my stomach and still be able to breathe, being able to cross my legs like I could when I was thin, stopping the short-term memory loss and headaches I get from sleep apnea, stopping acid reflux, being able to run to keep up with my younger grand-children, being able to squeeze between the network server cabinet at work and the shelves next to it without fearing I'll rip a button off my shirt, and feeling the excitement of wearing pants I haven't worn in 10 years. That's just a start of all the benefits I can think of that I would get from losing weight. If you'd like, you can start with my list and then add more benefits of your own or you can start fresh with your own list.

What about things that you fear that your being overweight might cause? To help you get started, I'll tell you a few of mine. I'm afraid that my being overweight will cause me to need knee and hip replacements, that my sleep apnea will get worse and I'll have to start using a CPAP machine, that I won't look handsome to my wife, that all my patients will abandon me as their medical provider because I can't stop from getting bigger and bigger, that I'll get a blood clot in my legs like my uncle, that I'll die and my wife will marry someone else (she says she won't), and that my varicose veins will pop while I'm walking in a warm rain storm and I won't know that I'm bleeding to death because the blood will just feel like rain running down my legs. Oh my, I'm revealing too much! Again, make your own list.

Then, list the things that you hate about your weight. And keep in mind that the hate we are using here is really a strong dislike that will motivate change for the better. I hate my weight for the times that people don't notice me first at counters and stores, because my wife has to lean over my belly to kiss me, because I can't reach around my back to scratch where my back itches, because so many of my clothes don't fit, because my knees hurt when I try to exercise, because I'm tired of not being able to walk up the stairs like all the skinny people, because I hate not looking like I want to look, etc. I think you get the picture.

Once you love the idea of weight loss enough, fear the consequences of not losing weight, hate what being heavy has already done to hurt you, and once you have quieted down other pressing priorities in your life, such as holidays, deaths, taxes, marriages, births, long hours at work, etc., then you will be raring to go to start a weight-loss attempt.

What do you do if you still are not ready to lose weight? First, you're not alone. There are many good people out there who just can't find the mental motivation to lose weight. Many of these people are successful in their careers, socially well-adjusted, and happy with their lives. They pay their taxes, keep their yards nice, and pay their bills. Yet, they're just not ready to lose weight. I challenge each one of you reading this book to carefully think through what I am presenting in this chapter. Weight loss is doable. While it is not fun or pleasant to diet, it's easier than you think, and the benefits are greater than you believe. I promise. Talk to your therapist, minister, or medical provider about the things keeping you from being ready to lose weight. Maybe you like going out to dinner with your friends and eating your favorite foods so much that you just can't see giving them up. Maybe desserts and sweets are such a need for you that you can't imagine not having them. Could it be that you fear losing weight because it will bring unwanted physical attention to your body? How about fear that you'll lose weight and just gain it back again, like you always have? Could it be worry that your spouse will get jealous of other people noticing how good you look when you're thinner? Are you afraid that you won't have the time to cook special meals or to exercise? Is there someone close to you that harasses you excessively every time you try to diet? Again, if these, or other reasons for not losing weight, are weighing so heavily on your mind that you just can't see past them to start a weight-loss plan, then please see a professional for help.

Once you are ready to lose weight, and I mean that you want to lose weight really badly, then you are ready for the next step.

2. Formulate a plan for change.

Before you run off to start any old weight-loss program, it is critical to formulate a plan for how you'll lose weight that maximizes your chance for success. The plan must be realistic, applicable to your current life situation, and goal oriented. It should also include self-monitoring as well as external monitoring by a diet coach and/or a support group.

To be realistic, a weight-loss plan must fit within the science of weight loss. For all self-directed diets, and there are hundreds, the average weight loss is about 10 pounds in six months with no subsequent weight loss. For diets that are run by diet companies and include in-person or online support, the average weight loss is about 15 pounds in six months with no subsequent weight loss. For a medication-assisted diet, the average weight loss is about 30 pounds in six months with no subsequent weight loss. For a very low-calorie diet (VLCD), the average weight loss is about 50 pounds in six months and about 100 pounds in a year, depending on how long a person remains on the VLCD and how much they had to lose to start with. For gastric banding, gastric sleeve, and gastric bypass, the average weight loss at one year is about 40 pounds, about 60 pounds, and about 100 pounds, respectively (Benefits of Bariatric Surgery, n.d.). The numbers above vary widely from study to study and from person to person, and how much weight is lost depends a lot on ideal weight, starting weight, and effort expended. For every weight-loss method out there, there are some that have lost 200 pounds and there are some that have lost nothing. To determine if your weight-loss goal is realistic, then determine how much weight you want to lose and be sure that the weight-loss method you have selected will result in the amount of weight you desire to lose. I caution you against assuming that you will be the rare person who will lose much more than the average person loses on any given method.

For a weight-loss plan to be applicable to your current life situation, it needs to be affordable, contain foods that you are willing to eat, fit into your lifestyle, and conform with the length of time that you're willing to diet. The cost of the diet options listed above varies widely. Self-directed diets cost the least with the only expense involved being the purchase of a diet book, if needed, and the higher cost of foods that are allowed on the diet. These foods usually include more vegetables and lean meats, which cost more per calorie, and less breads, starches, and desserts, which cost less per calorie. On the other end, the average price of gastric bypass performed in the US in 2017 was $25,571 (Average cost of gastric bypass surgery, n.d.). Hopefully, those who are considering weight-loss surgery will have insurance coverage, which will reduce the out-of-pocket expense related for the weight-loss surgery. The weight-loss method you are planning to use needs to contain foods that you are willing to eat. A vegan can't very well undergo a meat-based keto diet and a person with Celiac Sprue can't start a gluten-based diet. A person who doesn't like soy shouldn't try to do a diet that involves consuming soy products. The diet that you are planning needs to fit into your lifestyle. If you travel a lot, then a diet that involves frequent visits with diet personnel will not work. If you entertain for work, a diet that prohibits eating out at restaurants might not work. Last, the diet that you are considering needs to get the job done before you get tired with the whole thing and throw in the towel. I call this the diet attention span, and we all have a limit to how long we can diet before we mentally and emotionally just have to go back to eating regular quantities of regular food. If your weight-loss goal is to lose 50 pounds and the diet you are considering only causes about 2.5 pounds of weight loss per month for a total of 15 pounds of weight loss after six months, then that diet is not the diet for you.

For a diet to work well, it is best for the diet to be goal oriented. There needs to be both long-term and short-term goals. The foremost long-term diet goal on most of our minds is to lose all of our excess body weight down close to our ideal body weight. That is closely followed by the second long-term goal of not gaining back any of the weight that has been lost after the diet. Both of those goals can be daunting to take on. For most, lofty long-term goals are better conceptualized and achieved when broken up into a series of much smaller short-term goals.

Short-term goals during dieting are essential to be sure that the dieter can achieve incremental successes along the way to the ultimate long-term goal. Decide, for example, that your first goal is to lose the first 10 pounds. Additional supporting goals that might aid you in accomplishing your short-term goal of losing 10 pounds might be to avoid going to restaurants or fast-food joints during the time that you are losing the 10 pounds, to exercise five days a week for 30 minutes, to avoid all calorie-containing drinks and to drink more water instead, and to remove your favorite snacks from your places of residence and work.

Once the initial short-term goal of losing 10 pounds is achieved, it will be time to set a new short-term goal that is still easy to wrap your mind around and achieve, such as losing another 10 pounds. Adjustment of some of the supporting goals might also be needed, such as allowing diet drinks into the diet along with the water; permitting one trip to a restaurant once a month at which you will consume no more than 600 calories; allowing yourself to snack on pickles, celery, and carrots while at home and at work; and including more variety in your exercise.

Diet monitoring is a critical part of weight-loss success. Diet monitoring can be done by the dieter or by another person or entity. Self-monitoring by the dieter usually involves daily tracking of calorie, protein, and carbohydrate intake, supplement consumption, prescription medication use, and exercise. Dieters who track their calories lose more than dieters who don't track their calories (Baker R. , 1993). This can be accomplished by a pen and paper, or by apps on the dieter's phone or computer. Dieters who weigh themselves frequently while dieting lose more weight than their fellow dieters who don't weigh frequently (Shieh, 2016). Frequent weighing during a diet is defined as weighing at least weekly. I recommend that dieter's weights be tracked graphically, since a graphical representation of weight loss is a powerful tool in aiding with compliance. Graphing weight loss over time can be done by pen and paper, on a computer, or on an app on your phone.

External monitoring of weight loss over time by a third party can be helpful in improving weight loss (Samuel-Hodge, 2009) (Lemstra, 2016). External monitoring can be done by an individual, as long as your relationship with them can safely tolerate their monitoring of your weight loss, or a professional entity, such as a medical provider, diet clinic, dietitian, or personal trainer. I strongly recommend at least monthly contact with the person or entity doing the external monitoring of your weight loss, so that the external monitoring will be more likely to increase the amount of weight you will lose (Samuel-Hodge, 2009). To improve accuracy, the person or entity you have chosen to be your external monitor should weigh you in person on their scale. I also recommend that you use the person or entity that is monitoring your weight loss as your diet coach. I will loosely define a diet coach as any outside person or entity that will not only monitor your diet progress and compliance but will also give helpful advice and encouragement. There must be a positive relationship between you and your diet coach. Your diet coach needs to be able to make observations on your progress without incurring negative consequences from you for their efforts.

3. Maintain a positive attitude.

Dieters who have determined in their minds that they will succeed at weight loss and weight maintenance are more likely to succeed than dieters who are going to try to lose and maintain weight but are not sure in their minds if they will succeed (Williams G. , 1996). The theory behind this is the Self-Determination Theory, which basically says that if you believe that something will happen and you work to make it happen, it will happen. This sounds self-evident and even trite, until one realizes just how negative an overweight person can be about their weight and about themselves. Self-imposed and socially imposed negative views of their overweight body, combined with numerous past failed efforts at weight loss, can lead the overweight person to self-loathing and pessimism about their chance of success at weight loss. It takes a herculean effort on the part of many overweight individuals to even hope that they might lose some of their extra weight and keep it off.

To help to overcome negative attitudes about one's weight and about one's struggle to lose and maintain weight, I recommend both self-therapy and professional therapy. Self-therapy for negative thoughts about being overweight involves accepting the fact that as perversely pleasureful as negative thoughts about one's self are, they never have any positive benefits. They never make you happier. They don't make your life better in any way. They just leave you right where you started, mentally and emotionally exhausted, still unhappy with yourself about your weight, and too down on yourself to be able to find any motivation to do anything about it. A self-determined choice to have a positive attitude about your overweight body and your ability to lose the weight is not harmful at all. Even if being positive about weight loss doesn't result in much weight loss, at least you won't still be wallowing in the sticky quagmire of negative thoughts. Once you've determined to pull yourself away from the tar baby of negativity, how do you keep yourself from falling right back into the same black hole? By willfully pushing out all negative thoughts as they try to retake control of the stage of your mind. You'll have to push those thoughts out hundreds of times a day, if necessary, to keep your thoughts positive. Be ready to sing a happy song in your mind, to imagine the pleasure a favorite movie, to find someone positive to talk to, or to go somewhere where you don't feel as negative. Have pictures of when you were thinner and happy where you can easily see them, like on your bathroom mirror or in your car. Have positive affirmations about your weight memorized and ready to repeat to yourself, such as was written by Elizabeth Berg, "Nothing tastes as good as being thin feels," (Berg, 2008) or as was written by Deepak Chopra, "…it is never too late to begin creating the bodies we want instead of the ones we mistakenly assume we are stuck with." (Chopra, 2007)

Trust me, what I am suggesting that you do here is hard, really hard. There will be days where you do fall back into negative thoughts. Sometimes the only solution at the end of a negative day is to barely succeed in falling asleep amidst your negative thoughts and feelings, only to wake up to a new and decidedly better day, wondering why you let yourself fall into such negative thoughts again. But that's where the success will come here, when you keep getting up in the morning and deciding to again square your mental jaw against the negativity of the world and determine to be positive, especially about weight loss.

Don't be afraid to get professional help if, despite your best efforts, you just can't rise above the negative thoughts and feelings about yourself, your weight, and your past struggles with weight loss. A trusted therapist, dietitian, medical provider, or psychiatrist can really help.

4. Initiate the plan for change.

Once you are motivated to start your weight-loss plan, when is the right time to start? Although outside observers might say to start the plan immediately, it is best to initiate the plan to lose weight during a time when stressors are at a minimum and when there are no food-intensive holidays, vacations, or unavoidable dinners in the following few months that will likely derail your plan. Those events can be dealt with more successfully later in a diet than near the beginning.

5. Celebrate successes.

A common recommendation from experts in behavioral change is to celebrate successes in changing undesirable behaviors. This applies to weight-loss endeavors as well. Making a weight-loss plan with short-term goals that can be completed relatively easily throughout the diet allows for more frequent celebratory activities at the successful completion of each short-term goal. Of course, celebrations shouldn't be comprised of foods that a dieter is trying to avoid while dieting, or out-of-town trips with inevitable restaurant eating, for concern that they will create a setback which could become a weight-loss plateau. To celebrate completing a short-term goal of losing the first 10 pounds on a diet, the dieter could purchase a new article of clothing, buy a novel that they would like to read, go to a play, or attend an art show. The reward you give yourself will vary with your interests and with your financial resources. Involve family, friends, and your diet coach and/or support group in your celebration as you are able, either in person, by phone, via video chatting, or though social media.

6. Have a plan for setbacks.

Setbacks in the process of changing human behavior are common. Setbacks occur during weight-loss efforts as well. No one wants there to be a weight-loss setback, but to err is human and there are so many food temptations around us all day long. The nice thing about a diet setback is that it's never the end of the world if it happens. You can just stop yourself in the middle of your inappropriate food intake and get back on your diet program. It's not how many times you fail at your diet that causes the diet to fail, it's how many times you fail to get back on your diet plan that undermines the success of your diet.

If and when a diet setback occurs, self-reflection needs to occur to determine what led to the diet slipup, what can be changed to prevent the event from happening again, and what you learned about yourself from this occurrence. It's usually obvious why the diet slipup occurred. Either you were getting hungrier as the diet progressed and you just couldn't avoid eating something that looked so good, or someone brought one of the foods you crave to work or to your home. It could have been an invitation to a restaurant that you agreed to go to that served your favorite foods on the menu, or it might have been candy that someone gave you as a nice gesture or gift. Whatever it was, the next step is to determine how to not have the slipup occur again. Plan to remove the foods you can't resist from your environment. Ask your family and co-workers not to bring those foods to work or home unless they can be locked up where you can't get them. Plan to avoid restaurants as much as possible during your diet since most dieters overeat at most visits to their favorite restaurants. Ask friends, family, and co-workers to not make social events only about food. With respect to snack foods, ask friends and family to not give you calorie-containing treats while you're dieting. Most people are glad to help you with staying on your diet if you just ask them.

Make sure you have a plan in place, both as you start your diet and after slipups, for what to do if you are suddenly faced with situations that might put you at risk to stumble and mess up on your diet. Examples might be a birth, marriage, or death in the family that demands attendance at events where there will be a lot of food, or where you are expected to eat the food. Entertaining for work, or entertaining guests from out of town, can also frequently involve situations where the dieter will be expected to be present at meals. For these situations, your diet plan might be to eat a protein bar before an event that involves food to blunt your appetite, and then to only sip water or a diet drink during the meal. For other dieters, their diet plan for these situations might instead be to eat only the protein on the plate, and no carbohydrates of any kind.

7. Maintain the behavioral change.

Maintaining weight after a diet is the hardest step of the diet because it goes on for not just weeks or months, but for the rest of your life. See Chapter 11 of this book for my discussion about weight maintenance.

Breaking down the barriers that prevent a dieter from starting and successfully completing a diet are accomplished by following similar steps that are required to change any human behavior. Recognizing the need to diet is the first step and involves efforts to increase the level of emotional urgency of the need to lose weight and to recognize that successful weight loss is achievable for the dieter. A diet plan is then selected by the dieter and long- and short-term goals are established. A positive attitude is maintained by the dieter throughout the weight-loss process. The diet plan is initiated, and the dieter celebrates their successes and deals appropriately with diet setbacks. Once the long-term goal of weight loss is achieved, then long-term weight maintenance ensues.

CHAPTER 16

WEIGHT-LOSS SURGERY DO'S AND DON'TS

WEIGHT-LOSS SURGERY IS an essential tool in the treatment of obesity and can be necessary when individuals have tried unsuccessfully to decrease their weight by dieting. The three commonly performed weight-loss surgeries are quite safe and, when diets fail, are the most effective tools we have that result in significant and lasting weight loss. Weight-loss surgery can also be an important part of the treatment for the serious medical complications of obesity. At the same time, there is significant hesitance by patients to have weight-loss surgery and by medical providers to refer patients for weight-loss surgery, due to real and perceived risks, adverse effects, and fear of weight regain after surgery.

The three commonly performed weight-loss surgeries, listed in order of the frequency in which they are performed, as of writing of this book, are vertical sleeve gastrectomy (more commonly referred to as gastric sleeve), Roux-en-Y gastric bypass (more commonly referred to as gastric bypass), and adjustable gastric banding (gastric banding). From the website for the American Society of Bariatric and Metabolic Surgeons, it was estimated in 2018 that gastric sleeve comprised 61.4% of total bariatric surgeries, followed by gastric bypass 17.0%, and gastric band at 1.1%. The remainder of the bariatric surgeries occurred at a frequency of 15.4% for revisions of previous bariatric surgeries, 2.3% for other types of bariatric surgery, 2% for inflatable gastric balloons, and 0.8% for an uncommonly performed bariatric surgery called biliopancreatic diversion with duodenal switch (Estimate of Bariatric Surgery Numbers, 2011-2018, 2018).

Bariatric surgery is indicated for the following groups by the American Academy of Clinical Endocrinology (AACE, 2016) and the American Society of Metabolic and Bariatric Surgeons (Mechanick, 3013):

A. Body Mass Index (BMI) ≥ 40 with no obesity-related comorbidities. (A comorbidity is a medical complication.)

B. BMI ≥ 35 with one or more severe obesity-related comorbidities, including type 2 diabetes, high blood pressure, high cholesterol, obstructive sleep apnea (OSA), obesity-hypoventilation syndrome (OHA), Pickwickian syndrome (a combination of OSA and OHA), nonalcoholic fatty liver disease, acid reflux, asthma, venous stasis disease, urinary incontinence, debilitating arthritis, pseudotumor cerebri, or considerably impaired quality of life.

C. BMI ≥ 30 with type 2 diabetes or metabolic syndrome, although evidence is limited for this recommendation as of writing this book.

In addition, the patient must have failed previous non-surgical attempts at weight loss, be committed to adhering to postoperative care, not have a reversible cause for their obesity, not be abusing drugs or alcohol, not be suffering from uncontrolled and severe psychiatric illness, and not be too sick to tolerate surgery.

The benefits of bariatric surgery are amazing for the individuals it is indicated for. Diabetes completely resolves in 82% of patients and improves in 18%. Sleep apnea resolves completely in 74% and improves in 19%. Depression improves in 55%. Asthma improves in 82% (Schauer, 2003). In a 7.1-year-long study, the overall death rate was improved by 40%, with heart-disease-related deaths dropping 56%, diabetes-related deaths dropping 92%, and cancer-related deaths dropping 60% (Adams, 2007). Other diseases that are greatly improved are high cholesterol, high blood pressure, nonalcoholic fatty liver disease, acid reflux, stress urinary incontinence, degenerative joint disease, gout, venous stasis disease, and polycystic ovarian syndrome in women. It is well-known that patients with the highest BMIs have the greatest risks from each of the diseases mentioned above and therefore have greater improvement with weight loss. It cannot be assumed that patients with lower BMIs, especially those with BMIs less than 35, will have the same degree of benefit.

As I discuss the three most commonly performed bariatric surgeries, I want to point out that I will be reporting the average weight loss from bariatric surgery as the percentage of total weight lost and not as the percentage of weight loss of excess body weight. Bariatric-surgery literature typically reports weight lost after bariatric surgery as the percentage of loss of excess body weight, whereas weight loss by non-surgical means is reported as the percentage of loss of total body weight. Let's take, for example, an individual who weighs 300 pounds, but has an ideal body weight of 150 pounds, then loses 100 pounds. Weight-loss surgeons would report that the individual had lost 67% of his excess body weight, whereas non-surgical weight-loss providers would report that the individual had lost 30% of his total body weight. You can see the confusion that can result when trying to compare the degree of weight loss when the two different reporting methods are being used. To avoid confusion and to help with comparing surgical results with the results of non-surgical weight-loss methods discussed in Chapter 11, I will report weight loss by an individual as the percent of total weight lost, which would be the 30% answer in the example above.

Gastric sleeve has overtaken gastric bypass as of 2012 as the most commonly performed bariatric surgery. This surgery is most often performed laparoscopically.

BEFORE

SLEEVE GASTRECTOMY
WEIGHT LOSS SURGERY

AFTER

SLEEVE GASTRECTOMY
WEIGHT LOSS SURGERY

Gastric sleeve
section
(reduced stomach
area)

Surgically
removed
stomach
section

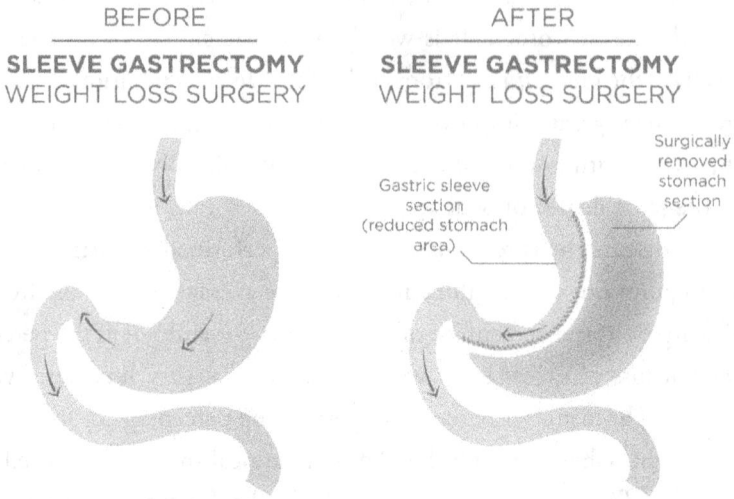

Figure 13 - Sleeve Gastrectomy

During gastric sleeve surgery, two-thirds of the stomach is removed, leaving only a small portion of the stomach that then causes a feeling of fullness much sooner at meals, as is shown in Figure 13. Removal of two-thirds of the stomach also markedly lowers ghrelin levels, thereby significantly reducing hunger.

The 30-day mortality, or death rate, from a laparoscopically performed gastric sleeve is 0.2%, or about one in 500 patients (Longitudinal Assessment of Bariatric Surgery, 2007). Patients who have a gastric sleeve lose about 30% of their total body weight in one year (Sjöström, Effects of Bariatric Surgery on Mortality in Swedish Obese Subjects, 2007) (Barzin, 2016) (Hoyuela, 2017). This is due in part to the restriction in the size of their stomach, which gives them a feeling of fullness, cramping and even nausea when the stretch receptors in the now-much-smaller stomach sense that the stomach is reaching its new and smaller maximum capacity. Most of the patients who meet the requirements for gastric sleeve are Muse Satiety Type 4s and 5s and have never felt full before on less than a half plate of food. This feeling of fullness is not the same as the painless feeling of fullness that individuals in Muse Satiety Types 1, 2, and 3 feel when they reach the exact point where they have eaten enough to meet their calorie needs. But this feeling of fullness still results in significant weight loss. Weight is also lost after a gastric sleeve due to the lower ghrelin levels that come from two-thirds of the stomach being removed. Ghrelin is produced by the lining of the stomach and the first part of the small intestine. The low ghrelin levels after gastric sleeve surgery leave the patients feeling less hungry, both at mealtimes and in between meals. The loss of hunger is somewhat like the loss of savor signal that Muse Satiety Type 1s feel, but the loss of savor in gastric sleeve patients is present 24 hours a day, while a Muse Satiety Type 1 will feel hungry on and off throughout the day when it is time to eat.

About two years after a gastric sleeve, ghrelin levels start to rise as the remaining stomach and the first part of the small intestine increase their production of ghrelin. Hunger worsens. After the first two years, the only defense a gastric sleeve patient has against increasing hunger is the fullness caused by the smaller volume of the stomach. Thankfully, the stomach is not able to stretch that much and patients who have had a gastric sleeve remain unable to eat a whole plate of food at one sitting. Unfortunately, many gastric sleeve patients learn that they can eat small amounts of food all day long and those small amounts of food add up to more calories than the patients are burning, which causes weight gain.

At five years from gastric sleeve surgery, on average, patients have gained back about 30% of what they had lost. This does not mean that gastric sleeve surgery is the wrong thing to do. The gastric sleeve surgery benefits are both real and beneficial over a long period of time. While we all wish that the average gastric sleeve patient didn't gain back 30% of the weight they had lost in five years, gastric sleeve patients are still significantly thinner than they were before surgery and therefore are still reaping the benefits of the weight they have lost. In addition, the years that they were thinner are believed to have lasting effects on preserving the function of insulin-producing cells in the pancreas and also on the cartilage in the knees, thereby preventing type 2 diabetes and knee arthritis needing knee replacement, respectively.

The long-term benefits of gastric sleeve surgery are improvements in type 2 diabetes, high blood pressure, high cholesterol, and sleep apnea. Some studies have shown a reduction in death due to improvement in these medical diseases after people have gastric sleeve surgery (Reges, 2018). Long-term side effects of gastric sleeve include stomach leaking at the surgery site, stomach narrowing due to scar tissue, acid reflux, stomach ulcers, abdominal-wall hernias at the surgery sites, bowel obstruction due to internal hernia, and symptomatic gallstones. While some of these side effects are easily treated, others can require surgery, can be serious, and, in rare cases, can result in death.

There are advantages of gastric sleeve over gastric bypass. The pyloric valve at the bottom of the stomach is not removed with gastric sleeve. This prevents dumping syndrome, which can happen in gastric-bypass patients. In addition, the gastric sleeve procedure doesn't bypass any of the small intestine, so deficiencies in micronutrients are infrequent. With gastric sleeve, a gastrointestinal specialist can still insert a lighted scope into the stomach to look for cancer, should the need ever arise. It is not possible to pass a lighted scope into the stomach in gastric-bypass patients.

Gastric bypass was overtaken by gastric sleeve in about 2012 and is now the second most commonly performed bariatric surgery. Gastric bypass is also most often performed laparoscopically.

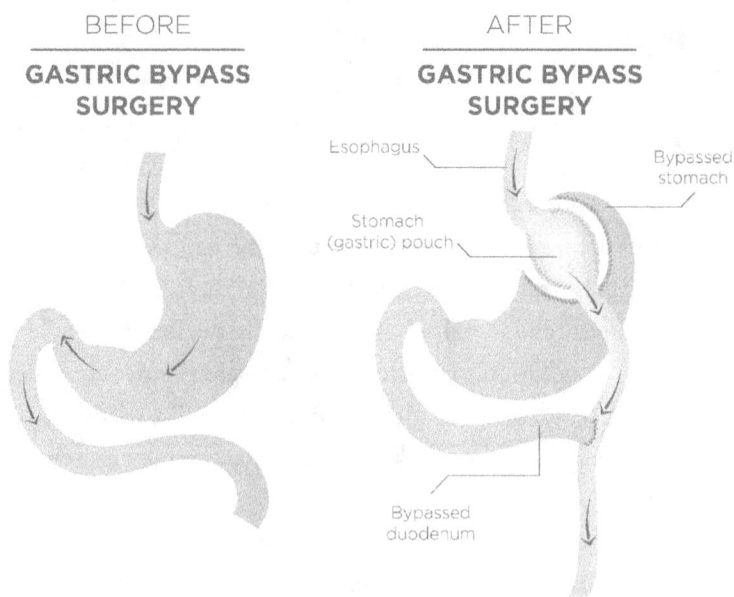

Figure 14 - Gastric-Bypass Surgery

During gastric-bypass surgery, the most proximal portion of the stomach that is just below the end of the esophagus is separated from the rest of the stomach, leaving behind just a tiny stomach attached to the esophagus. Then, the small intestine is cut at a point about one-third of the distance from the stomach to the colon. The distal end of the proximal third of the small intestine is attached at about the halfway point in the remaining small intestine. The distal two-thirds of the small intestine is attached to the tiny stomach. This is shown in Figure 14. This procedure results in significantly elevated GLP-1 levels, which markedly suppresses hunger. Gastric bypass does not lower ghrelin.

The 30-day mortality, or death rate, from a laparoscopically performed gastric bypass is 0.2%, similar to that of a laparoscopically performed gastric sleeve, or one in 500 patients (Longitudinal Assessment of Bariatric Surgery, 2007). Patients who have gastric-bypass surgery lose about 33% of their total body weight in one year (Sjöström, Effects of Bariatric Surgery on Mortality in Swedish Obese Subjects, 2007). This is due in part to the restriction in the size of the stomach, which gives them a feeling of fullness, cramping, and nausea when the stretch receptors in the now-much-smaller stomach sense that the stomach is reaching its maximum capacity. Most of the patients who meet the requirements for gastric bypass are Muse Satiety Type 4s and 5s and have never felt full before on less than a half plate of food. This feeling of fullness is not the same as the painless feeling of fullness that individuals in Muse Satiety Types 1, 2, and 3 feel when they reach the exact point where they have eaten enough to meet their calorie needs. But the feeling of fullness caused by gastric bypass still results in significant weight loss. Weight is also lost after gastric bypass due to the high GLP-1 levels that come from the first part of the small intestine. In spite of ghrelin levels rising steadily with each loss of 10 pounds in gastric-bypass patients, the elevation in GLP-1 blocks the effect of the elevated ghrelin levels and leaves gastric-bypass patients feeling less hungry, both at mealtimes and in between meals. The loss of hunger is somewhat like the loss of savor signal that Muse Satiety Type 1s feel on and off after meals throughout the day, but loss of sensation of loss of hunger in gastric sleeve patients is present all day.

About two years after gastric bypass, it is theorized that GLP-1 levels start to drop, and hunger starts to increase. Ghrelin levels have remained high for the previous two years as the body has been trying get the gastric-bypass patients to gain the weight back that they have lost. The resulting increase in hunger is only mitigated by the smaller volume of the stomach. Thankfully, the stomach is not able to stretch that much and at least the patients who have had a gastric bypass remain unable to eat a whole plate of food in one sitting. Unfortunately, many gastric-bypass patients learn that they can eat small amounts of food all day long and those small amounts of food add up to more calories than the patients are burning, which causes weight gain.

At five years from gastric-bypass surgery, patients have gained back an average of about a third of what they have lost. This does not mean that gastric-bypass surgery is the wrong thing to do. The benefits of gastric-bypass surgery are real, just like those of gastric sleeve, and they are beneficial over a long period of time. While we all wish that the average gastric-bypass patient didn't gain back a third of the weight they lost in five years, the patients are still significantly thinner than they were before surgery and therefore are still reaping the benefits of the weight loss. In addition, the years that they were thinner are believed to have lasting effects on preserving the function of insulin-producing cells in the pancreas and on the cartilage in the knees, thereby preventing type 2 diabetes and knee arthritis needing knee replacement, respectively.

The long-term benefits of gastric bypass are similar to those from gastric sleeve and include improvements in type 2 diabetes, high blood pressure, high cholesterol, and sleep apnea. Some studies have shown reduced all-cause mortality from gastric bypass due to improvement in these medical diseases (Reges, 2018). Long-term side effects of gastric bypass include stomach leaking at the surgery sites, stomach narrowing due to scar tissue, acid reflux, stomach ulcers, abdominal-wall hernias at the surgery sites, bowel obstruction due to internal hernia, symptomatic gallstones, dumping syndrome, and vitamin and mineral deficiencies. While some of these side effects are easily treated, others can require surgery, can be serious, and, in rare cases, can result in death.

The only advantage of gastric bypass over gastric sleeve is modestly greater weight loss.

Adjustable gastric-band surgery, which is also called gastric-band surgery or lap-band surgery, is the next most common weight-loss surgery, although in recent years the number of gastric-band surgeries have dropped significantly. In 2011, 35% of weight-loss surgeries were gastric-band surgeries. By 2018, it has now dropped to about 1% of weight-loss surgeries. Gastric-band surgery is also most often performed laparoscopically. During gastric-band surgery an adjustable plastic band is wrapped around the upper portion of the stomach and snapped into place, creating a small pouch of stomach above the band as is shown in Figure 15.

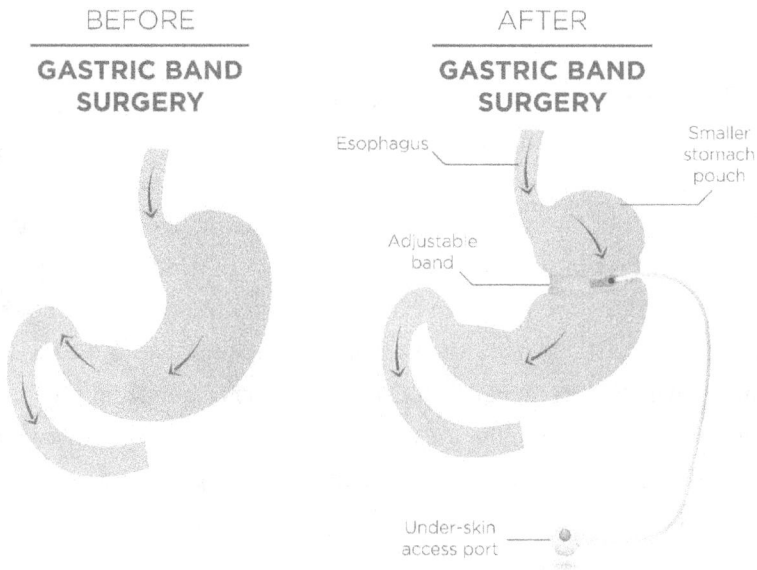

BEFORE

GASTRIC BAND
SURGERY

AFTER

GASTRIC BAND
SURGERY

Esophagus

Smaller
stomach
pouch

Adjustable
band

Under-skin
access port

Figure 15 - Gastric-Band Surgery

A tube attached to the band is then attached via a metal coupler to a tube from a port placed under the skin on the abdominal wall. The silicone portion of the port can then be accessed by a non-cutting needle to add fluid to the gastric band when needed to keep a consistent pressure against the wall of the stomach at the base of the small pouch.

After gastric-band surgery, patients are asked to consume a liquid diet for one to two months to allow the body time to form a fibrous capsule around the band, which will hold the band in place on the stomach's surface. About a month after gastric-band surgery, the patient returns to their surgeon to have their gastric band filled for the first time with a sterile salt-water solution, which is called a fill. Care is taken to avoid overfilling the gastric band, which can result in vomiting and the need for an urgent removal of some, or all, of the fluid in the gastric band, which is called an unfill. The patient then returns as often as once a month to have additional fills of the gastric band, to achieve a state where the patient can only eat two to four ounces of food, or about one-fourth to one-third of a plate of food, in one sitting. As long as the patient is compliant with the recommended diet of three small meals a day with little or no snacking between meals, then the patient will lose weight.

The 30-day mortality, or death rate, from a gastric-band surgery is 0.1%, or, one in 1,000 patients (Longitudinal Assessment of Bariatric Surgery, 2007). That is lower than the 0.2% death rate of laparoscopically performed gastric sleeve and laparoscopically performed gastric bypass. Patients who have gastric-band surgery lose an average of 22% of their total body weight in one year (Sjöström, Effects of Bariatric Surgery on Mortality in Swedish Obese Subjects, 2007). This is mostly due to the restriction in the size of the stomach, which gives them a feeling of fullness, cramping, and even nausea when the stretch receptors in the now-much-smaller stomach sense that the stomach is reaching its maximum capacity. The orexigenic and anorexigenic hormones of the body are not affected by gastric-banding surgery, so hunger levels are not decreased.

I have filled hundreds of gastric bands for patients and have learned a lot about doing fills. Even though gastric bands are much less popular recently, I'd like to still share what I have learned from filling bands. As I became more experienced with filling gastric bands, I began doing all of my fills with the use of a fluoroscopy machine (a low-dose real-time x-ray machine) that allows me to precisely insert the needle into the access port with ease, to determine that the band is still functioning properly, and to accurately assess the level of a patient's fill.

The advantages of gastric-band surgery over gastric sleeve surgery and gastric-bypass surgery include the ease of insertion of the gastric band, the fact that the gastrointestinal tract is not surgically altered by gastric-band surgery, a shorter time in the hospital after gastric-band surgery, a lower complication and death rate in the 30 days after surgery, the fact that the gastric band can be easily removed if side effects or complications develop, the ability to adjust the band as needed over time to help maintain weight lost, and less weight regain over time. The disadvantages of gastric-band surgery are less weight loss and the fact that a significant percentage of gastric-band patients need to have their gastric band removed due to side effects and complications, although the complications and side effects that do develop are rarely life threatening. Internationally, 25%-40% of gastric bands are removed within five years of gastric-band surgery (Longitudinal Assessment of Bariatric Surgery, 2007).

The side effects and complications related to a gastric band include paroxysmal burping; nausea and vomiting with eating too fast or with eating too much; uncontrolled vomiting from being overfilled; chronic pain around the band and port; slippage of the band; dilation of the pouch; micro-perforation of the stomach at the level of the band; malfunction of the band; damage to the port and port tubing by improperly performed fills; rotation of the port; and the tubing from the band becoming uncoupled from the tubing from the port. Aside from a malfunction of the band, chronic pain around the band and port, and a rotation of the port, the other side effects and complications can be mostly avoided by following the gastric-band surgeon's dietary instructions.

The side effect of paroxysmal burping refers to a spasm of the esophagus as it tries to push food from the esophagus into the tiny pouch above the stomach. The normal pouch after gastric-band surgery is only about two ounces in size and only holds about a quarter cup of food. It is common for band patients to eat more than two ounces of food at a meal because they are hungry, but then the additional food remains in the esophagus. The esophagus tries and tries to push the food into the pouch, which causes a sensation of recurrent burping. In addition, thinking that the food is stuck, the lining of the esophagus secrets a thick mucus in an effort to try to lubricate itself to make the passageway more slippery so the food will slide into the stomach. This thick mucus can well up into the back of the throat when the patient experiences paroxysmal burping. Paroxysmal burping can be prevented by eating slower, being sure that the food to be consumed is chopped small enough to pass slowly through the small opening in the band, eating smaller portions of food, and by the surgeon avoiding overfilling the band. Avoidance of overfilling the band will be discussed below.

The side effects of nausea and vomiting can occur with eating and drinking too much or too fast. The small pouch at the top of the stomach then becomes overfilled with food and drink. The muscles of the wall of the stomach begin to spasm. The recurrent spasming can lead to vomiting of the contents of the small pouch. This can be prevented by the same techniques I discussed with paroxysmal burping above.

Slippage of the band occurs in two different ways. First is a true slippage of the band down the wall of the stomach during the first weeks after surgery when a patient doesn't follow the prescribed liquid diet. Eating solid food fills the small pouch above the stomach with food, and then the wall of the small pouch starts to contract to push the food through the band and into the lower part of the stomach. This pushing effort can result in a freshly placed gastric band being pushed down farther into the body of the stomach, like a napkin ring being pushed from one end of the napkin toward the middle of the napkin. When the band finally scars in place farther down on the stomach, the pouch above the stomach is not as small as it should be, leaving the band patient able to eat more food before they feel full. Another result is that the amount of stomach wall encircled by the band is thicker, leaving little room for the band to be adjusted successively. A third result is that the larger pouch above the stomach fills with food, becomes quite heavy and then flops down the side of the stomach below the band, pulling the band and causing it to tilt downward. This can be seen on fluoroscopy of a patient's band while the patient is sitting up. A band in a proper position is at a 45-degree angle from the vertical axis of the patient's body. However, when the band is being pulled down by a large pouch full of food above the stomach, the band is then seen at 60 to 90 degrees from the vertical axis. I will discuss the management of a slipped band resulting in pouch dilation later.

Pouch dilation occurs when a patient's band is too tight and consumed food is retained for long periods in the pouch above the stomach, even until the next meal. Over time, the pouch begins to expand. Under fluoroscopy and with the use of a liquid suspension of barium that shows up dark on the fluoroscopy screen, pouches can be seen that exceed eight ounces in size. This leaves the band patient able to eat half, and even all, of a plate of food in a single sitting. The solution is for the provider performing band fills to avoid band overfills.

The complication of micro-perforation of the stomach at the level of the band occurs when the band is overfilled, which then causes both food and stomach acid produced by the wall of the small pouch above the stomach to sit for hours in the pouch. After weeks and months, this can result in the formation of tiny ulcers that then extend deeper and deeper until they open into the space around the band. This allows bacterial-laden liquid from the stomach to enter the space between the stomach and the scar tissue around the band, causing localized infection and pain. The stomach lining at the level of the band is thinner than the lining around the rest of the stomach because it has been squeezed tightly by the band for a long period of time, so it is more easily perforated by the stomach acid in the pouch. These micro-perforations are difficult to see even with an endoscope by a gastroen-terologist. Once a micro-perforation occurs, the only solution is to remove the band. Even though a micro-perforation of the stomach sounds like a life-threatening problem, it is most often not a serious problem because the space around the band is thickly covered by scar tissue. This prevents the infection from spreading into the abdominal cavity. Micro-perforations can be prevented by avoiding overfilling the band.

Sometimes the band itself can develop a leak, or the two ends of the band can come unattached, so the band no longer forms a tight band around the top of the stomach. A band with a leak can be suspected when a patient states that they were feeling that their band was adequately filled one day and that by the next few hours, or by the next day, the band didn't seem to be filled at all. At the time of the next fill and when the all the fluid is withdrawn from the band to check for the residual amount of fluid in the band, it will be discovered that there is a lot less fluid in the band than there should be. If there is still some uncertainty about a leak, then the band can be refilled and then rechecked a month later to see if the fluid has leaked out again.

A band with a leak doesn't look any different than a band that isn't leaking on fluoroscopy. However, a band in which the two ends of the band have become unattached can definitely be seen on fluoroscopy. When the ends of the band become unattached, the band stops working suddenly, and the patient suddenly doesn't feel filled at all. They immediately find that they can eat anything that they want, like they could before they had the band placed. At the time of an attempt to fill the band, the expected amount of fluid will be found in the band, and a provider attempting to fill the band without using fluoroscopy would not have a way of knowing that the band ends had become unattached. Once it is discovered that the band is either leaking or has become unattached, the patient should be referred to a band surgeon to discuss replacing the band. The surgeon might also be of assistance in determining if the manufacturer of the band might cover part, or all, of the band replacement.

A known complication of performing gastric-band fills with sterile saline is piercing the tubing that leads from the port to the band with the needle that is used to access the port. The port for the gastric band is hat-shaped and its vertical walls are made of hard plastic. The brim of the hat, so to speak, contains a circular metal plate that prevents the fill needle from passing completely through the port and into the deeper structures of the abdomen. The top of the hat is made of a thick silicone membrane. The outer edge of the brim of the hat contains four small eyes that allow the port to be sewn, brim down, against the muscular wall of the abdomen. Ports are usually placed in the left upper quadrant of the abdomen, although I have seen surgeons implant ports as low as the pelvic area and as high as just below the lowest rib. The tubing from the port is then attached via a coupler to the tubing coming from the band. When a gastric-band patient needs a fill, a medical provider prepares to insert a non-cutting needle though the silicone membrane until the tip of the needle comes to rest against the metal at the back of the port. Fluid can then be added to the band, as per manufacturer recommendations and as per the medical provider's judgment. Most medical providers localize the port by touch, place their index and middle fingers on each side of the port, visualize exactly in their minds where the silicone membrane is and then advance the needle through the skin and tissue between their fingers and into the port. It sounds easy, but it is frequently not, depending on the thickness of the fat over the port and on whether the port has come loose from the abdominal wall or if it has rotated a little or a lot. Some fill attempts require multiple tries at inserting the needle, with the tip of the needle being withdrawn partially back through the fat of the abdomen and then adjusting the angle of the before trying again to access the port. The provider pushes the needle in until they feel the tip of the needle against the firmness of the silicone cap of the port. A slightly harder push is then attempted to see if the needle is against the metal brim or hard-plastic side of the hat-shaped port, or if it is over the silicone membrane. If the needle doesn't slide into the silicone membrane with a distinctive give, then the needle is in the wrong position on the port. I have heard of fill attempts that have taken more than an hour for the provider to access the port, with the needle being pushed against various parts of the port until the membrane was finally accessed. Some fill attempts for some providers are unsuccessful even after an hour. In the process of the provider repeatedly attempting to find and insert the needle into the silicone membrane of the port, it is possible for the tip of the needle to be placed against the plastic tubing and then piercing the tube as the provider attempts to insert the needle. Once the port's plastic tubing has a hole in it, the port is permanently damaged, the fluid leaks out and the patient loses the tightness of their fill moments after the fill is done. The only solution when the tubing has been punctured is to replace the port and tubing and then reattach the new port and tubing to the tubing from the band. It is a minor surgery with a quick recovery, but the surgery could have been avoided if the provider doing the fill had been using fluoroscopy to aid in placing the tip of the needle right in the middle of the silicone port.

The silicone port can be damaged when the port is improperly accessed by a cutting needle. The difference between a cutting and non-cutting needle is best understood by seeing the two different needles side by side. A cutting needle is just a long and small steel tube that has been cut at a steep angle. The tip and edges around the angled opening are then sharpened. Since there is a hole in the center of the cutting needle, if inappropriately used on a gastric-band port, it cuts a tiny core out of the silicone membrane on the top of the port. Even using a cutting needle on the port one time can cause a permanent leak. A non-cutting needle looks exactly like a cutting needle until closer examination reveals that there is no opening in the beveled end of the needle; the opening is instead on the side of the needle just behind the sharp tip of the needle and opposite the bevel of the needle. The non-cutting needle can slip into the port through the silicone membrane without coring out a hole in the membrane. Providers that do gastric-band fills know to use non-cutting needles to access gastric-band ports. However, other medical providers sometimes don't know to use non-cutting needles and the port can be damaged, thus a replacement of the port needed.

As I already alluded to, the port of the gastric band can become unattached from the abdominal wall and can rotate to the point that it is upside down. In the case of an upside-down port, it takes extra skill and patience to successfully fill the band. In gastric-band patients who have lost a lot of weight, a fill can be accomplished with some effort by manually rotating the port back to its correct position through the skin and then holding it in place while the port is accessed. However, for heavier patients with a thicker abdominal wall, it can be nearly impossible to access the port when it is upside down, since the port can't be manipulated through the thicker skin. The provider doing the fill may suspect that the port has flipped when repeated attempts at accessing the port result in hitting the hard metal back of the port, without ever first feeling the needle go through the silicone membrane. With the use of a fluoroscopy machine, I can quickly determine if the port is upside down and then try my best to turn the port over so it can be accessed with the needle. If I can't turn it over, then the patient must return to their surgeon to resew the port to the abdominal wall.

Last of all, the coupling where the tubing from the band is attached to the tubing coming from the port can come unattached. Once again, when this happens, the patient suddenly loses the sensation of being filled and afterward can eat almost the same amount of food they could eat before getting the band. This can be seen with the fluoroscopy machine, since the coupling ends of each tube are visible on x-ray, and the ends will be seen lying apart from each other. The only solution is to return to a surgeon to have the two ends reattached.

This is not an exclusive list of all complications that can occur with a gastric band, but it does encompass the majority of the complications that I have seen in my gastric-band practice for the last decade. I have done all my gastric-band fills with the help of fluoroscopy for the last half of that decade. It is so helpful to always find ports, no matter how deep they are, in order to get the needle into the port successfully in about a minute (rotated ports take longer), assess whether the band has slipped and whether the pouch has become dilated, and accurately determine whether the band is overfilled or underfilled. Although it is more expensive to have gastric-band fills performed under fluoroscopy, I strongly recommend that all gastric-band fills be done under fluoroscopy to ensure safety, success, accuracy, and to avoid damaging the port and tubing.

Avoiding the temptation, by both the patient and the provider performing the gastric-band fill, to overfill the band in a misguided attempt to help the patient lose more weight is essential. Overfilled bands cause nausea, vomiting, paroxysmal burping, acid reflux, micro-perforations, and pouch dilation, which are all avoidable complications. When patients come in complaining about the above symptoms, I access their ports under fluoroscopy, and then, without adding any fluid to the band, I have them swallow barium under fluoroscopy to see if their anatomy is still normal and if the band is too tight. I can tell if the band is too tight by seeing a delay of more than 15 seconds for the barium in the pouch to empty into the lower stomach through the band, or by seeing a large pouch. For patients who aren't complaining of symptoms but are there because they feel like their band is not tight enough, I first ask how much of a regular plate of food they can eat before they have to stop for at least a few minutes because they are too full. If they answer less than half a plate of food, then I remind them that their band is working properly and that if they are not losing weight, it is because they are finding a way to consume the rest of the food on their plate, which they shouldn't be doing.

I will not be addressing biliopancreatic diversion with duodenal switch since it isn't commonly performed and is more dangerous than the above-mentioned weight-loss surgeries. I will also not be reviewing the gastric balloons nor the gastric and intestinal devices that cause weight loss by limiting intake of food and/or absorption of calories of consumed food.

These balloons and devices can be more dangerous and are most often less effective than the above-mentioned weight-loss surgeries. Time will tell if any of these balloons and devices will prove themselves to be a worthy alternative.

Long-term weight maintenance is much harder than weight loss, and this applies to surgical weight loss as well as non-surgical weight loss. However, there are important differences between weight maintenance after surgical weight loss and non-surgical weight loss. After non-surgical weight loss, an individual experiences more hunger due to elevated levels of ghrelin. Also, the individual's daily calorie burn is lower due to a drop in basal metabolism and due to a drop in non-exercise activity caused by fatigue. As a result, it is quite easy to eat more calories than are being burned per day. The satiety hormones that should have stopped the individual from overeating at a meal don't rise in response to overeating. That is because the body wants the individual to gain back the weight they have lost. It's like the body thinks the dieter has just survived a famine and now it's time to gain back the weight that was lost during the famine as quickly as possible so that the dieter will be ready to survive the next famine. The stretch receptors in the stomach wall don't signal the brain with a feeling of painful fullness and bloating until too many calories have been consumed.

In contrast to non-surgical weight loss, after gastric sleeve, gastric bypass and gastric banding, the stomach is much smaller, and a full plate of food cannot be consumed at one sitting. With gastric sleeve, ghrelin is lower after surgery, resulting in less hunger. After gastric bypass, the effect of rising ghrelin is suppressed by high levels of GLP-1, also resulting in less hunger. There isn't a change in hunger after gastric banding. As a result of these changes, it would seem that surgical weight-loss patients would be able to maintain weight more successfully than non-surgical weight-loss patients. However, studies don't support this theory very well. In a large study of surgical weight-loss patients, the average weight regain in six years was about 33% (Sjöström, 2007). A study of 268 non-surgical individuals who lost more than 100 pounds showed that the average weight regain in about two years was 35% (Anderson J. , 2006). A comparative study of 105 surgical weight-loss patients and 210 non-surgical weight-loss patients was completed in 2009. At the start of the study, both groups had lost an average of 123 pounds and had maintained that weight loss for 5.5 years. Both groups regained about four pounds during the one-year study. Of note, the surgical weight-loss patients reported less physical activity, more intake of fat and fast food, and less control over their eating (Bond, 2009). This study suggests that post-surgical patients were able to maintain weight successfully with less dietary restraint and less exercise than non-surgical patients.

Weight-loss surgery is a necessary and important tool for medical providers and surgeons who treat obese patients who meet the criteria for surgery and have failed to lose weight by dieting. Weight-loss surgery and its resultant weight loss can prevent a host of serious complications of obesity and can improve and even resolve a number of obesity-related diseases. If you feel that you have reached the point where weight-loss surgery is for you, then see your weight-loss provider to discuss the possibility of weight-loss surgery.

CHAPTER 17

EXERCISE, EXERCISE, AND EXERCISE

ANY BOOK ON weight loss is not complete without a chapter on exercise. Even though I have already touched on exercise as a critical tool in weight maintenance and as an integral part of a healthy lifestyle, these principles bear repeating. I will also discuss again the never-ending myths that exercise causes weight loss, and that low metabolism makes it impossible to lose weight.

Exercise alone rarely results in meaningful weight loss. Results of multiple studies have shown that exercisers on a healthy diet lose only a few pounds more than non-exercisers on the same diet after six months (Franz, 2007). In the National Weight Control Registry (Hill J. , 2005), less than 2% of the 10,000-plus members lost weight by exercise alone. In a 15-year study of 34,079 women on a usual diet, even those who exercised at a moderate- or a high-intensity level throughout the study didn't lose weight (Lee I.-M. , 2010). And yet, if you ask almost everyone you meet if exercise causes weight loss, they will say that it does. That is because our brains have been so flooded by convincing ads from gyms, exercise trainers, and infomercials for exercise equipment that we have been lulled into believing their claims.

Money drives advertising, and that money comes from the huge profits made by companies that have convinced us that exercise causes weight loss. When a study comes along that proves otherwise, it gets published in a medical journal that the general public never reads. At most, the study might be mentioned briefly once on a news channel, on the internet, or in the newspaper. Since the results of the study are not hammered into our heads day after day by advertisement after advertisement, people tend to ignore the results of the study. Humans tend to accept as true what they are told repeatedly over a long period of time by a supposed credible source. The massive amount of expert-endorsed advertising for the gyms and exercise equipment that we have been exposed to for most of our lives has led us to believe that what they are selling must be beneficial. In reality, they are just successful marketers. Almost subliminally, the frequency of the advertisements suggests to us that the exercise programs and equipment being touted are making lots of money for the companies because they really do work. Otherwise, how could they have the money to pay for the never-ending advertisements? Once again, it's all just marketing designed to lighten your pocketbook, but not necessarily your weight.

Our incorrectly placed belief in exercise as a weight-loss tool for the masses hasn't been helped at all by the astounding weight loss seen in the participants on *The Biggest Loser* TV show. Never mind that the long hours of trainer-supervised exercise on *The Biggest Loser* is all but impossible for full-time workers with families that have precious little time to exercise, or for those whose bodies can't handle that extreme of a level of physical activity. Ignore the fact that if they let the participants on the program return to their homes at night, they would be so hungry that they would eat thousands of calories per night. We see the participants in *The Biggest Loser* shed weight by what looks like exercise alone and we just add that to our belief system that exercise is a weight-loss tool.

Even when a major news source publishes a front-page article based on a study or studies that prove that exercise doesn't work well for weight loss, it still isn't enough to get our attention. *Time Magazine*'s August 9, 2010 cover pictured a thin woman walking on a treadmill while in her mind's eye she was seeing a frosted cupcake. The caption for the picture on the cover read, "The Myth About Exercise." The well-researched article, "Why Exercise Won't Make You Thin," by John Cloud, presented multiple studies that proved that exercise alone doesn't cause weight loss. He lamented in the article how frustrating it was for him to work out hard to lose weight only to succumb afterward to excess hunger triggered by the exercise. The comments by readers of his article in the comment section said that his article was incorrect, but their statements were based almost completely on dependence on beliefs held by supposed experts in the field and on personal experience with individuals who had supposedly lost weight with exercise alone. When I asked patients what they thought about the article when it came out, the ones that had read it said, "I read it, but I didn't believe it was true." The same thing happened again when the article, "Why So Many of Us Don't Lose Weight When We Exercise," was published by *The New York Times* in 2019.

When patients come to see me for help with weight loss, frequently the first question out of their mouths is what is wrong with their metabolism because they have been exercising their hearts out and haven't been losing weight. In helping them, I first address the often-mistaken laymen's concept of metabolism. Often, I start the discussion by mentioning that I want to anchor a blimp over every major city in the world that reads in the appropriate language, "It's Not Your Metabolism, It's Your Inactivity." Most people of the same age, sex, height, and body frame have about the same basal metabolic rate, which is the amount of energy spent by lying still in bed for 24 hours without moving a muscle. However, people have vastly different levels of non-exercise activity, which is everything that we do for 24 hours besides just lying in bed and not moving a muscle. Of course, non-exercise activity doesn't include exercise activity. Non-exercise activity is the sum of all the gestures, lifting, standing, and steps that we take at work and at home. It includes the steps needed to take the garbage out, the effort made in brushing our teeth, the calories spent in carrying around a purse or backpack, and the number of times we get up to turn the lights on and off. Figure 16 below shows an approximation of the calories burned from daily activities for a 170-pound person:

ACTIVITY	CALORIES BURNED PER HOUR[1]
Sleeping	77
Sitting	100
Standing	139
Walking	270
Running at a moderate pace	540
Light work	230
Moderate work	348
Heavy work	502

Figure 16 - Calories Burned per Hour of Various Activities

[1] *(Ainsworth, 2011)*

After reviewing the above chart, you can see how an active 70-year-old grandma can burn more calories per day than her 20-year-old grandson that sits on a couch all day long while playing video games and then goes to bed.

Overweight individuals burn a lot more calories per day than non-overweight individuals of the same age, sex, and body frame (Savoie, 2009). That is because they are carrying around a 50-to-100-pound backpack worth of weight all day long and not because they have a higher "metabolism". If the non-overweight individual put on a backpack that made his or her total weight the same as the overweight individual's weight, then they would burn about the same number of calories per day as the overweight person would burn as long as they were equally active.

People also have vastly different levels of exercise activity. Therefore, the wide range in calories burned per day by different individuals of the same age, sex, height, and body frame comes almost completely from differences in non-exercise activity and exercise activity.

So, why don't individuals lose weight when they burn more calories from exercise? First, if the human body didn't protect us from weight loss from exercise, then skinny individuals who exercised would lose weight and become emaciated. Second, the ideal human body is designed to burn calories and then eat back exactly what it has burned, so that the body's weight stays the same. It's that homeostasis thing, again. If there is even the slightest difference in calories burned per day and calories consumed per day, then the individual will gain or lose a lot of weight over a 10-year period. One 20-calorie bite of food more per meal for 10 years causes a 90-pound weight gain. One 20-calorie bite of food less per meal for 10 years causes a 90-pound weight loss. How much is food is 20 calories? It's a little more than one-square inch of peperoni pizza or one tablespoon of ice cream. When members of Muse Satiety Type 1 burn 500 calories by exercising, their hunger lasts longer at meals and they eat back exactly 500 calories over the next day. This happens for them time after time for their whole lives. Otherwise, they would be gaining or losing weight. Members of Muse Satiety Types 2 to 5 have appetite systems that are dysregulated. When they burn 500 calories through exercise and then have an appropriate increase in hunger, they eat the 500 calories back and then more, because they don't feel an appropriate sense of fullness, loss of savor, and nausea from overeating at exactly the right moment during a meal. The exact choice of food eaten doesn't make a big difference. Remember that many members of Muse Satiety Type 1 will suddenly stop in the middle of a favorite meal and ultimately end up throwing the rest away. Members of Muse Satiety Types 2 and 3 will stop appropriately in the middle of a plate of food but will save it and eat more later. Members of Muse Satiety Type 4 and 5 will finish the whole plate of their favorite meal and will look for more to eat.

The third reason that humans don't lose weight with exercise is that humans are designed to reduce their activity after exercise in an effort by the body to keep the body's weight the same. A rigorously scientific study on exercise for weight loss was performed on 11 sets of younger male twins that agreed to live in an isolated research station for four months. In order to establish their average daily caloric intake, for the first two weeks the twins were allowed to eat three meals a day until they were satisfied and were not given an exercise program. After the first two weeks, they were then fed the exact number of calories per day that they had consumed for the first two weeks for the rest of the four-month study. They were then started on a supervised two-hour per day exercise program for rest of the study. At the end of the study, the twins in each twin pair had lost an identical amount of weight, but there was a significant difference in weight loss from one twin pair to the next. One twin pair lost 90% of the weight loss that would have been predicted by subtracting the calories consumed from the calories burned. Another twin pair lost only 10% of the weight that they should have lost by subtracting their calories consumed from their calories burned. The other twin pairs were spread out between 10% and 90% of the weight loss that they had been predicted to lose. At first blush, it would appear that the young men had different metabolic rates, and therefore some lost more weight than others. However, further evaluation revealed that the twins that only lost 10% of the predicted weight loss became less active after exercise because they were tired, sore, and felt they deserved a rest after working so hard. Their decrease in activity after exercise partially to almost completely negated the extra calories that they had burned with exercise. On the other hand, the twins that lost 90% of the predicted weight loss finished exercise and kept on being active (Tremblay, 1997).

A similar finding was demonstrated in a study on 1,200 children attending 0 grade (equivalent to kindergarten) to 6th grade in Denmark in 2009 and 2010. The children were either attending schools where there were six weekly physical education (PE) classes, or schools where there were two weekly PE classes. Each child wore an Actigraph, a lightweight machine that measured total activity throughout the day, for two different time periods during the school year. At the end of the study, it was discovered that the calories burned through physical activity were the same for each group of kids, whether they had more PE classes at school or not. It was determined that the kids that did more PE at school were less active after school and that the kids that did less PE at school were more active once they got home (Møller, 2014).

Now that I have established that exercise doesn't cause weight loss, you might be wondering why I have titled this chapter "Exercise, Exercise and Exercise." That is because exercise is absolutely essential to weight maintenance after a diet. It is also essential to prevent the slow but sure weight gain that will occur throughout the lives of members of Muse Satiety Types 2 to 5. In addition, exercise promotes good health and longevity. I would like to see every patient in my practice exercising at least 30 minutes every day just to decrease the risk of death from heart disease. I would also like to see every patient in my practice exercising at least 60 minutes per day every day to prevent long-term weight gain. And I want my weight-loss patients to exercise 80 minutes per day every day to prevent weight regain after their diets. In my estimation, members of Muse Satiety Type 2 and 3 have a 70% chance or greater of regaining all the weight they have lost on a diet if they don't exercise during weight maintenance. Members of Muse Satiety Type 4 and 5 have a 90% chance or greater, in my estimation, of regaining all the weight they have lost in a diet if they don't exercise during weight mainte-nance. And people who don't exercise during a diet are usually not going to suddenly start at the end of their diet.

For most patients, brisk walking is the best exercise to achieve the bene-fits I have discussed above. While it is true that people who run for exercise have about the same reduction of risk for heart disease as those who walk (Williams P. , 2013) (Kyu, 2016), most of us don't have the knee and hip joints that would allow us to run for exercise on a regular basis. A recent study of about 4,800 adults 40 and older that wore accelerometers for 10 years indicated that the death rate from all causes was 77 out of 1,000 per year for people who took less than 4,000 steps per day, 21 out of 1,000 per year for people who took 4,000 to 7,999 steps per day, seven out of 1,000 per year for people who took 8,000 to 11,999 steps per day, and five out of 1,000 per year for people who took 12,000 or more steps per day. The speed of walking didn't make a difference in the death rate (Saint-Maurice, 2020). I read that article and immediately started walking 10,000 or more steps per day. As long as you're cleared by your medical provider to do so, I think that you should do the same.

Exercise has many other benefits and has been proven to improve self-im-age, depression, anxiety, back pain, fibromyalgia, type 2 diabetes, HDL cholesterol, osteoarthritis of the hip and knee, PMS, and cognitive function in older adults. Exercise decreases LDL cholesterol. Exercise increases lon-gevity and sexual prowess. Exercise prevents osteoporosis, breast and colon cancer, hypertension, and obesity.

Many obese individuals struggle to exercise due to pain in knees, hips, and feet, and due to significant shortness of breath. The shortness of breath can come from being out of shape and from the stress on the body of carrying around 100-300 extra pounds but can also come from more serious medical problems. Each patient should consult with their medical provider before starting an exercise program to be sure that they are healthy enough to do so.

Exercise is essential for weight maintenance. Exercise is critical to optimal health of all individuals. Everyone that has been cleared by their medical provider should exercise every day to profit from its many health benefits. However, as we all exercise, we should be aware that no amount of exercise will result in significant weight loss. That requires a diet.

CHAPTER 18
WHEN MEDICATIONS CAUSE WEIGHT GAIN

A NUMBER OF medications prescribed for various illnesses can cause weight gain. Some are more potent in their weight-gaining effect than others. For members of Muse Satiety Types 2 to 5 that are already struggling with their weight, anything that makes the desire to snack and overeat at mealtimes worse is potentially disastrous. In my observation, the magnitude of weight gain related to medications is most pronounced in Muse Satiety Type 4s and 5s and is negligible in Muse Satiety Type 1s.

Medications that cause weight gain don't have calories themselves. They just enhance the effect of ghrelin on the neurons in the appetite centers of the brain, which increases desire to snack and increases the quantity of food consumed at meals. This effect is not easily perceived by the person taking the medications, at least not until their weight begins to rise and their clothes become tight. That is because hunger and satiety are controlled almost subconsciously, as I have discussed in previous chapters. Since most humans eat when they are hungry and most only stop when they are satiated, an increase in craving for snacks and a delay in feeling full at mealtimes invariably results in consumption of extra calories, which in turn causes weight gain.

The first defense against medications that cause weight gain for those who already struggle with their weight is to ask their medical provider if the medications they are being prescribed are known to cause weight gain. If they are, then the medical provider should be asked if other medications can be prescribed for their medical conditions that don't cause weight gain, or at least cause less weight gain. If the medications causing weight gain can't be stopped for medical reasons, then sometimes the medical provider can reduce the doses, change the times of day the medications are taken, or add other medications that might reduce the weight-gaining effect of the offending medications.

Second, everyone should read package inserts and pharmacy handouts in order to be educated on whether the medications they are taking can cause weight gain. Individuals should not stop any medication that has been prescribed by their medical provider until they have checked with that provider to make sure it is safe for them to stop the medication.

The third defense against medications that cause weight gain is to redouble your efforts at weight maintenance while you are taking these medications. This is especially necessary when your medical problems are such that you have no choice but to take medications that cause weight gain. Effective weight maintenance is discussed in detail in Chapter 11 of this book.

Figure 17 below lists the generic and brand names of medications that, either in my opinion or based on results from clinical trials, have been associated with weight gain. They are organized in groups by one of the possible uses for the medications. The next column lists my perception of how strong the weight-gaining effect is for each medication, based on my clinical experience and upon the results of clinical trials, if referenced. My rating is on a scale of one to three, with three being the most potent effect. The final column lists possible replacement medications that don't cause weight gain, or that even cause weight loss. An individual can use this list to identify medications they are taking that might be causing weight gain and then to meet with their medical provider to ask if a change in medication might be appropriate. The figure lists only one brand name for each generic medication. If your brand name medication is not listed, then use the internet to look up the generic name of your medication before attempting to find it on the list by its generic name. This list is not meant to be all inclusive for all medications that cause weight gain.

Some of the medications listed cause weight gain by both increasing intake of calories that results in an increase in fat mass and by increasing fluid retention. The weight gain caused by the fluid-retention component is temporary and resolves quickly with cessation of the causal medication. The medications on this list that are known to cause fluid retention, as well as an increase of fat mass, are pioglitazone, amlodipine, diltiazem, birth-control pills, prednisone, hydrocortisone and insulin.

MEDICAL INDICATION	GENERIC/COMMON NAME	BRAND NAME	WT. GAIN INTENSITY (1-3)	POSSIBLE SUBSTITUTE MEDICATIONS THAT CAUSE NO WEIGHT GAIN, OR THAT CAUSE WEIGHT LOSS
Allergy (Ratliff, 2010)	Cetirizine	Zyrtec	2	Fluticasone spray (Flonase), Triamcinolone sp. (Nasacort), Mometasone spray (Nasonex)
	Cyproheptadine (Lavenstein, 1962)	Periactin	2	
	Diphenhydramine	Benadryl	2	
	Fexofenadine	Allegra	1	
	Loratadine	Claritin	1	
Anti-inflammatory steroids (Liu, 2013)	Hydrocortisone	Cortef	3	Consult with your medical provider
	Methylprednisolone	Medrol	3	
	Prednisone	Prednisone	3	

Bipolar disorder/ psychosis	Aripiprazole (White, 2013)	Abilify	1	Topiramate (Topamax), Lamotrigine (Lamictal), Zonisamide (Zonegran), Ziprasidone (Geodon), Aripiprazole (Abilify)
	Asenapine (White, 2013)	Saphris	1	
	Chlorpromazine (White, 2013)	Thorazine	2	
	Clozapine (White, 2013)	Clozaril	3	
	Olanzapine (White, 2013)	Zyprexa	3	
	Quetiapine (White, 2013)	Seroquel	2	
	Risperidone (White, 2013)	Risperdal	2	
	Ziprasidone (White, 2013)	Geodon	1	
Birth control	Depo-progesterone	Depo-Provera	3	Copper IUD (ParaGard), Barrier methods
	Ethinyl estradiol-progestins	Birth control pills, rings	2	
	Etonogestrel insert	Nexplanon	1	
	Levonorgestrel	Mirena IUD	1	
Blood pressure	Acebutolol	Sectral	2	Lisinopril (Prinivil), Ramipril (Altace), Losartan (Cozaar), Olmesartan (Benicar), Carvedilol (Coreg), Nebivolol (Bystolic), Others - consult with your medical provider
	Amlodipine	Norvasc	1	
	Atenolol	Tenormin	2	
	Clonidine	Catapres	2	
	Diltiazem	Cardizem	1	
	Metoprolol	Toprol	2	
	Propranolol	Inderal	2	
	Verapamil	Calan	1	
Cancer	Methotrexate	Trexall	2	Consult with your medical provider
	Tamoxifen	Nolvadex	2	

Chronic pain	Duloxetine	Cymbalta	2	Many - consult with your
	Gabapentin	Neurontin	2	medical provider
	Milnacipran	Savella	1	
	Pregabalin	Lyrica	2	
Depression	Amitriptyline	Elavil	3	Bupropion (Wellbutrin)
	Citalopram	Celexa	1	
	Desipramine	Norpramin	1	
	Doxepin	Sinequan	2	
	Duloxetine (Wise, 2006)	Cymbalta	1	
	Escitalopram	Lexapro	1	
	Fluoxetine (Ferguson J. , 2001)	Prozac	1	
	Fluvoxamine	Luvox	2	
	Imipramine	Tofranil	1	
	Mirtazapine	Remeron	3	
	Nortriptyline	Pamelor	2	
	Paroxetine (Ferguson J. , 2001)	Paxil	3	
	Sertraline (Ferguson J. , 2001)	Zoloft	2	
	Trazodone	Desyrel	2	
	Venlafaxine	Effexor	2	

Diabetes	Glimepiride	Amaryl	3	Metformin (Glucophage),
	Glipizide	Glucotrol	3	Sitagliptin (Januvia),
	Glyburide	Diabeta	3	Saxagliptin (Onglyza),
	Insulin aspart	Novolog	3	Linagliptin (Tradjenta), Canagliflozin (Invokana),
	Insulin degludec	Tresiba	2	Dapagliflozin (Farxiga),
	Insulin detemir	Levemir	2	Empagliflozin (Jardiance),
	Insulin glargine	Lantus	2	Exenatide (Byetta),
	Insulin glargine	Toujeo	2	Liraglutide (Victoza),
	Insulin glulisine	Apidra	3	Dulaglutide (Trulicity), Others - consult with your
	Insulin lispro	Humalog	3	medical provider
	Nateglinide	Starlix	1	
	Pioglitazone	Actos	3	
	Repaglinide	Prandin	1	
Infertility	Clomiphene	Clomid	2	Consult with your medical provider
Insomnia	Amitriptyline	Elavil	2	Suvorexant (Belsomra), ramelteon (Rozerem)
	Diphenhydramine	Tylenol PM	2	
	Doxepin	Sinequan	2	
	Nortriptyline	Pamelor	2	
	Trazodone	Desyrel	2	
Menopause	Estradiol	Estrace	3	Consult with your medical provider
	Conjugated estrogens	Premarin	3	
Migraine	Atenolol	Tenormin	2	Carvedilol (Coreg), Nebivolol (Bystolic)
	Metoprolol	Toprol	2	
	Propranolol	Inderal	2	
	Verapamil	Calan	1	
Seizures	Carbamazepine	Tegretol	2	Topiramate (Topamax), lamotrigine (Lamictal), zonisamide (Zonegran)
	Gabapentin	Neurontin	2	
	Lithium	Lithobid	3	
	Valproic acid	Depakote	3	

Figure 17 - Medications That Cause Weight Gain

I am aware there are people who have taken each one of these medications who have never gained a pound of fat mass. I am also aware there are high-quality studies that have shown that some of these medications don't cause weight gain.

I would like to explain these supposed conundrums from the perspective of the Muse Satiety Types. Again, and in my opinion, medications that cause weight gain do so by enhancing the effect of ghrelin. In individuals in Muse Satiety Type 1 that take medications that can cause weight gain, the counter-regulatory anorexigenic hormones are still able to stop food intake right at the point of meeting calorie needs, in spite of the elevated effect of ghrelin. In my practice, I don't ever recall a member of Muse Satiety Type 1 gaining appreciable fat mass on any of the drugs that cause weight gain. However, for Muse Satiety Types 3, 4, and especially 5, receptor resistance to the anorexigenic hormones results in a failure to oppose the enhanced effect of ghrelin. The partially, or completely, unopposed and enhanced effect of ghrelin then almost subconsciously causes individuals to eat more often and to eat greater quantities of food, resulting in weight gain.

In explaining why there are studies on some of these medications that have shown that the medications don't cause weight gain, I first need to give a little background on myself. I am a certified clinical researcher. I have performed more than 100 studies for the pharmaceutical industry on emerging, or not yet FDA approved, medications in various clinical areas. Some of these areas have been chronic pain, post-surgical pain, type 2 diabetes, weight loss, high blood pressure, high cholesterol, gout, endometriosis, migraine, post-injury pain, and opioid-induced constipation. I have also done many studies on not-yet-FDA-approved vaccines. Each of these studies has been carefully conducted in accordance with an exacting and lengthy study protocol. I have also reviewed many other protocols for studies in which I have not ended up participating. In each of the study protocols that I have participated in, or have at least reviewed, there is a section of the protocol called the inclusion and exclusion criteria. The inclusion and exclusion criteria define the exact type of patient that will be studied and exclude all other types of patients.

A common practice in many study protocols is to exclude individuals with a high BMI. Some protocols are more limiting than others and exclude anyone with a BMI of 30 or greater. A rare study allows individuals up to a BMI of 39. Some studies go one step further and exclude anyone who has had a change in weight of more than 5% in the preceding six months, which would be a weight gain or loss of 10 pounds, or more, for a 200-pound individual. The effect of these exclusions in most protocols is to exclude most members of Muse Satiety Types 4 and 5 from studies, since most are either over a BMI of 30, or they are frequently losing and gaining to stay under a BMI of 30. In other words, the individuals who are most likely to gain weight during these studies are excluded from the trials. Because these studies are then performed on patients who are lower risk for weight gain, the data from these studies can end up showing that the medications studied cause little or no weight gain. This information is then included in the submissions to the FDA for approval of these medications. If the medications are approved by the FDA, then FDA-approved package inserts are prepared and distributed with the newly approved medications which state that the medications showed little or no weight gain in trials. The pharmaceutical representatives from the drug companies then share with medical providers the supposedly proven fact that these new drugs cause little or no weight gain. The medical providers then begin prescribing the new medications to patients, some of which are members of Muse Satiety Types 4 and 5 that were underrepresented in the pre-approval trials. Sometimes, members of Muse Satiety Types 4 and 5 have gained a significant amount of weight on some new medications.

I have recently asked a few the pharmaceutical representatives for the inclusion and exclusion criteria for the studies that were submitted to the FDA for drug approval for medications that the representatives were touting as not causing weight gain. I have wanted to see if patients who struggled with their weight were excluded from the studies on the new drugs. As of yet, I have not been sent the inclusion and exclusion criteria from the studies.

I don't exactly know the reason why patients who struggle with their weight are excluded by the protocols for many clinical trials. When the topic has come up a few times in investigator meetings held before the start of clinical trials, the scientists from the pharmaceutical companies have stated that obese patients have a larger fat mass that might trap some of the medication, affecting drug levels in the blood, or that significantly obese patient have unstable medical problems that make them unsuitable for clinical trials, such as hard to control sleep apnea, type 2 diabetes, and heart failure. In addition, if overweight patients lost weight during a trial, that could make some medications look like they work better than they really do, such as in studies of diabetic medications, blood pressure medications, and cholesterol medications. Weight gain by overweight patients during a trial could make the medications look like they don't work, since weight gain makes a number of medical problems worse. I don't recall many studies done by pharmaceutical companies on exclusively obese patients that have been submitted to the FDA as a part of new-drug applications.

Years after FDA approval of these medications, practicing medical providers begin to suspect these medications are causing weight gain. Non-pharmaceutical-industry-sponsored studies are conducted that finally confirm what medical providers had already been observing, that the medications are causing excessive weight gain in patients who are prone to problems with weight gain. Are the drug companies purposely trying to hide the fact that some of their medications cause weight gain from the FDA and ultimately the public? I don't know.

I would like to call for all study participants in all trials to be classified as Muse Satiety Types 1 to 5 prior to trial participation and that members of all Muse Satiety Types be equally represented in clinical trials on emerging medications, regardless of their weight and regardless of their struggle to maintain weight. In addition, I would like for medical providers to determine their patient's Muse Satiety Types and then inform their patients of the possibility of weight gain before prescribing medications that could cause weight gain. Most patients who struggle with their weight will decline to take medications that could cause weight gain.

Medications that cause weight gain are commonly prescribed to patients who are high risk for weight gain. Often, an alternative medication could have been prescribed that causes less weight gain, no weight gain, or even weight loss. Patients need to educate themselves on the weight-gaining potential of their current medications and of any medication that they might be prescribed in the future. Patients can then ask their medical providers if there is an alternative medication that be prescribed. Medical providers need to avoid prescribing medications that cause weight gain as much as possible to their patients who are already overweight or are high risk for weight gain due to their Muse Satiety Type.

CHAPTER 19

OBESITY WILL ONLY BE CURED WHEN IT IS TREATED AS A CHRONIC DISEASE

OBESITY IS A chronic disease. It is similar to many other chronic diseases of the human body, such as type 2 diabetes, high cholesterol, and high blood pressure, with respect to the need for long-term treatment and regular follow-up to help patients to maintain long-term control of the disease.

In previous chapters, I have established that obesity is a genetically based disease that is comprised of three disease processes:

1. Muse's Satietopathy, or a failure to experience one or more of three protective satiety signals at mealtimes and with snacking.

2. Maximum weight memory, or the body incorrectly determining that an individual's new maximum and clearly unhealthy weight is now to be defended as the person's ideal weight.

3. Food craving, or the irresistible and consuming desire to ingest favorite foods above and beyond a person's calorie needs for the day.

A number of environmental, behavioral, and psychological factors play a role in the degree of expression of these three genetic diseases in individuals. The way that a person's body functions and looks is the result of their environment being focused through the lens of the person's genetics. Just as with type 2 diabetes, high cholesterol, and high blood pressure, the degree of expression of the disease of obesity is lessened by appropriate education, medication, and lifestyle changes, along with close follow-up with well-trained and supportive medical providers.

Misunderstanding that obesity is a disease can lead to patterns of treatment that are not adequately helpful to overweight individuals. One such misunderstanding that is held by many medical providers and patients is that obesity is a disease of bad behavior and there that there is no abnormal genetic component. This misunderstanding can lead to patients feeling ashamed and guilty over their obesity and to medical providers feeling frustrated by the patient's supposed lack of self-control. Another misunderstanding that is held by many medical providers and patients is that additional treatment is not needed at the end of a successful diet. Medications are stopped and weight-specific follow-up visits with the medical provider cease. A slow erosion of the patient's lifestyle changes occurs. As the individual gains back the weight they lost, the provider is puzzled at the lack of long-term success and the patient is disappointed. The patient often then looks for another diet, believing erroneously that a successful diet should result in permanent weight loss. After repeated failures at weight maintenance by multiple patients, medical providers become disenchanted and quit trying, assuming that their efforts are of no value.

As presented in Chapter 11, consistent long-term changes in lifestyle, long-term use of weight-loss medications, and long-term follow-up with a medical provider are essential for the majority of patients to achieve long-term weight maintenance. However, with the high cost of medical care, long-term follow-up with a medical provider, and long-term use of appetite suppressants will be difficult to achieve for the majority of patients unless these services are covered by insurance. Many studies have demonstrated that patients without insurance coverage for type 2 diabetes care and for high blood pressure treatment have worse control of their respective diseases and have worse long-term outcomes. The same certainly applies to obesity. Failure to offer effective and accessible treatment for obesity will result in spiraling health care costs for the treatment of obesity-related diseases.

I implore medical providers to begin treating obesity as a disease that responds well to proven medications and diets. Medical providers should either learn how to use these proven medications and diets or should refer their patients to providers that are trained in their use. I also call upon private and public insurers nationwide to immediately begin covering proven weight-loss treatments and long-term regular follow-up visits with medical providers who are adequately trained in the proven principles of weight loss and weight maintenance. Readers of this book are encouraged to contact their elected officials and their insurance companies to demand coverage for these needed services.

CHAPTER 20

ENDING PREJUDICE TOWARD OVERWEIGHT PEOPLE

OVERWEIGHT INDIVIDUALS ARE the largest group in the human population towards which prejudice at many levels and many extremes is tolerated and even condoned by some. In opposition to the indignant reactions of many people when they are subjected to prejudice, overweight people just hang their heads in shame, having been taught since an early age by much of society that obesity is completely the fault of the dietary habits of the overweight individual.

Prejudice against any individual or group for any reason has always been injurious to the moral fiber and productivity of the society that commits the prejudice. The group or individual who is singled out for prejudice is often repeatedly humiliated, sometimes forced to suffer loss of freedom of activity, and occasionally a target of violence. The history of humanity is full of examples of the extensive injury caused by prejudice, such as the oppression of the early Christians by the Romans, the North and South American Indians by the European settlers, and the African Americans by many of the citizens of the United States. However, never has there been a larger group of individuals who has been the target of prejudice like the overweight individuals of the world. Based on my in-office study, approximately 40% of the world population are members of Muse Satiety Types 4 to 5 and are gaining weight at an alarming rate. Over half of the members of Muse Satiety Types 2 and 3 are gaining some weight every year, and many are already overweight or obese, making more than half of the world's population obese and a potential target for weight-based prejudice.

It is true that significantly overweight individuals have a number of physical characteristics that cause them to look different than normal-weight individuals. These characteristics include a round face with large cheeks, a shorter neck, male breast enlargement, a larger and even pendulous abdomen, absence of a waist, and larger thighs and calves. However, the problem runs much deeper because the body shape of the overweight individual has been inappropriately associated in our society with laziness, slothfulness, gluttony, self-neglect, and a lack of self-control. These strongly negative associations induce strongly negative emotions in the observer that can result in disdain toward the overweight individual. When a large portion of a population feels the same disdain, prejudice can easily occur.

Overweight people experience prejudice in many forms. Socially, they are alienated by their schoolmates starting as early as elementary school (Deitz, 1998). They are often chosen last for impromptu competitive games on the playground, and they are excluded from many team competitive sports because they can't compete with their peers. Weight-challenged women are less likely to be accepted to college than thin women (Canning, 1966). They are less likely to have their parents pay for their college expenses than their thinner siblings. Overweight people are less likely to marry than their thin counterparts. Female job applicants that are significantly overweight are less likely to be hired than thin applicants, even if they are equally qualified for the job. Significantly overweight women make $5 to $10 thousand less per year than thin women. People with other physical disabilities don't experience these same losses of opportunity (Gortmaker, 1993). In my experience, when a significantly overweight and a non-overweight person arrive simultaneously at the reception counter of a business, more often than not, the thin person gets helped first. Even worse are the all too frequent reports of cruel teasing, mean physical pranks, and outright physical violence towards the overweight.

As individuals, groups, and societies, we can choose to be more tolerant and accepting of overweight individuals. Pretty much each one of us suffers from at least one genetically or misfortune-related defect. Many of these defects are not as visible as others and often no one knows the burden of pain and suffering that we carry because of them. The overweight individuals of this world are no different than the rest of us with respect to the pain and suffering that their disease brings to them. The only difference is that their obesity is so clearly visible.

In my opinion, obesity, even without any other medical complications, is a disabling disease. I say this because it has been well established that obesity prevents sufferers from achieving equal opportunities in education, in the workplace, and in relationships. Obesity is also a genetically ordained disease. Try as hard as they might, most members of Muse Satiety Types 4 and 5 that have failed to inherit some or all of the signals of satiety, will be obese. The Americans with Disabilities Act (ADA) does not specifically make occupational discrimination against obese people illegal in the workplace. I propose that the ADA be updated to include obesity as a disease for which occupational discrimination is illegal. Employers should be required by law to accommodate overweight people in the workplace by making sure they are not discriminated against in the hiring process, they are not mistreated by co-workers, hallways and doors are wide enough, elevators are in work-ing order, task chairs and lunch-room chairs are rated as being capable of comfortably and safely supporting overweight individuals, and desks are comfortable to work at.

Overweight people need to stop hanging their heads in shame when they are targets of social and occupational prejudice. When an appropriate and safe opportunity presents itself, they need to point out to those who are committing prejudice that their actions are inappropriate. If necessary, they need to seek legal help from competent and sympathetic attorneys. If and when overweight people are targets of physical violence, they need to report the illegal acts to the police.

Prejudice against overweight people needs to stop. Individuals need to examine their speech and behavior to be sure to avoid derogatory remarks about and to overweight people and make certain that they are avoiding mistreatment of overweight people. Producers of entertainment need to avoid portraying overweight individuals as anything less than normal, well-adjusted, and successful individuals who have a disease that makes it almost impossible to control their body weight. Societies need to enact laws that protect overweight people from discrimination in education and in the workplace. Overweight people need to stand up for themselves, as they are able, to insist that they not be treated with prejudice.

CHAPTER 21
CAUSES OF THE OBESITY EPIDEMIC

AS I NEAR the completion of this book, I can't resist writing a chapter on the causes of the obesity epidemic. Clearly there is a strong genetic basis for obesity. Maximum weight memory, food craving, and the absence of satiety signals that determine a person's Muse Satiety Type are genetically based. In addition, there are number of other non-genetic causes of obesity, some of which have been more validated by research than others. These additional causes of obesity can be grouped into behavioral, economic, societal, obesity-related, medical-illness-related, and environmental causes.

Most of the studies on the causes of obesity are less than reliable. Almost all past studies are potentially flawed because the researchers didn't know to control for the percentages of Muse Satiety Types in their study populations. Even a slight increase in percentages of Muse Satiety Types 4 and 5 versus Muse Satiety Type 3 in study populations could have skewed the data, due to the greater difficulty that Muse Satiety Types 4 and 5 have with weight maintenance. In addition, most studies done on causes of obesity are observational studies and not randomized placebo-controlled trials. Observational trials can show that a certain behavior or trait is associated with obesity, but don't prove that the certain behavior or trait is the cause of obesity. Last, many of the studies done on the causes of obesity have been done only in animals, mostly rats and mice, and are difficult to apply to humans.

As I discuss the causes of obesity in this chapter, it is important to remember that about 20% of Americans are not becoming overweight and obese, despite the causes of obesity that I will discuss below. The 20% of Americans that are not becoming obese are most certainly Muse Satiety Type 1s, along with a few Muse Satiety Type 2s, that are successfully resisting snacking. When most, or all, of the satiety signals are present, such as in members of Muse Satiety Type 1, then the external influences discussed below are not powerful enough to overcome the genetically ordained resistance to weight gain of the members of Muse Satiety Type 1. On the other hand, the causes of obesity discussed below magnify the trends toward weight gain over time experienced by members of Muse Satiety Types 2 to 5, resulting in weight gain earlier in life and weight gain to a greater degree for each decade of life. In no group is this tendency more profound than in the members of Muse Satiety Type 5.

Put simply, those gaining weight are either expending too little energy each day for the number of calories they are consuming or are consuming too many calories each day for the amount of energy they are expending, or both. For each of the causes of obesity listed in Figure 18 to Figure 23 below, I have noted whether the cause of obesity results in reduced energy expenditure, increased intake of food at mealtimes, or increased intake of food in between meals. Many of the causes of obesity contribute to more than one of these three items. In addition, for each cause of obesity, I have listed whether state and federal government intervention, government-supported education, or both, could change the magnitude of the effect of the causes of obesity. It is in the government's best interest to aggressively prevent obesity, to avoid the massive burden obesity places on the government due to the cost of treating obesity-related illness, loss of productivity in the workforce, disability payouts, and a shrinking pool of non-obese military recruits.

Finally, I have listed my opinion of the magnitude of the effect of each cause of obesity on the obesity levels of the whole population. Without question, some of the causes listed are more powerful causes for obesity in one individual over another, but I am considering the effect of the causes of obesity on the whole population. A ranking of 4 means I consider the effect to be very strong, 3 to be a strong effect, 2 to have a moderately strong effect, and 1 a weak effect.

BEHAVIORAL CAUSES OF OBESITY

Behavior that causes obesity is a behavior that an individual or group does volitionally in response to their environment. With the causes of obesity discussed in this section, the individual or group largely has a choice to participate in the behavior or to avoid the behavior. The behavioral causes of obesity that I think are at least in part responsible for the obesity epidemic are listed in Figure 18.

BEHAVIORAL CAUSES OF OBESITY	Decreased Energy Expended	Increased Mealtime Intake	Increased Snack Intake	Mitigated by Direct Government Intervention	Mitigated by Government-Sponsored Education	Magnitude of the Effect of the Cause of Obesity
Larger portions at meals		X		X	X	4
Increase in juice and sugar-sweetened beverage intake		X	X	X	X	4
Loss of social norms against public snacking			X	X	X	4
Larger portions of snacks			X	X	X	3
Increased sugar intake		X	X	X	X	3
Dessert served with lunch and dinner		X		X	X	2
Longer mealtimes		X			X	2
Decreased activity due to too much screen time	X			X	X	2
Increased fast-food intake outside of mealtimes			X	X	X	2
Higher stress levels			X	X	X	1
Reduced sleep hours per night	X		X		X	1

Figure 18 - Behavioral Causes of Obesity

Larger Portions at Meals

Americans are eating meals at home on larger plates and are serving themselves larger portions from larger serving dishes (Benton, 2015). Restaurants are serving more food on larger plates (Young, 2002) and often with free refills on breads, soups, and calorie-containing beverages. Fast-food restaurants are serving more food in larger containers with the opportunity to purchase even larger portion sizes for a nominal fee. For Muse Satiety Type 1s that are overserved, all that happens is that they stop eating right when they meet their calorie needs and then they discard more food than in the past, or they take home more leftovers for other members of the household to eat later. For the members of Muse Satiety Types 2 to 5 that are prone to overeat, larger meal sizes are a disaster, because they will most often result in overconsumption. The fact that Americans are overserving themselves is compounded by the simultaneous presence of additional causes of obesity that I will discuss later, including food being considerably less expensive for families to purchase, food having enhanced palatability, dessert being served with many meals, and food having a higher sugar content.

In my opinion, overconsumption of food at mealtimes is the second most powerful cause of obesity in America, second only to excess snacking. I have listed it as a level 4 on a scale of 1 to 4.

I have indicated in Figure 18 that direct government intervention can help with this problem, but that applies only to sit-down restaurants and fast-food restaurants. The government has already helped somewhat by mandating that the calories in each menu item be printed on the menus, although this law only applies to food-serving business that have 20 or more locations (Fox, 2018). Also helpful is the requirement for listing the total calories in whole containers of snack foods in large type on the front of the containers. However, the listing of calorie content in menus and on packages of foods is destined to help only the minority of people who are trying to follow the rules of weight maintenance. Most people get used to the calories listed for each item on menus and on the front of food labels and end up reading right past them.

The government can help even more by passing laws that increase the cost and decrease the portion size of foods that are highly palatable and irresistible, and also increase the cost of food additives that make food highly palatable and irresistible. As has already been evidenced in New York City when former Mayor Michael Bloomberg tried and failed to institute a law that limited fast-food beverage sizes, this not a popular option (Grynbaum, 2014). But the reason for doing so is clear. Members of Muse Satiety Types 2 to 5, which make up about 85% of our population, do not have the ability to consciously control their calorie intake and will almost always overconsume any type of highly palatable food they are served. They just don't know that they are doing it. They are not the guilty party in this matter. The food industry is just a business that profits from selling its wares. It has no interest in causing obesity in its customers. It's just interested in selling more and more food to increase profits. Remember that Muse Satiety Type 1s are not becoming obese in response to the success of the food industry in selling more food to the public, unlike what is happening to members of Muse Satiety Types 2 to 5. Is it the food industry's fault that their customers overconsume the food they sell? No. Should the food industry itself decrease portion sizes, remove the sugar and other flavor enhancers from the foods they make, and raise the prices on foods so they are less likely to be overconsumed? No. It is not economically possible, because if one company tries to do it and their competitors don't, then they will lose business, which is not acceptable to any company. The root problem is the genetically based disease of Muse's Satietopathy. Since the consumer is largely unable to control their overeating and the industry can't act out of concern for loss of profits, then the only solution is for the government to do what has to be done, even though it will be unpopular and difficult to do.

Government legislation should:

1. Stop government subsidies for the ingredients used to make highly palatable foods, such as beef, sugar, corn, and white flour. Instead, the government should subsidize non-starchy vegetables and fruits that are not as prone to overconsumption.

2. Impose additional taxes on highly palatable foods in an effort to reduce the frequency and quantity of purchases of those foods. Foods

that should be immediate targets are sugar-sweetened and corn-syrup-sweetened sodas and drinks, fruit juice, ice cream, milk shakes, French fries, candy, and dessert foods.

3. Mandate a reduction in portion sizes of all items that are prone to overconsumption at sit-down and fast-food restaurants. The average restaurant meal with beverages and dessert can easily exceed 2,000 calories. I estimate that less than 1% of the population burns enough calories per day to justify such a large meal.

4. Mandate the listing of calories of each menu item at all sit-down and fast-food restaurants, no matter the number of locations. In addition, the confusion created by listing a range of calories for a food item on a menu to which the diner can then add additional condiments needs to be stopped. Exact calories need to be listed for the food item without additions and the number of calories added by each option need to be listed separately. In restaurants where the diners add their own condiments to their food after receiving it from the kitchen, the calories in each condiment needs to be listed at the location where the condiments are served.

5. Impose additional taxes on food additives that make food highly palatable, namely sugars and saturated fats, since they have little nutritional value. Highly unsaturated oils, such as olive oil, should not be taxed since they lower heart disease and they reduce the likelihood of overconsumption of a high-carbohydrate sugar-laden diet.

The taxes I am recommending must be significant enough to change behavior, but not high enough to promote a black-market for the items being taxed. I believe that doubling or tripling the prices of the foods and food additives that I have mentioned above would be a good place to start, with studies done after a few years to determine the effect of the higher prices on the consumption of sugars and saturated fats.

Direct government intervention can't help with meal sizes at home, but government-funded education could have some benefit. The public needs to be educated on:

1. The fact that more than 85% of the population is missing at least one satiety signal, and therefore individuals and caregivers just can't purchase, prepare and consume food with abandon.

2. Controlling portion sizes at home and at restaurants using external clues, since most people don't have the complete slate of satiety signals found in the members of Muse Satiety Type 1.

3. Meal planning to prevent over production of food in the home.

4. Establishing rules in the home that prohibit taking seconds at meals and snacking in between meals, except for those who are at their ideal body fat percentage and are very active.

5. The fact that some sacrifice must be made by those who are at their ideal body weight. They can often be heard to say to the obese members of their households, "It's not fair that I have to limit buying my favorite foods just so you won't eat too much." This response comes as a reply to a request by their obese household members to stop buying the foods that the obese members of the household can't help from overeating. I'd like to respectfully point out that this type of response by those at their ideal weight is shortsighted. The obese family members have almost no choice but to gain weight if their most addictive foods are in their household environment. The consequences of worsening obesity to the obese members of the household are severe and have already been discussed in this book. The correct answer to the obese household members is a hard one to have to say for household members that are thin, but it should be that they'll help by consuming their favorite foods outside the home, and that they will lock up their favorite foods if they bring them home. In the case of ice cream, since there aren't locking freezers in most homes, the only answer can be to consume ice cream outside the home.

Increase in juice and sugar-sweetened beverage intake

Americans are some of the highest consumers of soda per person per year in the world, at about 148 liters per person per year, according to data from 2018 (Bedford, 2020). If that soda is sugar sweetened, that works out to an extra 60,000 extra calories per year, or about 17 pounds gained per year, if food intake is not reduced to compensate for the increase in calorie consumption from the soda. Not everyone in the US drinks soda, and soda consumption has been dropping since it peaked in 1998 (Holodny, 2016). However, many of those who don't drink soda instead drink sugar-sweetened coffee and tea, fruit juice, sports drinks, energy drinks, sweetened milk products and other beverages, many of which have the same number of calories, or more, than soda. From 2005 to 2008, half of the people in the US consumed a sugar-sweetened beverage of some kind every day (Ogden, 2011).

Before you think that the rest of the world is off the hook, most of the countries in the Western Hemisphere have a per capita consumption of soda that is between 70 to 148 liters per person per year. In most of Western Europe, the per capita consumption of soda averages about 94 liters per person per year (Wunsch, 2019).

By my observation, most sweetened beverages consumed in the US are consumed outside of mealtimes, with a smaller amount being consumed with meals. With the less-than-effective satiety centers of members of Muse Satiety Types 2 to 5, their brains fail to warn them that they are overconsuming calories when they are drinking calorie-containing beverages, either with meals or in between meals. Their brains also fail to signal them to stop eating earlier at the next meal to compensate for calorie-containing beverages consumed since the last meal, like what happens with Muse Satiety Type 2s to Type 5s snacking between meals.

Just like soda consumption, fruit juice consumption in the US has been declining slowly and steadily for the last decade. This is felt by some to be due to health-conscious consumers switching to beverages containing less sugar. However, at the same time, consumption of sweetened teas and energy drinks have increased steadily (Mintel, n.d.) (Euromonitor International, n.d.).

In addition to the obesity caused by overconsumption of fruit juice and sugar-sweetened beverages, there are other health concerns related to overconsumption of these beverages. Dental caries and dental disease are well-known risks. As previously explained, most fruit and fruit juices, table sugar, high-fructose corn syrup, honey and agave nectar contain higher amounts of fructose, as compared to lower amounts in vegetables, proteins and grains. In susceptible individuals, excess fructose consumption can cause fatty liver, which in turn can cause insulin resistance, and then can lead to type 2 diabetes with all its potential complications. The World Health Organization (WHO) has recommended that intake of all sugars should not exceed 10% of total calories per day, or about 50 grams of sugars a day for an average adult (WHO calls on countries to reduce sugars intake among adults and children, 2015). In addition, the WHO has proposed lowering intake of sugars even more to less than 5% of total calories per day, or about 25 grams of sugars a day for an average adult, but this has not become an official recommendation as of yet (WHO calls on countries to reduce sugars intake among adults and children, 2015).

In my opinion, the increase in juice and sugar-sweetened beverage intake is a major contribution to the obesity epidemic, and I have rated it as a 4 in a scale of 1 to 4.

Again, the consumer and the companies that sell the calorie-containing beverages are mostly powerless to change the level of calorie-containing beverage intake. The government can make the tough decisions needed to regulate and reduce the intake fruit juice and sugar-sweetened beverages.

Government legislation should:

1. Stop government subsidies for the sugar and high-fructose-corn-syrup industries.

2. Impose new or additional taxes on fruit juice, sugar-sweetened beverages and corn-syrup-sweetened beverages that are monetarily high enough to meaningfully reduce the frequency and quantity of purchases of those beverages.

3. Mandate a reduction in portion sizes of fruit juice, sugar-sweetened beverages and corn-syrup-sweetened beverages at sit-down and fast-food restaurants.

Direct government intervention can't help with sweetened-beverage serving sizes at home, but government-funded education could have some benefit. The public needs to be educated on:

1. The fact 85% of the population is missing at least one satiety signal and is prone to overconsumption of sweetened beverages, therefore individuals and caregivers just can't purchase, prepare and serve sweetened beverages with abandon.

2. Controlling beverage portion sizes at home and at restaurants.

3. Establishing rules in the home that prohibit drinking sweetened beverages, even in those who are at their ideal body fat percentage and are very active. Excess intake of sugars increases the risk of type 2 diabetes in everyone, obese or not (Basu, 2013).

4. The fact that some sacrifice must be made by those who are at their ideal body weight, as I have already discussed above. Sugar and high-fructose-corn-syrup sweetened beverages should be consumed in small quantities even by those at their ideal weight and should not brought into the home where there are members of Muse Satiety Types 2 to 5 that will overconsume them. A possible solution might be to keep sugar-sweetened beverages locked up in the home.

Loss of social norms against snacking

Snacking in between meals has exploded in quantity in just the last 100 years. In the Victorian Era, or most of the 19th century, snacking between meals was considered socially improper and even unhealthy. The earliest American snacks, peanuts and popcorn, got their starts in the 19th century. They were messy and were associated with the working class, less-than-clean street vendors, Vaudeville Theater, and sporting events, where the cheaper and rowdier upper seats were called the "peanut galleries." The public in general rarely snacked.

What changed? The food industry, ever searching for ways to sell more of its products, found ways to package and advertise highly palatable food that slowly overcame social norms against snacking. In 1904, Dr. Pepper, waffle cones for ice cream, hot dogs, hamburgers, and cotton candy became popular after being introduced at the Saint Louis World's Fair. The Oreo was introduced in 1912 and Life Savers Pep-O-Mint candy was released in 1913. The 1920s brought us Baby Ruth, Oh Henry!, Butterfinger, Heath Bars, Nestle Drumsticks, 7-UP, and popsicles. The 1930s heralded Twinkies, Snickers, Tootsie Pops, Fritos, 3 Musketeers, Ritz Crackers, and Lay's Potato Chips. Even though snacking was diminished in the 1940s due to World War II, still M&Ms, Tootsie Rolls, Almond Joys, Junior Mints, Smarties, and Cheetos were introduced during that decade. The post-war 1950s brought fast-food franchises, including McDonald's, Jack in the Box, Taco Bell, Denny's, Burger King, Kentucky Fried Chicken, and Pizza Hut. Sprite, Pop-Tarts, Pringles, Lucky Charms, Doritos, Starburst and Gatorade were introduced in the 1960s (Holmes, n.d.). Many more snack foods have been introduced since then.

Slick marketing ignited the national love affair with snacking, along with packaging and preservatives that prevented spoiling and maintained taste. However, it was really the unsuspected presence of Muse Satiety Types 2 to 5 in the US population that got the snacking ball rolling. Once members of Muse Satiety Types 2 to 5 started snacking, the sky was the limit. As the decades went by and more and more snack foods were rolled out, members of Muse Satiety Types 2 to 5 snacked more and more. Snacking slowly became a normal occurrence at churches, at schools, on the playground, on public transport, at sporting and entertainment events, and libraries. The snacks were so pleasant and plentiful that almost no one could resist overeating them. They became an integral part of birthday parties, school gatherings, and church events. They became gifts and rewards for good behavior and good performance. Recently, for a growing number of people, they have become the only food consumed all day long.

There is no question that snacking in between meals increases daily intake of calories and causes weight gain. A study in 2011 indicated that average American consumed nearly a third more calories per day in the 2000s versus the 1970s. This was shown in the study to be due to a 29% increase in the number of eating episodes per day (from 3.8 per day in the 1970s to

4.9 per day in the 2000s) and a 12% increase in portion size at those eating episodes. Energy density, or the number of calories in each bite of food, declined slightly during the same time period (Popkin, 2011). Other studies have also confirmed that increased snacking is directly linked to weight gain (Levitsky, 2004) (Nicklas, 2003).

In my opinion, the loss of social norms against snacking is a major contributor to the obesity epidemic, and I have rated it as a 4 in a scale of 1 to 4.

Since excess snacking is causing obesity, then the solution for everyone seems to be simple. Everyone needs to stop snacking. However, that well-meaning solution is not going to work if members of Muse Satiety Types 2 to 5 are in an environment that is rich in snack foods. Once again, the companies that make the snacks, the people who buy and serve the snacks, and the people who eat the snacks are not the guilty parties. The government needs to step in to aggressively control this problem by:

1. Stopping government subsidies for the corn, high-fructose corn syrup, and cane and beet sugar industries.

2. Impose significant new or additional taxes on candy, ice cream, sugar-sweetened baked goods, chips, fruit snacks, popcorn, pudding, crackers, pretzels, nuts, snack bars, etc., in an effort to reduce the frequency and quantity of purchases of these snacks.

3. Impose new or additional taxes on sugar, high-fructose corn syrup, chocolate chips, chocolate powder, etc., since these items are often used to make irresistible snacks to be consumed in the home.

Government-funded education could also have some benefit. The public needs to be educated on:

1. The fact that about 85% of the population is missing the loss of savor signal, and therefore individuals and caregivers just can't purchase, prepare and consume snack food with abandon.

2. Controlling portion sizes of snacks at home.

3. Meal-size planning to prevent between-meal consumption of leftover food as snacks.

4. Establishing rules in the home that prohibit snacking in between meals, except for those who are at their ideal body fat percentage and are very active.

5. The fact that some sacrifice must be made by those who are at their ideal body weight. I have already discussed this above. In this era of plentiful and tasty meals and snacks, even Muse Satiety Type 1s are taking an extra bite of food here and there, even when they are not hungry, resulting in a weight gain of 10 to 15 pounds over 10-20 years. In addition, some evidence indicates that excess sugar consumption, even by those who are at their ideal weight, significantly increases risk for type 2 diabetes (Lim, 2010). If some household members insist on bringing irresistible snacks into the home, then they must keep them locked up.

Larger portions of snacks

Portion sizes of snack foods have been increasing steadily since the 1970s. The FDA recommended serving size for snacks foods is one ounce (FDA, 2014). Since portion sizes of snack foods have increased, most packages of snack foods now contain multiple 1-ounce servings. However, Americans that are Muse Satiety Type 3s to 5s are consuming the whole package. Even if they buy smaller packages of snack foods, they end up eating more than one package. Increased portion size of snacks leads to increased daily calorie consumption (Nielsen, 2003). For Muse Satiety Types 2 to 5, this leads to weight gain. The effect of larger portions of snacks on obesity, in my opinion, is a strong effect, a 3 on a scale of 1 to 4.

In addition to what I have already listed above under "loss of social norms against snacking," the government can help by reducing the number of servings in packages of snack foods. Government-funded education could also have some benefit and was discussed in the section on "the loss of social norms against snacking."

Increased sugar intake

Sweet-sugar intake from all food sources by American adults, which I define as intake of any fructose-containing sugar, has gone from an average of about 20 grams per day in 1800, to about 100 grams per day in 1900, and then to about 180 grams per day in 2000 (Johnson, 2007). The fructose-containing foods that are of concern are fruit and fruit products, cane- and beet-sugar-sweetened products, products containing high-fructose corn syrup, honey, and agave nectar. Gratefully, sweet-sugar consumption has declined a little since 2000, with American adults consuming about 150 grams of sugar per day in 2012, per one source (Nursing Your Sweet Tooth, n.d.). American teens are consuming even more sweet sugar, with teen's sweet-sugar intake in 2012 being estimated to be more than 180 grams per day (Sugar: The Bitter Truth, 2012). It is difficult to determine exactly how much sweet sugar the average American is consuming per day, because sweet sugar is coming from so many different sources. Many estimates of sugar consumption don't include intake of fruit. Recently, manufacturers have been adding concentrated fruit juice to their products so that on the label it looks like their products have less added sugar in them.

The increase in sweet-sugar consumption over the years has largely been caused by an increase in refined sweet-sugar intake, which comes through the foods we eat, the sweetened beverages we drink, and the desserts and snacks we consume. It is also related, to a smaller degree, to a rise in consumption of fruit and fruit products. To repeat what I have explained earlier, sweet sugar describes both mixtures of fructose and glucose, such as is found in fruit and fruit products, honey, high-fructose corn syrup, and sucrose, which is commonly known as table sugar and is chemically one fructose molecule attached to one glucose molecule. The sweetener agave nectar is like any other fruit and contains a mixture of fructose and glucose.

Humans, as well as all other mammals, find sweet sugar to be irresistible, and even addictive. When sweet sugar is added to foods, we eat more of them. When offered sweet-sugar-based snacks, most of us will eat them beyond our daily calorie needs. This is particularly true of members of Muse Satiety Types 2 to 5.

In my estimation, increased sweet-sugar intake contributes significantly, but less so, than other behaviors discussed thus far in this section. I have given it a magnitude of effect rating of 3 on a scale of 1 to 4.

Once again, I want to stress that the companies that refine and distribute sweet sugar and sweet-sugar-containing foods are not able to alter their behavior in a free market, unless they are all required by law to do so.

I recommend that governments:

1. Stop subsidies for producers of high-fructose corn syrup, cane sugar, and beet sugar.

2. Impose significant new or additional taxes on high-fructose corn syrup, cane sugar and beet sugar. I personally would like to see a bag of table sugar selling for three to four times what it sells for now.

3. Add grams of fructose to all food labels, instead of grams of sugar. That will quell any argument about added versus natural sugar. There is little difference between added sugar that is refined from natural sources, and naturally occurring sugar in fruits and vegetables. The consumer just needs to know how much fructose is in the foods they are buying, since excess fructose consumption is harmful to our bodies. The glucose in sweet sugars is not harmful to the human body, unless it is overconsumed. Glucose is the body's main energy source. Since the US government and the World Health Organization recommend no more than 50 grams of sugar per day for adults, then this would be no more than about 25 grams of fructose per day for adults. Since both organizations recommend no more than 25 grams of sugar a day for children 12 and under, then that would mean no more than about 12 grams of fructose per day for children 12 and under.

Government-funded education would also be beneficial. The public needs to be educated on:

1. Encouraging preparation of foods in the home that are low in sweet sugars.

2. Which foods contain large amounts of sweet sugars.

3. The harms of excess intake of sweet sugars.

Dessert served with lunch and dinner

Dessert after meals has been around since man began, although consumption of dessert prior to the 20th century occurred much less often and in much smaller quantities. The term *dessert* is defined as, "A usually sweet course or dish, usually served at the end of a meal." (Merriam-Webster, n.d.) Consumption of sweet foods at the end of a meal became much more common in the early 1900s and continued as such through most of the 20th century. However, the number of dinners per week served in the home where dessert was served has declined steadily in the recent past, with 23% of dinners including a dessert in 1986, and just 13% of dinners including a dessert in 2014. This is felt by some to be due to increasing consumer concern about overconsumption of sugar. However, for those who do consume dessert after meals, it almost always becomes extra calories eaten for that meal and is most often overconsumed by members of Muse Satiety Types 4 and 5, and not members of Muse Satiety Types 1 to 3, because they are too full to eat more than just a little bit of dessert at the end of a meal. In addition, the declining number of dinners that don't end in the consumption of a dessert could also be explained by an increase in sugar-sweetened food consumed during the meal, such as large amounts of added sugar in ketchup, salad dressing, barbeque sauce, sweet-and-sour sauces, sweetened drinks and milk, Jell-O salads, jams, and honey.

In my estimation, consumption of dessert with meals contributes significantly, but less so, than other behaviors discussed in this section. I have given it a magnitude rating of 2 on a scale of 1 to 4.

As previously explained, the companies that sell pre-packaged desserts, the companies that sell the ingredients to make home-prepared desserts, and the individuals who eat them are not able to easily change their behavior. However, government can help to reduce dessert consumption both in the home and when eating out by doing the things discussed under the snacking section above.

In addition, government-funded education again could also have some benefit. The public needs to be educated on:

1. The fact that about 85% of the population is missing the loss of savor signal, and therefore individuals and caregivers just can't purchase, prepare, and consume dessert after meals with abandon. For members of Muse Satiety Types 3 to 5, dessert consumption after meals will always result in excess calorie intake for the meal and subsequent weight gain.

2. If dessert is served with a meal in the home, then portion sizes of the meal should be significantly decreased.

3. Dessert purchasing, or dessert preparation in the home, should aim to have only enough dessert for small servings at the intended meal, with no dessert left over to be consumed later as snacks.

Longer mealtimes

In my estimation, Americans are spending more time at the meal table in recent years, and it is increasing daily calorie intake. I cannot find any references to support this, but I do know that the average American eats out 4.5 times per week. When Americans do eat out, they eat for longer than they would eat if they were eating at home, due to the length of time it takes for each course to be served at restaurants. While it was hard to find statistics for mealtimes in the US, an estimate of 60 to 80 minutes for a sit-down dinner at a restaurant fits with what I have read and observed. For members of Muse Satiety Types 1 and 2, the length of the meal doesn't affect the calories consumed at the meal, since the Muse Satiety Type 1s eat until full and then most often don't eat another bite. Muse Satiety Type 2s eat until full, take a few more bites a little later and then don't eat another bite. Muse Satiety Type 3s will put their fork down for five to 10 minutes in the middle of a meal, but then can pick the fork back up and continue eating, resulting in overconsumption. When members of Muse Satiety Types 4 and 5 sit at a meal of highly palatable and plentiful food, they just keep eating for the whole 60 to 80 minutes without stopping, resulting in significant overconsumption.

In my estimation, longer mealtimes contribute significantly, but less so, than other behaviors discussed in this section. I have given it a magnitude rating of 2 on a scale of 1 to 4.

In my opinion, there is not a lot that governments can do to help to shorten mealtimes, although decreasing meal sizes at sit-down and fast-food restaurants would decrease mealtimes due to it not taking as long to consume smaller meals. This was already discussed in the section on larger portions at meals earlier in this chapter.

Government-funded education would be beneficial. The public needs to be educated on:

1. Encouraging preparation of smaller amounts of food cooked at home that is consistent with the number of people who will be eating the meal with a single serving for each.

2. Changing back to smaller 10-inch plates that were commonly used in the 1970s and before. Humans have been proven to eat less when served on smaller plates.

3. Having a rule in the home that seconds are not allowed at mealtimes, except for individuals who are at their ideal weight and are exercising an hour or more a day.

4. Not serving calorie-containing drinks, except for white milk when it is part of the two servings of a milk product per day that is recommended for adults. Children's medical providers should be consulted on the proper number of servings of milk products per day.

5. Serving all the food at once at meals, and not one course at a time, so that those who are prone to sit at the table a long time and keep eating will be less likely to do so.

6. Limiting the serving of dessert after meals to only special occasions, and then only in small serving sizes.

Decreased activity due to too much screen time

There is no question that humans all over the world are using their electronic devices with screens so much that it significantly decreases their activity levels and thereby adversely affects their health. In the US in 2018, adults 18 and older spent more than 11 hours per day watching, listening, or interacting with media (The Nielsen Total Audience Report: Q1 2018, 2018). I am certain that the viewers were at rest 99% of the time while they were viewing the various forms of media. Inactivity is strongly associated with risk for obesity later in life (Pietilainen, 2008).

Not all risks of inactivity are due to obesity. Multiple studies have shown that sedentary people have a 1.2-fold to 2.0-fold higher chance of dying over the 10-20 year observation periods of the studies (Slattery, 1988) (Leon, 1991). Physical inactivity is also associated with increased risk for coronary heart disease, type 2 diabetes, breast cancer, and colon cancer (Lee I. , 2012).

In my estimation, decreased activity due to too much screen time contributes significantly, but less so, than other behaviors discussed in this section. I have given it a magnitude rating of 2 on a scale of 1 to 4.

I recommend that governments:

1. Mandate more organized and supervised activity time for elementary school children and require daily physical education for all junior high, high school, college, and advanced degree students.

2. Mandate that employers allow at least 30 minutes of organized exercise per workday for all able-bodied employees that have been cleared by their medical provider.

Government-funded education would also be beneficial. The public needs to be educated that:

1. The minimum amount of exercise per day for able-bodied adults is 30 minutes a day for most days or at least 150 minutes per week.

2. Walking is the best choice of exercise for most people.

3. Screen time for entertainment purposes should be cut in half.

4. Caregivers should help children and teens to be more active by having the whole family turn off their screens at times of the day when they are only being used for entertainment.

Increased fast-food intake outside of mealtimes

There is no question that fast-food intake is increasing in the United States. Fast-food intake is defined as food that can be purchased ready to eat with little wait time. It can come from fast-food restaurants, bars, cafés, snack bars, and quick-food establishments. Fast-food consumption at mealtimes causes weight gain. Fast food eaten outside of mealtimes as a snack only compounds the problem.

On any given day 37% of US adults consume fast food. Young adults age 20 to 39 consume fast food more frequently with 45% consuming fast food daily. About 23% of all adults reported consuming fast food as a snack outside of regular meals every day (National Health and Nutrition Examination Survey 2013 to 2016, n.d.). Multiple studies have shown that the greater the fast-food consumption, the more that a person is at risk for obesity. A 2008 meta-analysis, which combined the results of multiple studies, showed unequivocally that there is a correlation between increasing fast-food intake and increased body weight (Rosenheck R. , 2009). A 2017 United Kingdom study of 2,083 adults showed that fast-food consumption was associated with a 30% increased chance of obesity (Penney, 2017).

Consuming fast food outside of mealtimes, such as late-night stops at the drive-throughs, leads to additional weight gain. I again propose that Muse Satiety Type 1s will not gain weight from increased visits to fast-food restaurants, because they'll just leave their excess fast food uneaten, both at mealtimes and during late-night snack attacks. All other Muse Satiety Types will at least have a bite or two extra of the fast food, and the Muse Satiety Types 4 and 5 will definitely overeat.

In my estimation, increased fast-food intake outside of mealtimes contributes significantly, but less so, than other behaviors discussed in this section. I have given it a magnitude rating of 2 on a scale of 1 to 4.

I recommend that governments:

1. Mandate that all eating establishments, no matter the number of locations, list the calories of each item sold on their menus, including the condiments that the diner can add to the meal.

2. Mandate reduction of portion sizes of food served at fast-food restaurants, including all calorie-containing beverages.

3. Consider mandating limited operating hours for fast-food restaurants to prevent late-night consumption of additional food.

Government-funded education would also be beneficial. The public needs to be educated:

1. Not to purchase more fast food than is needed for a single serving for each person in the family that will be fed at the meal.

2. To purchase healthier fast-food meals that are lower in calories, contain more non-starchy vegetables and less red meat, sugar, and highly refined carbohydrates.

3. Educate the public to stop buying any calorie-containing drinks with their fast-food meals, with the exception of white milk. For white milk, the recommendations of the American Academy of Pediatrics are that children age one to eight have no more than two 8-ounce cups of milk, or servings of a milk product, per day, and that older children and teens age nine to eighteen should have no more than three 8-ounce cups of milk, or servings of a milk product, per day (Gidding, 2006). Parents should check with their medical provider for additional information on the types of milk and milk products that are appropriate for their child.

4. Teach the public to avoid buying fast food outside of mealtimes.

Higher stress levels

If you stop about anyone on the street and ask them if stress and anxiety are worse now in the US than decades ago, most often the reply will be "yes." In our modern world, there are more things to potentially be stressed about than in past decades, such as maintaining our image on social media; the widening gap between the poor and rich; 24/7 news coverage that brings more peoples' pain, angst, and suffering to our attention; fake news; the increasingly visible and ugly side of politics; loneliness, or the fear of being lonely; the loss of nuclear families; and more media emphasis on individual success and less on the success of family and community. I'm sure that both you and I could go on listing other modern causes of stress. Add these modern stressors to the age-old stressors of finding enough money to pay the bills, providing a living space and food for ourselves and those we love, working long hours for not enough pay, increasing medical and mental health problems, relationship problems, coping with aging parents, raising children, etc., and it's a miracle that we're all still sane.

A major stressor for many of us is being overweight. But could that very stress about our weight be causing us to gain more weight, especially when stress over our weight is added to all of our other stressors? Recent research suggests that stress does play a role in weight gain. A four-year observational study on 56,622 women in 2017 indicated that job stress contributes to weight gain (Fujishiro, 2017). A 2009 nine-year observational study of 1,355 US adults showed that stress was related to weight gain, but only in those who were already heavy to start with. In this study, both sexes of heavier adults gained weight when they experienced demanding jobs, problems paying bills, depression, and anxiety. Heavier men also gained weight when they felt trapped in jobs that didn't allow them to use their skills and when they had no authority to make decisions at work. Heavier women also gained weight when faced with strain in family relationships and with perceived constraints in life, such as not having enough time in a day and not being able to be everywhere at once. In contrast, thin men and women in this study tended to lose weight with the above stressors (Block, 2009).

Two randomized controlled trials have confirmed that treating stress causes weight loss. In the first study, 45 adults with obesity were randomized to receive only standard instructions for a healthy lifestyle, or standard instructions for a healthy lifestyle plus an 8-week stress-management program. After eight weeks, the subjects in the stress-management program group lost 1.36 BMI points, or about three to five pounds, more than the healthy-lifestyle group (Xenaki, 2018). In the second study, 49 overweight children and adolescents age 9 to 15 were all placed on a low-calorie diet by a clinical nutritionist and instructed to exercise by a physical trainer. They were then randomized to either a control group or a stress-management group.

The 23 patients in the stress-management group lost 1.08 BMI points, or about two to four pounds, more than the control group after eight weeks (Stavrou, 2016).

Taken together, these studies strongly suggest that stress does cause weight gain for those already struggling with their weight. In addition, stress reduction causes a modest increase in weight lost from a diet. In my estimation, increased stress contributes significantly, but less so, than other behaviors discussed in this section. I have given it a magnitude rating of 1 on a scale of 1 to 4.

While government regulation can't impact stress in the home, at church, in relationships, etc., the government can help with work-related stress. I recommend that governments:

1. Consider designing and implementing mandatory tools to screen for harmful work-place stressors.

2. Consider using an existing or a new government agency to help businesses to remediate harmful levels of work-place stress.

3. Consider putting in place penalties for businesses that fail to improve harmful work-place stress.

4. Legislate improved coverage for and access to mental health care by both public and private insurance.

Government-funded education would also be beneficial. The public needs to be educated on:

1. The harmful effects of excessive stress on body weight for those who are already struggling with their weight.

2. Aggressively counting calories, avoiding purchasing binge foods, controlling portion sizes, and avoiding snacking outside of meals during stressful times of life.

3. Effective methods of reducing stress that individuals can do for themselves, or in other words, self-therapy.

Reduced sleep hours per night

It is well-known that many people are not sleeping enough. The National Sleep Foundation recommends that adults under 65 sleep seven to nine hours per night and adults over 65 sleep seven to eight hours per night (Hirshkowitz, 2015). However, 35.2% of US adults sleep less than seven hours per night (CDC, 2014). The average American adult sleeps 6.8 hours per night, which is one hour less than in 1942 (Gallup, 2013).

Does sleeping less than seven hours a night cause obesity in adults? Yes. Approximately 33% of US adults who sleep less than seven hours per night are obese, compared to 26.5% of adults who sleep seven or more hours per night (CDC, 2014). Sleep-deprived individuals have increased levels of ghrelin, a hormone that directly increases food consumption, and decreased leptin, a hormone that decreases food consumption (Cooper, 2018). Dieting adults who get seven or more hours of sleep per night are 33% more likely to lose at least 10% of their body weight than dieters sleeping less than seven hours per night. Adults who are trying to maintain weight after a diet are 38% more likely to be successful if they sleep seven or more hours per night (Thomson, 2012).

There are many reasons why US adults sleep less than they should. Some have primary insomnia, which is difficulty falling asleep without any associated medical illnesses. Others have medical problems that keep them awake, such as arthritis, chronic pain, acid reflux, stress, anxiety, depression, asthma, etc., or they take medication that keeps them awake. The previously mentioned individuals should see their medical provider for help with their lack of sleep. Some sleep poorly due to an uncomfortable mattress, an uncomfortable pillow, or a bedroom that is too hot, cold, or noisy. These causes of poor sleep can be improved, as finances and ability allow.

Finally, many spend what should be sleep hours watching and interacting with media, whether on big screens or small screens. Be it online gaming, gaming at a console, interaction with social media, binge-watching movies and TV series on streaming services, or just watching live TV, media cuts into the hours allotted for sleep in our busy schedules and decreases the quality of our sleep. Almost all of these devices that we interact with produce blue light, which has been shown to delay onset of our night-time circadian rhythm and to suppress the release of melatonin, a hormone that promotes sleep (Why Electronics May Stimulate You Before Bed, n.d.). The solution is to turn off these devices, except for those that don't emit blue light, at least 30 minutes before you plan to sleep and to interact instead with printed pages under lamplight, such as reading a book, writing in a journal, or doing crossword puzzles.

> In my estimation, reduced sleep hours contribute to obesity significantly, but less so, than other behaviors discussed in this section. I have given it a magnitude rating of 1 on a scale of 1 to 4.

While government regulation can't increase sleep hours, government-funded education would be beneficial. The public needs to be educated on:

1. The harmful effects of reduced sleep hours, including difficulty with weight loss and weight maintenance.

2. The importance of turning off screens in the bedroom that emit blue light at least 30 minutes before planned sleep.

ECONOMIC CAUSES OF OBESITY

For the purposes of this book, economic causes of obesity are those that are related to companies' needs to increase profits through the preparation and sale of food. Again, I don't blame any company that wants to make more money legally and ethically by selling more of the products that they produce. These businesses must make a profit from their sales or they risk ceasing to exist. As a nation, we can tell these businesses that we want them to improve the nutrition of and decrease the serving sizes of their products, but for any one or two companies that try to do so, their new product's smaller size and decreased savor due to lower amounts of sugar, fat, and carbs will make their products less appealing to the average consumer than the products of their nonconforming competitors. This will result in a decrease in sales for the compliant companies and could ultimately lead to the end of those companies. One possible way to change the behavior of companies is for the community to stop buying their less healthy products, but efforts in this direction have been largely ineffective (Do Boycotts Work?, 2017). In my opinion, the only way to change the behavior of food-producing companies fairly and effectively is government regulation and government-sponsored education. With the causes of obesity discussed in this section, the individual or group largely has a choice to participate in the behaviors encouraged by the food industry or to avoid those behaviors.

The economic causes of obesity that I think are at least in part responsible for the obesity epidemic are listed in Figure 19.

ECONOMIC CAUSES OF OBESITY	Decreased Energy Expended	Increased Mealtime Intake	Increased Snack Intake	Mitigated by Direct Government Intervention	Mitigated by Government-Sponsored Education	Magnitude of the Effect of the Cause of Obesity
Cheaper food		X	X	X	X	4
Commercially preserved food available 24/7		X	X	X	X	4
Increased palatability of food		X	X	X	X	3
Increased production of highly processed foods		X	X	X	X	3
Increased restaurant eating		X		X	X	3
Increased food advertising		X	X	X	X	2

Figure 19 - Economic Causes of Obesity

Cheaper food

In the US, people spent about a fourth of their disposable income on food in 1930. By 2010, that cost had dropped to a tenth of disposable income in the US. From 1970 to 2009, the consumption of calories per day in the US increased by 20% (Sturm, 2014). While cheaper food is not the only cause of the increase in calorie consumption, cheaper food is one of the more significant drivers of calorie overconsumption and the resulting obesity in the US and in the world.

Who is gaining weight from cheaper food in the US? Almost everyone. Even residents of Colorado and those of Asian descent are gaining weight, even though folklore has repeatedly told us that these two populations are resistant to obesity. The mild weight-gain differences over time between races, education levels, sex, and the state of residence is smaller than weight gained by every demographic in the US during the same time period (Sturm, 2014).

An easy solution might seem to be increasing the cost of all foods so that people will buy less food. However, this will mostly only affect the poor and could have serious repercussions for the economy. In addition, evidence is weak on whether taxing unhealthy food, or subsidizing purchases of healthier food, will change food consumption as much as desired. However, a study in South Africa that was published in 2013 indicated that a 25% reduction in the price of healthier food resulted in a 9.3% increase in healthier-food expenditure and a 7.2% reduction in less-healthy food expenditure (Sturm, 2013).

In my opinion, cheaper food is a major contributor to the obesity epidemic, and I have rated it as a 4 in a scale of 1 to 4.

I recommend that governments do the following to reduce excess calorie consumption from cheaper food:

1. Stop subsidies for foods that provide more calories per dollar spent, such as grains, sugar, and fat, and instead subsidize foods that provide less calories per dollar spent, such as fruits and vegetables. In this subsidization process, care must be taken to avoid excessively increasing the daily food cost for low-income families that are paying more than 10% of their household income for food and are already

stretching their limited household income by buying foods that have a high calorie amount per dollar spent, such as grains, sugar, and fat. Removing subsidies for grains, sugar, and fat and then failing to subsidize fruits and vegetables will force these families to just pay more for the grains, sugars, and fats, since they won't be able to afford the unsubsidized fruits and vegetables.

2. Mandate reduction of portion sizes of food served at all types of restaurants, including all calorie-containing beverages.

Government-funded education would also be beneficial to reduce the calories eaten per day of cheaper food. The public needs to be educated on:

1. Not purchasing more food than is needed for a single serving for each person in the family that will be fed at each meal. Since cellphone use is almost universal for almost all demographic groups in the US, encourage shopping with free or inexpensive recipe apps that tell the shopper exactly how much of each food to buy for the planned meal, or a week of planned meals.

2. Avoiding the purchase of desserts to be eaten after a meal and snack foods to be eaten between meals.

3. Trying to avoid shopping when hungry, which might promote excess buying of food.

4. Purchasing and making healthier foods that are lower in calories, contain more non-starchy vegetables and less red meat, sugar, and highly refined carbohydrates.

5. Avoiding buying any calorie-containing drinks, except for white milk, as previously discussed.

6. Avoiding buying fast food outside of mealtimes.

7. What to do when you're hungry between meals and feel like snacking. Appropriate behaviors in this situation might be to drink water or a calorie-free beverage, eat a pickle or celery which has almost no calories, go for a walk, or go to the gym.

Commercially preserved food available 24/7

Along with cheaper food, the availability of highly palatable packaged and preserved food that is ready to eat immediately, or if not immediately, then within 10 minutes or less, has significantly contributed to overconsumption of calories in the US, in my opinion. The major contributor to food becoming much more quickly available in the last century is the vast improvement in man's ability to keep food fresh by canning, packaging, refrigeration, and freezing. While the bottling of food as a food preservation method was invented as early as 1809 by Nicolas Appert (Britannica, n.d.), it wasn't until the mid-nineteenth century that canned food began to be increasingly popular. The first refrigerators for home use were invented in 1913 and by the 1920s were increasingly popular (Heldman, 2003). Separate freezers were introduced in the 1940s. Plastic packaging of foods became widespread in the 1950s.

The availability of canned, packaged, refrigerated, and frozen foods has allowed households to store large quantities of food in their home that is available for immediate, or almost immediate, consumption. It has also enabled households to keep leftover food from past meals and snacks immediately available for later consumption. This has not made as much of a difference in calories consumed per day for members of Muse Satiety Type 1, since they stop eating when they have reached their exact calorie need at each meal. However, it has opened new avenues for in-between meal snacking and late-night snacking for Muse Satiety Types 2 to 5.

Studies of commercially packaged and preserved foods on weight gain have failed to confirm my opinion that such foods are a significant cause of obesity. However, in my opinion, studies that have failed to show a connection between these foods and overconsumption didn't control properly for Muse Satiety Types and weren't conducted on Muse Satiety Types 4 and 5 alone, who make up 40% of the US population and are at the highest risk for weight gain.

In my opinion, commercial preservation of food so that it is readily available for consumption 24-hours a day is a major contributor to the obesity epidemic, and I have rated it as a 4 in a scale of 1 to 4.

I recommend that governments do the following to reduce excess calorie consumption from commercially preserved foods:

1. Strengthen existing regulations so that all commercially preserved food labels identify how many calories there are in a serving of the food in the package and how many total servings there are in the package in large letters on the front of the package, can, or bottle.

2. Mandate reduction of portion sizes of commercially preserved foods that are most likely to be overconsumed, such as frozen desserts, chips, pastries, candy, juice, and sugar-sweetened drinks, and reduce the number of servings allowed to be purchased in a single package.

3. Mandate hefty price increases on commercially preserved foods that are most likely to be overeaten.

Government-funded education would also be beneficial to reduce the calories eaten per day of readily available packaged and preserved foods. The public needs to be educated on:

1. Purchasing foods as raw ingredients and then preparing them efficiently and nutritionally.

2. Limiting the purchase of packaged preserved foods as much as possible.

3. Avoiding buying larger packages of food than needed for one serving per person at each meal.

4. Avoiding the purchase of commercially preserved foods that are designed to be eaten outside of mealtimes as snacks.

5. Trying to avoid shopping when hungry, which might promote excess buying of packaged snack foods.

6. Avoiding buying any calorie-containing drinks, except for white milk, as previously discussed.

Increased palatability of food

It is human nature that people are attracted to foods that taste good to them. The better foods taste, the more of those foods people will eat. In recent years, food science, food processing, and food esthetics have created myriads of highly palatable and attractive foods that can border on irresistible for many.

However, I propose that weight gain does not occur when members of Muse Satiety Types 1 and 2 are exposed to highly palatable foods. This is also mostly true for members of Muse Satiety Type 3 in their first two to three decades of life. These three groups make up about 60% of the US population according to the study at my clinic.

Studies in the area of food palatability are hard to interpret since many are done on animals and not in humans. The few that are done on humans are small, or epidemiologic in nature, making the study results unreliable. Some studies have showed that increased palatability increases weight (Louis-Sylvestre, 1984) (Wene, 1982) and others have not shown this effect (Tordoff, 2017) (Naim, 1986). Without question, lack of ability to identify and control for the distribution of members of the Muse Satiety Types in these studies, both animal and human, could have contributed to their inconsistent results.

Lacking conclusive study evidence, I will stick with my personal assessment that highly palatable foods are a significant cause of modern obesity due to their undeniable effect on members of Muse Satiety Types 4 and 5, at least until further studies can be performed. I have rated the effect of an increase in highly palatable foods on the obesity epidemic as a 3 on a scale of 1 to 4.

It would be impossible for governments to mandate laws to reduce the palatability of food, and it would be unwise to do so for foods that are considered nutritious. However, governments can take steps to reduce human consumption of highly palatable and less nutritious foods by educating the public about the items I have listed in previous sections of this chapter.

Increased production of highly processed foods

A lot of attention has been given to the explosion in the availability of highly processed foods in the modern age, which has been suggested to be a major cause of food overconsumption. Highly processed foods are manufactured by the food industry to be highly palatable and calorie dense so they will sell well. Highly processed foods can be irresistible to members of Muse Satiety Types 2 to 5, resulting in excess consumption and subsequent weight gain.

When it comes to categorizing foods as to their degree of processing, I will use the four categories proposed by the Center for Epidemiological Studies in Health and Nutrition at the University of Sao Paulo, Brazil, and that is called the NOVA Food Classification System (Monteiro, 2016):

1. Unprocessed or minimally processed foods that are either available just as harvested from nature or are altered only by removing inedible or unwanted parts and then dried, crushed, ground, pasteurized, roasted, boiled, refrigerated, frozen, etc., with no added foods or chemicals.

2. Processed culinary ingredients that are pressed, refined, ground, milled, or dried, but otherwise not chemically altered, to make food ingredients. Examples are salt, oils, flours, starches, and vinegars.

3. Processed foods, which are made from ingredients from the first two categories and are preserved mostly for durability and maintenance of sensory quality during distribution and storage, but don't contain additives from the food industry. Examples are canned and bottled vegetables, fruits, legumes, and meats, as well as salted nuts, cheeses, fruits in syrup, and freshly made foods.

4. Highly processed foods, as I call them, or ultra-processed foods, as they are called by the authors of the NOVA System, are altered by the food industry by removing fiber and many other nutrients, and then salt, refined sugars, refined fats, synthetic flavors, synthetic coloring agents, preservatives, non-sugar sweeteners, chemically processed food extracts, etc., are added. Highly processed foods are designed to outsell foods from the first three categories and are inexpensive,

energy dense, nutrition poor, highly palatable, and attractively packaged. The food industry manufactures almost all highly processed foods and spends billions of dollars a year in advertising and store placement to coax you into purchasing their products instead of the healthier foods from the first three categories.

A number of studies have indicated that consumption of highly palatable high processed foods leads to overconsumption and to weight gain (Poti, 2107).

In my opinion, the strength of the effect of consumption of widely available, highly palatable, and energy-dense foods, or ultra-processed foods, is a 3 out of 4.

I recommend that governments do the following to reduce excess consumption of highly processed foods:

1. Change the status of all energy-dense highly processed foods to their own food category, separate from calorie-containing drinks (excluding milk, formula, and weight-loss products), dessert, and snack foods (excluding unprocessed natural foods, such as nuts and berries, in small portion sizes). Call this category highly processed, or ultra-processed foods, and tax this category heavily in an effort to decrease its sales.

2. Label foods that are in the category of highly processed foods as harmful to human health, leading to obesity, type 2 diabetes, heart disease, stroke, and cancer, similar to labels on foods that are still on the market that contain additives that are suspected to cause harm to humans. Foods containing saccharine are an example.

Government-funded education would also be beneficial to reduce consumption of highly processed foods. The public needs to be educated on:

1. Purchasing foods as raw ingredients and then preparing them efficiently and nutritionally.

2. Limiting the purchase of highly processed foods as much as possible.

3. Making the difficult choice between highly palatable and highly processed snacks and minimally processed snacks at the grocery store, since once they are in the home, it is hard for most family members to resist highly palatable and highly processed snacks.

Increased restaurant eating

Americans are in the middle of a long-standing love affair with eating at restaurants that is only getting deeper and deeper. Restaurant industry sales have grown from $43 billion per year in 1970 to as high as $863 billion per year in 2019. During that same period, the population of the United States grew from about 205 million to about 329 million people. In 1955, 25% of household expenditure on food went to the restaurant industry; in 2019 about 51% of household expenditure on food went to the restaurant industry. Nine in 10 consumers say they enjoy going to restaurants and four in 10 consumers say that restaurants are an essential part of their lifestyle (2019 Restaurant Industry Factbook, 2019). For this section of this chapter, the word restaurant will include restaurants that are sit-down, buffet, and fast food.

According to a 2016 study, average restaurant meals contained between about 800 to 1,700 calories (Urban, 2016), which can be more than half the total daily calorie need for many people. Restaurants serve calorie-dense and highly palatable meals more quickly than we can make in our homes. Often, restaurant meals contain foods that we don't have the skills or ingredients to make at home. Restaurant ambiance is designed to put us at ease and to help us leave our stressors at home. For many, restaurant meals are part of their social structure. The length of restaurant meals is longer than meals at home. This all can lead to overeating and weight gain, especially at fast-food restaurants (McCrory, 1999) (Anderson B. , 2011) (Rosenheck R. , 2008). Finally, based on my observation, overeating at restaurants is especially a problem for members of Muse Satiety Types 3, 4, and 5.

In my opinion, the strength of the effect of increased restaurant eating is a 3 out of 4.

I recommend that governments do the following to reduce unhealthy restaurant eating:

1. Expand the law requiring calorie listing on menus to include all restaurants, no matter how many locations, as I have discussed previously.

2. Mandate nutritional quality labels for all restaurant menu items that grades the nutritional quality and calorie content of that item with a "A" grade for the most nutritionally healthy menu items and a "D" grade going to the least healthy items. An easy-to-read legend should be placed in menus that explains the health risks associated with eating menu items that are labeled with a grade less than "A".

3. Mandate that restaurants track the number of calories ordered by each diner through all courses of a meal and then be required to issue a printed health warning to any diner that attempts to order more calories of food than what is recommended for good health. The diner would still be able to order and be served the additional food, but only after signing a consent form. Serving meals family style at restaurants would be strongly discouraged by this mandate.

Government-funded education would also be beneficial to reduce unhealthy restaurant eating. The public needs to be educated on:

1. Avoiding purchasing meals at restaurants that contain more calories in all the courses of the meal than an individual should consume per meal, based on their sex, age, height, and activity level.

2. Include the calories in all beverages to be consumed at a meal in the total calories consumed for the meal.

3. Avoid eating at restaurants that don't serve a good selection of "A grade" menu items, or items that are nutritionally sound and are lower in calories.

4. Limit restaurant eating to no more than once a week.

Increased food advertising

Given the profit-driven nature of the food industry, it is no surprise that advertising to increase the use of food products comes at consumers through many different media and at an ever-increasing pace. Not only does the food industry want us to use their products and frequent their establishments, but they also want us to become emotionally attached to their brands, to make their brands part of our family and social life. They start on us when we can barely talk and don't stop until we've uttered our last word.

With upwards of $10 billion spent per year on all forms of food advertising in the US, the food industry ranks second only to the auto industry in total advertising dollars spent per year (Frazão, 1999). The ad industry estimates that we are directly or indirectly exposed to some kind of advertising 4,000 to 10,000 times a day, including seeing brand names on products in our environments (Marshall, 2015). Of course, we don't notice the vast majority of these ads. The few that we do notice are the most engaging, creative, and personalized. That is why food companies spend so much on ads that will get noticed. To get their ads noticed, the ads contain superheroes, sports heroes, entertainment superstars, brand-specific mascots, logos, and icons, as well as humor, state-of-the-art graphics, catchy tunes, vibrant colors, and louder audio. TV commercials are still louder sometimes due to sporadic non-compliance with the CALM act of 2012 that specified that TV commercials are not to be louder than the program during which they air. The CALM act does not apply to radio and internet ads (Loud Commercials, n.d.).

Most food ads are for foods that are considered less healthy. Less than 1% of food ads are for vegetables, whole fruits, and healthy protein. Half of all ads during children's shows are for food, and all of those ads are for foods that are considered less healthy (Gantz, 2007).

While there is no question that food advertising increases sales, it is harder to prove that increased food sales leads to greater calorie intake per day and subsequent obesity. A 2016 meta-analysis of 45 studies with 3,292 participants indicated that when presented with food cues, such as pictures of snack foods, there was a moderate increase in craving, eating, and weight gain related to food cues (Boswell, 2015). Another 2016 meta-analysis of 22 studies showed a moderate increase in food consumption after exposure to food advertising in children, but not in adults (Boyland, 2016). The second study did not assess whether the increase in food consumption led to weight gain over time.

Children are at a greater risk than adults in regard to excess calorie consumption resulting from food advertising. Most children who are five or younger can't distinguish between programming and advertising. Many children five to seven-years old don't understand the persuasive intent of advertising. For these reasons, the advertising of food to children of these ages is unfair and exploitative. Children don't easily forget the content of food ads and it affects what they request for food, which then affects their parents' purchases (The impact of food advertising on childhood obesity, 2010). Children are bombarded with advertisements. Children two to seven-years old are viewing about 12 ads of all kind per day; those eight- to 12-years old view 21 ads per day; and those 13- to 17-years old view about 17 ads per day (Gantz, 2007). While I am not able to find studies that directly prove that food advertising causes obesity in children, in my opinion, and in the opinion of many experts, it does. Quebec, Canada, banned food advertising via print and electronic media to children under age 13 in 1980. Chile, France, Ireland, Mexico, Norway, Taiwan, and the United Kingdom all have laws that limit or ban food advertising to children.

In my opinion, members of Muse Satiety Type 1, whether adult or child, won't gain weight from the effect of food advertising, since an increase in consumption of an advertised food will just result in an identical decrease in consumption of other foods. Once again, it pays to be born a Muse Satiety Type 1. The effect of food advertising would be a little larger on members of Muse Satiety Types 2 and 3 and would cause significant weight gain in members of Muse Satiety Types 4 and 5.

In my opinion, the strength of the effect of food advertising on increasing daily calorie intake and causing obesity is a 2 out of 4.

I recommend that governments do the following to reduce the effect of food advertising:

1. Ban all food advertising in print and electronic media where the intended audience is children 12 and under.

2. Place a clearly visible black box warning on all print and electronic media ads for highly processed calorie-dense foods, stating that, "Consumption of this/these food/s has/have been associated with weight gain and its harmful effects."

3. Reclassify all highly processed energy-dense foods to their own food category and tax this category heavily in an effort to decrease sales and to encourage the food industry to produce healthier products that wouldn't be in this category.

4. Subsidize advertisement of healthier foods from NOVA categories one, two, and three to offset excess advertising for foods that are in NOVA category four.

Government-funded education would also be beneficial to reduce the effect of food advertising. The public needs to be educated on:

1. Redirecting children's requests for unhealthier highly advertised foods to healthier choices.

2. Choosing advertisement-free print and electronic media for children to view.

3. Helping children to understand the advertising goals of the food industry, which are almost never in their best interest.

4. Limiting the purchase of highly processed foods as much as possible.

5. Making the difficult choice between highly palatable and highly processed snacks and minimally processed snacks at the grocery store, since once they are in the home, it is hard for most family members to resist highly palatable and highly processed snacks.

SOCIETAL CAUSES OF OBESITY

Societal causes of obesity are society-wide changes in behavior that have resulted in either increased calorie intake or decreased energy expenditure, with increasing obesity across the society as a result. Societal changes in behavior that cause obesity can occur for a number of reasons, such as the influence of one society on another, the influence of a perceived harm of a behavior, the influence of a perceived benefit of a behavior, the influence of changes in technology, the influence of changes in the economy, etc. It is difficult for individuals to choose to behave contrary to societal norms due to a real and perceived societal pressure to conform, as well as a personal desire to conform. Without question, societal beliefs and values can be based on good quality information, poor quality information, or completely wrong information.

The societal causes of obesity that I think are at least in part responsible for the obesity epidemic are listed in Figure 20.

SOCIETAL CAUSES OF OBESITY	Decreased Energy Expended	Increased Mealtime Intake	Increased Snack Intake	Mitigated by Direct Government Intervention	Mitigated by Government-Sponsored Education	Magnitude of the Effect of the Cause of Obesity
Decreased non-exercise activity thermogenesis	X		X		X	2
Kids are kept at home more for safety	X		X	X		1
Reduction in variability of ambient temperature	X					1
Decrease in smoking		X	X		X	1
Low-fat dietary guidelines		X	X		X	1

Figure 20 - Societal Causes of Obesity

Decreased non-exercise activity thermogenesis

Non-exercise activity thermogenesis, or NEAT, is the energy that a person burns on top of their basal metabolic rate that doesn't include planned exercise or the energy spent digesting food. NEAT is all the energy that a person burns from walking here and there, lifting, pushing or pulling this and that, getting out of chairs, gesturing, tapping their feet, etc. In my opinion, NEAT has decreased over the past century due to longer work hours, loss of blue-collar jobs, machine-performed tasks at work and in the home, as well as increasing screen time. Like many processes in the body, with a reduction in NEAT, the body compensates perfectly in members of Muse Satiety Types 1 and 2 and exactly reduces the calories consumed for each day to equal the reduction in NEAT, resulting in no weight gain. This does not occur for members of Muse Satiety Types 3 to 5. As NEAT decreases for them, there is little or no mechanism in place to prevent them from eating the same amount of food they always have at meals and snacks. As a result, the calorie excess for the day increases as NEAT decreases, resulting in weight gain.

It is important to stress that I can't find any studies that prove that NEAT has been decreasing over the last century, or that decreasing NEAT causes weight gain. In my opinion, the strength of the effect of decreasing NEAT on the obesity epidemic is a 2 out of 4.

I can't think of anything that governments can do to reduce the effect of decreasing NEAT in our modern society. However, government-funded education would be beneficial in an effort to increase NEAT. The public needs to be educated on:

1. Staying as active as possible by trying to be the one that takes out the garbage, helps with meals, cleans up after meals, does yard work, does the shopping, and walks to the store instead of driving, as long as it is medically and environmentally safe to do so.

2. Limiting entertainment screen time as much as possible and trying to be active during entertainment screen time. Ideas on being active while viewing entertainment on screens are to stand instead of sit, to do isometric exercises, and to use exercise equipment. Also, make an effort to choose entertainment screen time that burns more calories,

such as virtual reality games, games that interact with the real world (like the popular character-finding games), and games that directly involve activity (like exercise or dancing). As I mention these activities, please be sure to perform each one of them safely. Also, see a medical provider before starting exercise if you have any concern about being able to exercise safely.

3. Using standing and walking desks, balance ball chairs, posture improvement stools, under-the-desk bikes, and under-the-desk elliptical trainers at work.

4. Trying to be the one that volunteers for activities at work that involve standing or walking as much as possible.

Kids are kept at home more for safety

A number of articles have been published which indicate that children who live in neighborhoods that parents deem unsafe gain more weight when compared to children in neighborhoods deemed safe by parents. The cause for the extra weight gain has been shown to result from a reduction in playtime outside in the unsafe neighborhoods. A meta-analysis of 22 studies on this topic was published in 2017. The meta-analysis indicated that children living in unsafe neighborhoods had a reduction of activity of eight minutes per day as compared to children living in safe neighborhoods, which did result in a small increase in weight. As with all meta-analyses, the authors called for more studies to further advance research in this area (An, 2017).

In my opinion, children and adults in Muse Satiety Types 4 and 5 are at the greatest risk for weight gain in unsafe neighborhoods. I recommend that the studies above be done again with equal numbers of study subjects from each Muse Satiety Type in each group. In my opinion, the strength of the effect of children and adults staying home more in unsafe neighborhoods and being less active on the obesity epidemic is a 1 out of 4, with the lower effect being due to most Americans not living in unsafe neighborhoods.

Governments can help with reducing crime rates, improving lighting, and improving sidewalks, which can help increase adults' perception that their neighborhoods are safe.

Reduction in variability of ambient temperature

Human bodies function optimally within a temperature range of 97.7 and 99.5, although body temperature does vary by as much as one and a half degrees from person to person and from midday to the middle of the night. When our body is in an environment that is cooler or warmer than the body's optimal temperature, then the body has to burn calories to either cool off by sweating and radiating heat from our skin or to heat up by turning on mitochondria in fat cells that convert fat to heat. It has been proposed by some that if humans live in temperature-controlled environments where the temperature of the rooms is always at about 72 degrees, then their bodies burn less energy per day to maintain proper body temperature (Moellering, 2012). If a person doesn't then consume less calories per day to compensate, this could lead to weight gain and obesity.

I am not able to find any current literature that proves whether our temperature-controlled environments are lowering our daily calorie expenditure and resulting in obesity. My opinion is that members of Muse Satiety Types 1 and 2 will have little or no weight gain due to the reduction in variability of ambient temperatures, since they will just compensate for the reduced energy expenditure by feeling full sooner at meals, causing them to exactly match their calorie consumption to their calorie burn. This is not true for members of Muse Satiety Types 3 to 5, and they will continue to eat the same amount of food despite burning less calories per day, resulting in weight gain. In my opinion, the strength of the effect of the reduction of variability of ambient temperature on the obesity epidemic is a 1 out of 4.

I can't think of anything that governments can do to reduce the effect of the reduction in variability of ambient temperatures in our modern society by legislation or by education. Humans are not going to spend a lot of excess time in significantly cold or hot environments when they don't have to.

Decrease in smoking

As a doctor, I have been thrilled to witness a marked drop in the number of people in the US that smoke cigarettes during my career. Smoking rates were even higher before I was born. In 1954, 45% of Americans smoked. The rate had fallen to about 28% when I began my medical practice in 1989. It had dropped to 16% as of 2018 (McCarthy, 2018). Yearly rates of lung cancer, the leading cause of cancer death, have been dropping as the number of smokers drop (Henley, 2014).

As much as I am glad to see smoking in the US decline, stopping smoking is associated with weight gain. The average smoker gains 10 pounds in the year after they stop smoking (Aubin, 2012). Weight is gained after stopping smoking due to a loss of the appetite-suppressing properties of nicotine, which is the stimulant in tobacco. In my opinion, it is mostly members of Muse Satiety Types 3 to 5 that gain weight after stopping smoking.

In my estimation, the strength of the effect of stopping smoking on the obesity epidemic is a 1 out of 4. I can't think of anything that governments can do to reduce the effect of stopping smoking causing weight gain by legislation, although education of the public on the risk of weight gain after stopping smoking would be helpful, along with educating the smoking public on tools that are available to prevent weight gain from stopping smoking.

Low-fat dietary guidelines

Based on poor-quality evidence, mostly expert opinion, and despite skeptics' objections, in 1977 the US government began recommending a low-fat diet for everyone to prevent heart disease. The American Heart Association began recommending a low-fat diet to prevent heart disease a few years later. Almost immediately, the food industry responded by increasing sugar in prepared foods to compensate for the reduction of fat in their products. At first, as I recall, commercially manufactured low-fat foods didn't taste as good as higher-fat foods. As time went on, more and more foods appeared that were pleasant to eat and were still low in fat. America's romance with an almost unlimited intake of sugar was in full swing. At the same time as the widespread adoption of low-fat diets to prevent heart disease, there was also an upswing in the rate of increase in obesity across the country. While it is true that Americans have been gaining weight slowly since about 1900, the rate of increase did worsen starting in the 1980s and hasn't tapered off since (Berge, 2008).

Was turning to a low-fat diet the cause of the increase in the rate of weight gain for Americans? No one knows for sure. Most Americans didn't follow a low-fat diet very well, but they still gained more weight. As a country, we have moved away from low-fat diets in the last 15 years, but the rate of increase in obesity has not lessened. Studies for and against the effect of a low-fat diet on weight gain have been mostly epidemiologic in nature and therefore not reliable. Expert opinion is all over the place and confusing. Amidst the confusion, however, one thing is for sure. We are eating more calories per day in the US than before the 1980s, and we aren't doing enough exercise and non-exercise activity to compensate for it.

In my estimation, the strength of the effect of shifting to a low-fat diet in the 1980s on the obesity epidemic is a 1 out of 4, and I'm not even sure of that. I can't think of anything that governments can do to reduce the effect of the shift to a low-fat diet in the 1980s, which then mostly ended in the 2000s, since it already has happened. Governments can help with education, but caution needs to be taken to ensure that the dietary guidelines being taught are based on good quality evidence.

OBESITY-RELATED CAUSES OF OBESITY

Obesity itself places the person who is already suffering from being overweight at risk for additional weight gain. The three diseases I have listed can create a vicious cycle of additional weight gain worsening a disease that causes more weight gain. This list is not meant to be all inclusive.

The obesity-related causes of obesity that I think are at least in part responsible for the obesity epidemic are listed in Figure 21.

OBESITY-RELATED CAUSES OF OBESITY	Decreased Energy Expended	Increased Mealtime Intake	Increased Snack Intake	Mitigated by Direct Government Intervention	Mitigated by Government-Sponsored Education	Magnitude of the Effect of the Cause of Obesity
Insulin resistance		X	X			3
Decreased activity from obesity-related chronic pain	X					2
Increased sleepiness from obstructive sleep apnea	X		X			1

Figure 21 - Obesity-Related Causes of Obesity

Insulin resistance

Insulin therapy for those with type 1 and type 2 diabetes is well-known to cause weight gain (Hartman, 2017). Any diabetes treatment that raises insulin production from the pancreas also causes weight gain (Cheng V. , 2011). It follows that any disease that raises insulin production from the pancreas will also cause weight gain, and this is the case for the disease of insulin resistance.

After a meal is digested, all of the different carbohydrates that can be digested are broken down into fructose and glucose and are absorbed into the blood stream. Fructose mostly can't be used directly by any cell of the body for energy and therefore is taken up by the liver to be converted first into free fatty acids and then to triglycerides. The uptake of fructose by the liver doesn't require insulin from the pancreas. The triglycerides produced from the fructose are released into the blood stream from the liver and then can be used by the body for energy or stored as fat.

Glucose levels in the blood stream, in contrast to fructose levels, are tightly regulated by insulin released from the pancreas, since high levels of glucose are toxic to the body. Even before glucose levels begin to rise after a meal, insulin from the pancreas begins to rise in anticipation of the need to stimulate the cells of the liver, muscles, and fat to take up and store any excess glucose that is not used by other cells of the body. Muscle cells throughout the body can store up to 2,000 calories of glucose as glycogen to be used later for energy to drive muscle activity or released later in between meals as glucose. The liver can store 400 to 500 hundred calories of glucose as glycogen to be released in between meals as glucose. Additional glucose taken up by the liver is converted to triglycerides and then released back into the blood stream for use in energy production or for storage in fat cells. Fat cells can also take up extra glucose, which is directly converted to fat and is stored.

In the disease of insulin resistance, the liver, muscle, and fat cells don't respond to normal levels of insulin from the pancreas and don't take up the excess glucose from the blood stream. Glucose levels in the blood stream rise abnormally. Sensing this, the pancreas then produces more and more insulin until the liver, muscle, and fat cells finally take up the extra glucose.

The exact cause of insulin resistance is not known and is still being debated by experts, but it is related at least in part to genetics, obesity in general, belly fat, aging, lack of exercise, smoking, and a high carbohydrate diet. For a person at risk for insulin resistance, the heavier they are, the worse the insulin resistance gets. The higher levels of insulin required to properly process glucose from meals results in weight gain. If not offset by weight loss, a lower carbohydrate diet, exercise, and/or stopping smoking, these two processes can cause an upward spiral to marked obesity and type 2 diabetes.

How big of a problem is insulin resistance? It's big, really big. As of 2012, one half of all Americans have either diabetes or insulin resistance, which is also called pre-diabetes (Menke, 2015).

In my estimation, widespread insulin resistance is a significant driver of the obesity epidemic. I have given it a magnitude rating of 3 on a scale of 1 to 4.

I recommend that governments:

1. Stop subsidies for producers of high-fructose corn syrup, cane sugar, and beet sugar.

2. Subsidize fruit growers, but only those that sell whole fruits and that don't sell their fruit to the food industry for juice production, the refining of fruit to be used as added sugar for other products, or for the manufacture of fruit products that contain added sugar and/or no fiber.

3. Impose significantly higher taxes, or new taxes, on table sugar and on sweeteners made from fruit. I personally would like to see a bag of table sugar selling for three to four times what it sells for now. Table sugar needs to be relegated back to being used as a spice to enhance flavor and not as a major source of calorie intake.

4. Impose significantly higher taxes, or new taxes, on products containing high-fructose corn syrup, cane sugar, and beet sugar. I personally would like to see all sweets selling for 10 times what they sell for now.

5. Add grams of digestible glucose and fructose to all food labels, instead of trying and failing to display grams of added sugar to food labels. That will quell any argument about added versus natural sugar. While there might be a difference in fructose consumed from whole fruit versus fructose consumed from refined fruit products and sweeteners (Astley, 2018), the consumer needs to know how much glucose and fructose is in the foods they are buying. Although controversial, I hold to the opinion that glucose intake is not harmful to the human body as long as it is not in excess, and that excess intake of fructose is the major problem in insulin resistance. Since the US government and the World Health Organization recommend no more than 50 grams of sugar per day for adults, then this would be about no more than 25 grams of fructose per day for adults. Since both organizations recommend no more than 25 grams of sugar a day for children under 12, then that would be about no more than 12 grams of fructose per day for children.

Government-funded education would also be beneficial. The public needs to be educated on:

1. Encouraging preparation of foods in the home that are low in sweet sugars, whether the sweet sugars are naturally occurring or added.

2. Educating the public on which commercially prepared foods contain large amounts of sweet sugars.

3. Educating the public on the harms of excess intake of sweet sugars.

Decreased activity from obesity-related chronic pain

Obese individuals are more likely than the general population to have chronic pain, including joint pain, back pain, and fibromyalgia, and the heavier they are, the more likely they are to have chronic pain (Smuck, 2014) (Stone, 2012) (Hitt, 2007). There is some evidence that elevated inflammatory proteins and elevated leptin in obese individuals causes chronic pain (Okifugi, 2015). Chronic pain is a cause of weight gain (Loevinger, 2007) (Ferguson S. , 2013). It is postulated that chronic pain causes obesity indirectly by causing decreased activity, which results in less calories burned per day, increased use of medications for pain control that cause weight gain, and decreased sleep due to interruption by pain. In my opinion, the largest effect of chronic pain on obesity is related to increased inactivity, and this is particularly a problem for individuals from Muse Satiety Types 3 to 5 that don't decrease food intake with dropping levels of activity.

In my opinion, the strength of the effect of decreased activity from obesity-related chronic pain on the obesity epidemic is a 2 out of 4. I can't think of anything that governments can directly do to help with this cause of obesity.

Increased sleepiness from obstructive sleep apnea

Obstructive sleep apnea (OSA) occurs when an individual's airway is closed off during sleep, most commonly by the palate or tongue, resulting in the individual having to partially or completely wake up in order to take a breath. As a person gains weight, their tongue gets larger and the diameter of their airway gets smaller, making it easier for obstruction by the palate or tongue to occur. If OSA occurs and breathing stops five or more times per hour of sleep, it is mild OSA. Moderate OSA is defined as OSA occurring 15 or more times per hour of sleep, and severe OSA is defined as occurring 30 or more times per hour of sleep (The Dangers of Uncontrolled Sleep Apnea, n.d.). Due to increasing interruption of sleep, the more severe the person's OSA, the more they are likely to feel sleepy during the day. The sleepier a person is, the more likely they are to overeat to stay awake, which results in weight gain, leading to a worsening of the OSA. A vicious circle can occur, with increasing weight making OSA and sleepiness worse, and vice versa.

OSA does affect 2%-4% of the general population and about 30% of obese individuals (Panossian, 2012). Since most people don't have OSA, the strength of effect of increased sleepiness from OSA is, in my opinion, a 1 out of 4 for the population as a whole. I can't think of anything that governments can directly do to help with this cause of obesity that hasn't already been discussed above.

MEDICAL-ILLNESS-RELATED CAUSES OF OBESITY

Medical-illness-related causes of obesity are different than the diseases in the previous section, in that the diseases below cause obesity, but the diseases don't typically worsen as the individual gains weight. This list is not meant to be all inclusive.

The medical-illness-related causes of obesity that I think are at least in part responsible for the obesity epidemic are listed in Figure 22.

MEDICAL-ILLNESS-RELATED CAUSES OF OBESITY	Decreased Energy Expended	Increased Mealtime Intake	Increased Snack Intake	Mitigated by Direct Government Intervention	Mitigated by Government-Sponsored Education	Magnitude of the Effect of the Cause of Obesity
Adverse life experiences		X	X			2
Psychological illness	X	X	X			2
Increased use of medications that cause obesity		X	X	X		2
Endocrine disorders	X	X	X			1

Figure 22 - Medical-Illness-Related Causes of Obesity

Adverse life experiences

Adverse life experiences are a part of human existence. Some adverse life experiences are more severe than others and adverse life experiences affect different people differently. We each have either experienced adverse life experiences or know of others who have experienced them. Children have a particularly hard time coping with adverse life experiences. Adverse life experiences include sexual abuse, sexual assault, physical abuse, emotional abuse, neglect, bullying, and witnessing or being part of a terrible accident or crime. There are many potential consequences of these and other adverse life experiences, including psychological illnesses such as PTSD, depression, anxiety, social isolation, chronic pain, substance abuse, cardiovascular disease, eating disorders, and obesity (Signs and Symptoms of Posttraumatic Stress Disorder, n.d.).

Adverse life experiences do cause obesity (Palmisano, 2016). In one study, 42% of female victims of childhood sexual abuse are obese as adults in comparison to 28% of non-abuse females (Noll, 2007). In another study, adult women who had experienced moderate to severe emotional abuse were 2.4 times more likely to be obese than women who had not experienced that level of emotional abuse. In the same study, adult women who had experienced moderate to severe physical abuse were also 2.38 times more likely to be obese than women who had not experienced that level of physical abuse (Hollingsworth, 2012). In a study of 20,013 adult men and women, 32.6% of those with PTSD from an adverse life experience were obese and 24.1% of those without PTSD were obese, with no difference by gender (Pagoto, 2012).

My heart truly does break for the pain and suffering that so many people go through, and especially for the children. Adverse life experiences most often don't cause weight gain in members of Muse Satiety Types 1 and 2. They cause can cause significant obesity in members of Muse Satiety Types 3 to 5. Even then, Muse Satiety Type 5s have the greatest risk for obesity from past adverse life experiences, since they are the only Muse Satiety Type that can binge eat.

In my opinion, the effect of adverse life experiences on the obesity epidemic is a 2 out of 4. I can't think of any new legislation that governments could enact to directly decrease the obesity caused by adverse life experiences. However, governments must continue efforts to reduce the incidence of each of the adverse life experiences listed above by both legislation and by education. An especially important target for reducing adverse life experiences is keeping our children safe.

Psychological illness

Psychological illnesses do cause weight gain. Depression causes weight gain in both women and men (Sutin, 2012). Generalized anxiety disorder causes weight gain in both sexes as well (Staiano, 2016). Weight gain also occurs in men and women with bipolar disorders (Goldstein, 2011). In addition to the weight gain caused by psychological illnesses, many of the medications used to treat these illness cause weight gain, which adds to the problem. Again, and in my opinion, the effect of mental illness and the medications used to treat them on weight gain is more pronounced in members of Muse Satiety Types 3 to 5, with the most profound weight gain occurring in members of Muse Satiety Type 5.

In my estimation, the effect of psychological illness on the obesity epidemic is a 2 out of 4. I can't think of any new legislation that governments could enact to directly decrease obesity caused by psychological illnesses, except to mandate better coverage for treatment of mental illnesses. In my opinion, additional government-sponsored education would not help with this cause of obesity.

Increased use of medications that cause obesity

I devoted Chapter 18 in this book to the discussion of medications that cause weight gain. In my opinion, the effect of increased use of medications that cause obesity on the obesity epidemic is a 1 out of 4.

I recommend that governments:

1. Mandate warning labels on the bottles of medications that cause weight gain, like what is already on labels for medications that cause falls and accidents.

2. Mandate stronger warnings in the package inserts for medications that cause weight gain. The warnings should include the observed weight gain per year for individuals in each Muse Satiety Type.

3. Increase funding for research into medications that don't cause weight gain.

4. Prevent pharmaceutical companies from designing self-serving studies for FDA approval of new drugs that exclude the very people who might gain weight from the medications. New medications should

be studied in each Muse Satiety Type before they are approved by the FDA, with effects on weight gain reported for each Muse Satiety Type.

Besides the above recommendations, as far as I can determine, additional government-sponsored education would not help with this cause of obesity.

Endocrine disorders

There are a number of hormone abnormalities associated with weight gain. Low thyroid, testosterone deficiency, and excess cortisol production from the adrenal gland (Cushing's Syndrome) will be discussed below. Less common hormone abnormalities, such as growth hormone deficiency, insulin-secreting tumors, and brain lesions of the thalamus and hypothalamus are examples of rare hormone abnormalities and diseases that can cause weight gain, but that I will not discuss here due to their negligible effect on the obesity epidemic.

A common question asked by patients in my practice is if low thyroid, or hypothyroidism, is causing their difficulty with being overweight. I do check each new weight-loss patient for hypothyroidism, but it is rare that I find overtly low thyroid levels in my overweight patients. It is a fact that having overtly low thyroid causes weight gain (Sanyal, 2016). However, sub-clinical hypothyroidism, or a thyroid level that is only mildly low and is not associated with any symptoms of low thyroid, appears not to cause weight gain (Garin, 2014). The actual number of people with overtly low thyroid is small at about 0.4% (four out of every 1,000 people) and the number of people who have borderline low thyroid is about 6% (60 out of every 1,000 people) (Garber, 2012). The treatment of overtly low thyroid causes a modest weight loss and treatment of sub-clinical hypothyroidism appears not to cause weight loss (Garin, 2014). Thyroid disease in obesity is even more confusing since obesity causes high TSH, the very hormone that is high in low thyroid. The borderline elevated TSH of obesity does revert to normal with weight loss, whereas the elevated TSH of overtly low thyroid doesn't improve with weight loss. It is important to state that current guidelines do not recommend thyroid hormone therapy solely for weight loss.

Low testosterone can cause weight gain in men (Wang, 2011). Low testosterone in women as a cause for weight gain has not been adequately studied to draw a reliable conclusion. One study did indicate increased abdominal fat in women who had low testosterone (Janssen, 2010). Weight gain in men causes testosterone levels to drop and weight loss in men causes testosterone levels to rise (Fui, 2014). While some weight-loss providers do use testosterone therapy for weight loss, it is important to state that current guidelines do not recommend testosterone therapy for men or women solely for weight loss.

Cushing's Syndrome does cause weight gain (Nieman, 2015). However, Cushing's Syndrome is even less common than overtly low thyroid disease. The number of people in the general population that are affected by Cushing's Syndrome is 40 in every million people. Treatment of Cushing's Syndrome does prevent further weight gain and can cause weight loss (Positive, long-term outcomes in fight against Cushing's syndrome, 2014). There is no medication that lowers cortisol that is approved for the treatment of obesity.

In my opinion, the effect of endocrine deficiencies on the obesity epidemic is a 1 out of 4, mostly because they are not common in the general population. I can't think of any legislation that governments could enact, or any government-sponsored public education, that would decrease obesity caused by endocrine disorders.

ENVIRONMENTAL CAUSES OF OBESITY

The human mind is a fascinating thinking machine that is driven to find answers to observed occurrences in our world. The observation that more people are becoming obese in the world then begs an answer, and yet the answers we have so far are complex and incomplete. Is the answer to the obesity question so multifaceted that the single mind can barely comprehend it, or is there one hidden cause that explains it all? Is there just one process that could be altered to change all members of Muse Satiety Types 2 to 5 into Muse Satiety Type 1s? With that in mind, let's now turn to some of these emerging, but as of yet unproven, causes of obesity.

The environmental causes of obesity that might in part be responsible for the obesity epidemic are listed in Figure 23.

ENVIRONMENTAL CAUSES OF OBESITY	Decreased Energy Expended	Increased Mealtime Intake	Increased Snack Intake	Mitigated by Direct Government Intervention	Mitigated by Government-Sponsored Education	Magnitude of the Effect of the Cause of Obesity
Changes in gut microbiota		X	X			?
Past infection with certain viruses		X	X			?
Intrauterine environment		X	X			?
Environmental obesogens		X	X	X		?

Figure 23 - Environmental Causes of Obesity

Changes in gut microbiota

The human body contains about as many bacterial cells externally and internally as there are cells in the body. The colon contains 99% of these bacterial cells, with the remaining bacterial cells being found in much smaller quantities in the rest of the gastrointestinal tract, the skin, and the genitourinary tract (Sender, 2016). With so many bacterial cells residing in and on our bodies, it has been proposed that changes in the number of different species of bacteria in our gastrointestinal tract could change the amounts of the chemical byproducts, or toxins, produced by these bacterial cells to the point where they would alter normal human body processes and promote disease. The term *gut microbiota* is defined as all the bacteria that inhabit the human intestinal tract.

It has been observed in the past that obese individuals have a greater number of the bacteria *firmicutes* and smaller numbers of the bacteria *bacteroidetes* in their small intestines (Ley, 2006). It has been postulated that the higher number of *firmicutes* bacteria would break down undigestible polysaccharides in the small intestine, rendering them digestible and allowing for greater absorption of calories from food. This theory was bolstered by the observation that bacteria-free mice don't develop obesity when fed a high-fat, high-sugar diet until they are transplanted with *firmicutes*-rich, small-intestinal bacteria from obese mice (Rabot, 2016). However, other similar studies in mice have failed to show the same results. Also, results of human studies in this area have not been consistent (Castaner, 2018).

In summary, there is not enough evidence to prove that changes in gut microbiota is a cause for obesity.

Past infection with certain viruses

Some scientists have proposed that past infection with as many as 10 different viruses might lead to obesity in animals and humans. Only two have been shown to cause obesity in humans: SMAM-1 and adenovirus 36.

SMAM-1 is an avian adenovirus from chickens and is named in part after the Asian Indian veterinary pathologist that first described it (Tara, 2016). A researcher tested 52 obese humans in Bombay, India, and found that about 20% of the individuals were positive for past exposure to SMAM-1. Those who were positive for past exposure to the SMAM-1 virus were about 33 pounds heavier than the other non-infected subjects (Dhurandhar, 2012). SMAM-1 has not been studied in humans in the US and without additional studies, it is not certain that past SMAM-1 infection causes obesity in humans.

The most studied virus associated with obesity in humans is adenovirus 36 (Adv36). Adv36 is a human virus that can also infect animals. In a study of 502 obese and non-obese human subjects in 2005, 30% of the obese subjects and 11% of the non-obese subjects were positive for Adv36 (Atkinson, 2005). Since then, additional studies have demonstrated weight gain in humans infected in the past with Adv36, but others have failed to demonstrate the same (Shirani, 2017). There is not yet adequate evidence that Adv36 causes obesity in humans.

It is not ethical to infect humans with SMAM-1 and Adv36 in randomized double-blind studies, so most of the research on SMAM-1's and Adv36's contribution to obesity will need to be performed in animals. We'll have to make an educated guess from the results of these animal studies on how much these viruses contribute to the human obesity epidemic. There is not a vaccine to prevent infection with SMAM-1 or Adv36. In addition, there is not a medication to treat these viruses if a person has been found to have been infected by them in the past.

Intrauterine environment

It has been shown in a number of studies that the intrauterine environment that a fetus inhabits for nine months of growth can affect the fetus's risk for obesity later in life. Studies have shown that women who gain excessive weight during pregnancy, or develop gestational diabetes during pregnancy, have offspring that are heavier at birth and also are heavier later in life compared to infants born to mothers that don't struggle with these problems during pregnancy (Dijk, 2015). It has also been shown that women who smoke during pregnancy have smaller babies at birth, but then the babies are more likely become obese as adults (Reynolds, 2019). The theory is that the expression of genes related to obesity was altered by the adverse intrauterine environment in a process called epigenetics. The structure of the fetus's DNA is not altered in the process, but the expression of genes is altered, so genes that have been silent in the fetus's ancestors become active in the fetus, and vice versa. In the process of epigenetics, a carbon and three hydrogens, called a methyl group, are added to the promoter genes for a section of the fetus's DNA which has been inactive in the fetus's ancestors. Methylation of the promotor gene then turns on expression of that gene for a period of time, potentially for the rest of that fetus's life. The activated gene can even be passed on to future offspring in the activated state.

The intriguing theory of epigenetic changes causing obesity in humans is far from proven. I will list just a few of the difficulties encountered in proving this theory. Many individuals who are thin have the epigenetic changes that are suspected to cause obesity and many who are obese don't have those epigenetic changes. Weight-gain studies that start with the testing of newborns are difficult to perform, since it takes 20 to 30 years for obesity to develop in more than half of the infants. Obesity itself causes epigenetic changes, and therefore it is difficult to determine if the observed epigenetic changes occurred during the prenatal period or afterward.

Environmental obesogens

Without question, our bodies are being bombarded with synthetic chemicals day in and day out for our whole lives. Almost all of these chemicals have at least a few proven side effects in animals if the dose is high enough. Some are suspected to have side effects in humans. A discussion on the effects of all of the synthetic environmental chemicals that pass through the human body is beyond the scope of this book. However, some of these chemicals are suspected to cause obesity in humans and will be briefly presented below.

One of the most studied potential environmental obesogens is tributyltin, which is widely used in industry and agriculture. While mice studies have shown that tributyltin increases obesity, studies in humans are poor quality and few in number. It is not known for certain if tributyltin causes obesity in humans (Heindel, 2018). Other environmental obesogens that are suspected to promote weight gain are the fungicides triflumizole and tolylfluanid; the plastic-softening agents bisphenol A and diethylhexyl phthalate; the preservatives based on p-hydroxybenzoic acid (parabens); the flame retardants based on polybrominated diphenyl ether;, the surfactant 4-nonylphenol; and the phytoestrogens from soy, legumes, lentils, and chickpeas. About 50 total chemical potential obesogens have been identified but have not been studied adequately to determine if they cause obesity in humans (Heindel, 2018) (Darbre, 2017).

In summary, the proposed environmental causes of obesity are inadequately studied to allow me to determine if they are adding to the multi-factorial disease of obesity. If they are adding to the obesity epidemic, then there is insufficient information available for me to determine the potency of their effect or to determine whether government intervention would be of help.

After discussing the above 33 causes of obesity, have I answered the question of what is causing the obesity epidemic in the US and in the world? The answer is yes, I partially have. There are many causes, both genetic and environmental, each with different levels of culpability. Still, there are still so many unknowns. Reliable dietary studies on real-world humans are exceedingly difficult to perform. We many never completely understand the true cause of the obesity epidemic.

CHAPTER 22
NEXT STEPS

I WROTE THIS book to be a call to action for overweight people, medical providers, governments, and people who don't have a weight problem. We all must act now to stop the rapid increase in obesity in our families, communities, states, and countries. It is injuring people, weakening societies, and threatening our nations. It will not just go away by ignoring it.

For those who are overweight, we must face up to one of the hardest challenges we will face in our lifetimes, and that is the challenge of losing weight and keeping it off. I have educated you on the disease that you suffer from, so that knowledge will give you the power to do something about being overweight. Since being overweight is a disease and not a lack of character or self-control, you can hold your head up, banish negative self-talk, and get to work. The many ways to lose weight have been laid out for you. Chose the one that will achieve your weight-loss goals and don't settle for a highly advertised program that will only get you part way there. Read and reread Chapter 11 on weight maintenance. Weight maintenance won't be successful for most dieters if they don't either exercise 500 minutes per week, take a medication, or do both. Ideally, I would like to see each of you consult with a board-certified obesity specialist for help with weight loss and weight maintenance. Lacking that opportunity, use what you have learned in this book to educate your medical provider on what they can do to help you achieve your goals.

Medical providers, it's time to make obesity medicine a part of your practice. Your patients need you to do it. Just telling patients to lose weight has hardly worked for the decades that we've been doing it. Educate yourself on what I have discussed in this book and then seek further education through the OMA. Take one of their training courses. Consider becoming a member of the OMA and even possibly become board certified in obesity medicine through the American Board of Obesity Medicine. Don't just start giving out medication and then seeing your patients in three or six months. It takes encouragement and hand holding to help overweight people lose weight. All the studies I have presented on medication for weight loss have all stipulated that their study subjects return every month for the duration of the studies. Trust me, you can't hope to get the same results by not seeing your patients monthly for visits that are primarily dedicated to weight loss.

For those who can help to make government policies and regulation, there is an uphill battle ahead. It will be exceedingly difficult to change decades of inertia with respect to the lack of policy and regulation that could slow and maybe stop the obesity epidemic. Individual people and companies that make up the food industry can't make the difficult changes that need to be made. Our state and federal governments need to make these changes that I have called for. I'm aware that I've proposed some stiff changes in this book, but a lot is at stake here. The staggering cost of treating obesity-related diseases, the staggering cost of obesity-related disability, the loss of productivity, and the inability in the near future to admit almost half of the young adults in the US into the military because of obesity are serious problems which will weaken our nation.

Obesity prevention must be started early for children who are members of Muse Satiety Types 4 and 5, before they start to gain weight. Part of that prevention will need to include aggressive changes in our national food environment and extensive and ongoing education for parents. It's much easier to keep a person from becoming overweight than it is to have them lose weight after they become obese.

For those of you who are members of Muse Satiety Type 1, I implore you to be a part of the solution. I'm asking you to give up freedoms with food that you enjoy. However, with worsening obesity throughout the world, please step forward and support limiting portions sizes of meals, calorie-containing drinks, fast-foods, and snacks in your homes and communities. Treat the overweight people with just as much respect and dignity as you would any other thin person. Teach the members of your family and community to do the same.

For those researchers that have spent countless hours and so much precious money on trying to answer the many questions that we all have about obesity, I'm asking you to reconsider the studies on obesity you have done in the past and to consider repeating those studies while controlling for the presence or absence of each of the Muse Satiety Types in your study populations. I strongly recommend that research on new medications not be restricted to the thinner members of our population and that all new medications should only be approved after being studied in each Muse Satiety Type.

I would be thrilled to see the disease of obesity eradicated in all age groups in the next 50 years. Our children need us to eradicate the disease of obesity in their age group now. The ability to do so exists. We just need to roll up our sleeves and get the job done.

APPENDIX 1

ESTIMATING IDEAL WEIGHT BASED ON BODY FRAME

THIS METHOD IS ONLY VALID FOR ADULTS WITH HEIGHTS FROM 5'0" TO 6'2", THAT ARE NOT TRIPLE-LARGE FRAME AND THAT DON'T HAVE MODERATE TO SEVERE DEFORMITY OF THE WRISTS OR FINGERS.

1. Obtain the patient's sex and height in inches.

2. Estimate the patient's frame size by having them encircle either wrist with their opposite thumb and middle finger at the narrowest part of their wrist. Find the frame size from the chart below:

THE TIP OF THE THUMB:	FRAME SIZE
Is three nail beds away from the tip of the middle finger	Large x 3
Is two nail beds away from the tip of the middle finger	Large x 2
Is one nail bed away from the tip of the middle finger	Large x 1
Is touching the tip of the middle finger	Medium
Overlaps the middle finger to the base of the nail bed	Small x 1
Overlaps the middle finger to the first knuckle	Small x 2
Overlaps the middle finger to a point halfway to the second knuckle	Small x 3

Figure 24 - Calculating Frame Size

3. Starting with 100 pounds, then add five pounds for every inch of height over five feet.

4. Add an additional 10 pounds for male patients.

5. Then add or subtract the amount below based on frame size:

FRAME SIZE	ADD OR SUBTRACT
Large x 3	Add 30 pounds
Large x 2	Add 20 pounds
Large x 1	Add 10 pounds
Medium	Don't add anything
Small x 1	Subtract 10 pounds
Small x 2	Subtract 20 pounds
Small x 3	Subtract 30 pounds

Figure 25 - How Much to Add or Subtract for Different Frame Sizes

6. The result is the low end of the patient's ideal weight range and correlates with approximately 10%-12% body fat for a male and approximately 18%-20% body fat for a female.

7. Multiply the low-end weight from number 6 above by 1.15. This result is the high end of the patient's ideal weight range and correlates with approximately 16%-18% body fat for a male and approximately 24%-26% body fat for a female.

8. Using the low-end weight from number 6 above, multiply by 1.3. This number is the weight at which the patient is obese and correlates with approximately 22%-24% body fat for a male and approximately 30%-32% body fat for a female.

BIBLIOGRAPHY

(n.d.). Retrieved from Mintel: http://reports.mintel.com/sinatra/oxygen/list/
id=590610&type=RCItem#0_1___page_RCItem=0

(n.d.). Retrieved from Euromonitor International: http://www.euromonitor.com/
sports-and-energy-drinks-in-the-us/report

2019 Restaurant Industry Factbook. (2019). Retrieved from National Restaurant
Association: https://www.restaurant.org/Downloads/PDFs/Research/SOI/
restaurant_industry_fact_sheet_2019.pdf

AACE. (2016). *Bariatric Surgery.* Retrieved from American Association of
Clinical Endocrinologists: https://www.aace.com/disease-state-resources/
nutrition-and-obesity/slide-library/34-bariatric-surgery

Adams, T. (2007). Long-term mortality after gastric bypass surgery. *New England
Journal of Medicine,* 753-761.

Adipex-P, F. P. (1959). *Phentermine Full Prescribing Information.* Retrieved from
Phentermine Full Prescribing Information: http://www.accessdata.fda.gov/
drugsatfda_docs/label/2012/085128s065lbl.pdf

Adolphus, K. (2013). The effects of breakfast on behavior and academic
performance in children and adolescents. *Frontiers in Human Neuroscience,*
425.

Ainsworth, B. (2011). 2011 Compendium of Physical Activities: a second
update of codes and MET values. *Medicine & Science in Sports & Exercise,*
1575-1581.

Al-Assal, K. (2018). Gut microbiota and obesity. *Clinical Nutrition Experimental,*
60-64.

AMA Resolution On Obesity. (2013, May 16). Retrieved from NPR: https://www.
npr.org/documents/2013/jun/ama-resolution-obesity.pdf

An, R. (2017). Influence of Neighborhood Safety on Childhood Obesity: A Systematic Review and Meta-analysis of Longitudinal Studies. *Obesity Reviews*, 1289-1309.

Anderson, B. (2011). Fast-food consumption and obesity among Michigan adults. *Preventing Chronic Disease*.

Anderson, J. (2001). Long-term weight-loss maintenance: a meta-analysis of US studies. *The American Journal of Clinical Nutrition* , 579–584.

Anderson, J. (2002). Bupropion SR Enhances Weight Loss: A 48-Week Double-Blind, Placebo- Controlled Trial. *Obesity Research*, 633-641.

Anderson, J. (2006). Weight loss and long-term follow-up of severely obese individuals treated with an intense behavioral program. *International Journal of Obesity*, 488-493.

Anderson, J. W. (1999). Long-term weight maintenance after an intensive weight-loss program. *Jounal of the American College of Nutrition*, 620-627.

Anderson, S. (2016). Lixisenatide in type 2 diabetes: latest evidence and clinical usefulness. *Therapeutic Advances in Chronic Disease*, 4-17.

Andriani, H. (2015). Parental weight changes as key predictors of child weight changes. *BMC Public Health*.

Apolzan, J. (2019). Long-Term Weight Loss With Metformin or Lifestyle Intervention in the Diabetes Prevention Program Outcomes Study. *682-690*, 682-690.

Apovian, C. (2010). Effects of Exenatide Combined with Lifestyle Modification in Patients with Type 2 Diabetes. *The American Journal of Medicine*.

Apovian, C. (2013). A Randomized, Phase 3 Trial of Naltrexone SR/Bupropion SR on Weight and Obesity-related Risk Factors (COR-II). *Obesity*, 935-943.

Arch, J. (2005). Central regulation of energy balance: inputs, outputs and leptin resistance. *Proceedings of the Nutrition Society*, 39-46.

Astley, C. (2018). Genetic evidence that carbohydrate-stimulated insulin secretion leads to obesity. *Clinical Chemistry*, 192-200.

Astrup, A. (2004). Topiramate: long-term maintenance of weight loss induced by a low-calorie diet in obese subjects. *Obes Res.*, 1658-69.

Atkinson, R. (1989). Low and very low calorie diets. *Med Clin North Am*, 203-215.

Atkinson, R. (2005). Human adenovirus-36 is associated with increased body weight and paradoxical reduction of serum lipids. *International Journal of Obesity*, 281-286.

Aubin, H. (2012). Weight gain in smokers after quitting cigarettes: meta-analysis. *The BMJ*.

Austin, J. (2009). Hormonal Regulators of Appetite. *International Journal of Pediatric Endocrinology*.

Average cost of gastric bypass surgery. (n.d.). Retrieved from Obesity Coverage: https://www.obesitycoverage.com/insurance-and-costs/how-much/average-laparoscopic-gastric-bypass-prices

Avigan, M. (2016). Scientific and Regulatory Perspectives in Herbal and Dietary Supplement Associated Hepatotoxicity in the United States. *International Journal of Molecular Sciences*.

Azad, M. (2017). Nonnutritive sweeteners and cardiometabolic health: a systematic review and meta-analysis of randomized controlled trials and prospective cohort studies. *Canadian Medical Association Journal*, 929-939.

Baker, R. (1993). Self-monitoring may be necessary for successful weight control. *Behavior Therapy*, 377-394.

Baloch, H. (2018). Combination of Phentermine/Topiramate ER and Liraglutide 3 mg for Intensive Therapy of Severe Obesity & T2DM: A Case Series and Brief Review. *AACE Clinical Case Reports*, e482-e486.

Barzin, M. (2016). Safety and effectiveness of sleeve gastrectomy versus gastric bypass: one-year results of Tehran Obesity Treatment Study (TOTS). *Gastroenterology and Hepatology from Bed to Bench*, S62-S69.

Basu, S. (2013, February 27). *The Relationship of Sugar to Population-Level Diabetes Prevalence: An Econometric Analysis of Repeated Cross-Sectional Data.* Retrieved from U.S. National Library of Medicine, National Institutes of Health: http://www.ncbi.nlm.nih.gov/pmc/articles/PMC3584048/

Bays, H. (2014). Canagliflozin: Effects in overweight and obese subjects without diabetes mellitus. *Obesity*, 1042-1049.

Bedford, E. (2020, January 23). *U.S. per capita consumption of soft drinks 2010-2018*. Retrieved from Statista: https://www.statista.com/statistics/306836/us-per-capita-consumption-of-soft-drinks/

Benefits of Bariatric Surgery. (n.d.). Retrieved from MidMichigan Health: https://www.midmichigan.org/conditions-treatments/bariatric/benefits-risks/

Benton, D. (2015). Portion Size: What We Know and What We Need to Know. *Critical Reviews in Food Science and Nutrition*, 988-1004.

Berg, E. (2008). *The Day I Ate Whatever I Wanted: And Other Small Acts of Liberation*. New York: Random House. Retrieved from Goodreads: https://www.goodreads.com/quotes/489648-nothing-tastes-as-good-as-being-thin-feels

Berge, A. (2008). How the Ideology of Low Fat Conquered America. *Journal of the History of Medicine and Allied Sciences*, 139-177.

Block, J. (2009). Psychosocial Stress and Change in Weight Among US Adults. *American Journal of Epidemiology*, 181–192.

Bond, D. (2009). Weight loss maintenance in successful weight losers: surgical versus non-surgical methods. *International Journal of Obesity*, 173-180.

Borga, M. (2018). Advanced body composition assessment: from body mass index to body composition profiling. *Journal of Investigative Medicine*.

Boschmann, M. (2003). Water-Induced Thermogenesis. *The Journal of Clinical Endocrinology & Metabolism, 88*(12), 6015-6019.

Boswell, R. (2015). Food cue reactivity and craving predict eating and weight gain: a meta-analytic review. *Obesity Reviews*, 159-177.

Boyland, E. (2016). Advertising as a cue to consume: a systematic review and meta-analysis of the effects of acute exposure to unhealthy food and nonalcoholic beverage advertising on intake in children and adults. *The American Journal of Clinical Nutrition*, 519-533.

Brinkworth, G. (2009). Long-term effects of a very-low-carbohydrate weight loss diet compared with an isocaloric low-fat diet after 12 mo. *American Journal of Clinical Nutrition*, 23-32.

Britannica, E. (n.d.). *Nicolas Appert*. Retrieved from Encyclopaedia Britannica: https://www.britannica.com/biography/Nicolas-Appert

Broomfield, P. (1988). Effects of ursodeoxycholic acid and aspirin on the formation of lithogenic bile and gallstones during loss of weight. *New England Journal of Medicine*, 1567-72.

Byrne, N. (2018). Intermittent energy restriction improves weight loss efficiency in obese men: the MATADOR study. *International Journal of Obesity*, 129-138.

Canning, H. (1966). Obesity — Its Possible Effect on College Acceptance. *The New England Journal of Medicine*, 1172-1174.

Carral, F. (2018). Beneficials Effects of Canagliflozin in a Weight-Centered Management in Patients with Type 2 Diabetes Mellitus in Real Practice. *Endocrinology & Metabolic Syndrome*.

Castaner, O. (2018). The Gut Microbiome Profile in Obesity: A Systematic Review. *International Journal of Endocrinology*.

CDC. (2014). *Short Sleep Duration Among US Adults*. Retrieved from Centers for Disease Control and Prevention: https://www.cdc.gov/sleep/data_statistics.html

Cheng, J. (2000). *Volume Of A Human Stomach*. Retrieved from The Physics Factbook: https://hypertextbook.com/facts/2000/JonathanCheng.shtml

Cheng, V. (2011). Weight Considerations in Pharmacotherapy for Type 2 Diabetes. *Journal of Obesity*.

Chopra, D. (2007). *Perfect Health—Revised and Updated: The Complete Mind Body Guide*. Potter/Ten Speed/Harmony/Rodale.

Clifton, P. (2017). Assessing the evidence for weight loss strategies in people with and without type 2 diabetes. *World Journal of Diabetes*, 440-454.

Cohen, A. (2013). Education and obesity at age 40 among American adults. *Social Science & Medicine*, 34-41.

Contrave Package Insert. (2014, September). Retrieved from FDA: https://www.accessdata.fda.gov/drugsatfda_docs/label/2014/200063s000lbl.pdf

Cooper, C. (2018). Sleep deprivation and obesity in adults: a brief narrative review. *BMJ Open Sport & Exercise Medicine*.

Counting Calories: Get Back to Weight-Loss Basics. (2018, March 18). Retrieved from Mayo Clinic: https://www.mayoclinic.org/healthy-lifestyle/weight-loss/in-depth/calories/art-20048065

Cummings, D. (2002). Plasma ghrelin levels after diet-induced weight loss or gastric bypass surgery. *The New England Journal of Medicine*, 1623-30.

Daniels, M. (2010). The impact of water intake on energy intake and weight status: a systematic review. *Nutrition Reviews*, 505–521.

Darbre, P. (2017). Endocrine Disruptors and Obesity. *Current Obesity Reports*.

Das, S. K. (2003). Long-term changes in energy expenditure and body composition after massive weight loss induced by gastric bypass surgery. *The American Journal of Clinical Nutrition*, 22-30.

Das, S. K. (2007). Long-term effects of 2 energy-restricted diets differing in glycemic load on dietary adherence, body composition, and metabolism in CALERIE: a 1-y randomized controlled trial. *The American Journal of Clinical Nutrition*, 1023-1030.

Degen, L. (2005). Effect of Peptide YY3–36 on Food Intake in Humans. *Gastroenterology*, 1430-1436.

Deitz, W. (1998). Health Consequences of Obesity in Youth: Childhood Predictors of Adult Disease. *Pediatrics*, 518-525.

Dhurandhar, N. (2012). Association of adenovirus infection with human obesity. *Obesity Research*, 464-469.

Dietary Supplements for Weight Loss. (2019, October 17). Retrieved from NIH: https://ods.od.nih.gov/factsheets/WeightLoss-HealthProfessional/

Dijk, S. J. (2015). Recent developments on the role of epigenetics in obesity and metabolic disease. *Clinical Epigenetics*.

Do Boycotts Work? (2017). Retrieved from Northwestern IPR: https://www.ipr. northwestern.edu/about/news/2017/king-corporate-boycotts.html

DPP. (2012). Long-Term Safety, Tolerability, and Weight Loss Associated With Metformin in the Diabetes Prevention Program Outcomes Study. *Diabetes Care*, 731-737.

Estimate of Bariatric Surgery Numbers, 2011-2018. (2018, June). Retrieved from American Society for Metabolic and Bariatric Surgery: https://asmbs.org/ resources/estimate-of-bariatric-surgery-numbers

Ewbank, P. P. (1995). Physical activity as a predictor of weight maintenance in previously obese subjects. *Obesity Research*, 257-263.

FDA. (2005, April). *Dietary Supplement Labeling Guide: Chapter VI. Claims.* Retrieved from FDA: https://www.fda.gov/food/ dietary-supplements-guidance-documents-regulatory-information/ dietary-supplement-labeling-guide-chapter-vi-claims#6-44

FDA. (2014, April 1). *Code of Federal Regulations 21CFR101.12 - Reference amounts customarily consumed per eating occasion.* Retrieved from U.S. Food and Drug Administration: http://www.accessdata.fda.gov/scripts/cdrh/ cfdocs/cfcfr/cfrsearch.cfm?fr=101.12

FDA approves first oral GLP-1 treatment for type 2 diabetes. (2019, September 20). Retrieved from FDA: https://www.fda.gov/news-events/ press-announcements/fda-approves-first-oral-glp-1-treatment-type-2-diabetes

Ferguson, J. (2001). SSRI Antidepressant Medications: Adverse Effects and Tolerability. *The Primary Care Companion to the Journal of Clinical Psychiatry*, 22-27.

Ferguson, S. (2013). Self-reported Causes of Weight Gain: Among Prebariatric Surgery Patients. *Canadian Journal of Dietetic Practice and Research*, 189-192.

Field, A. (2003). Relation between dieting and weight change among preadolescents and adolescents. *Pediatrics*, 900-906.

Field, A. E. (2009). Weight Cycling and Mortality Among Middle-Aged or Older Women. *Archives of Internal Medicine, 169*, 881.

Flegal, K. (2016). Trends in Obesity Among Adults in the United States, 2005 to 2014. *JAMA*, 2284-2291.

Flint, S. (2016). Obesity Discrimination in the Recruitment Process: "You're Not Hired!". *Frontiers in Psychology*.

Foster, G. (1992). A controlled comparison of three very-low-calorie diets: effects on weight, body composition, and symptoms. *American Journal of Clinical Nutrition*, 811-817.

Fothergill, E. (2016). Persistent Metabolic Adaptation 6 Years After "The Biggest Loser" Competition. *Obesity*, 1612-1619.

Fowler, S. (2016). Low-calorie sweetener use and energy balance: Results from experimental studies in animals, and large-scale prospective studies in humans. *Physiology Behavior*, 517-23.

Fowler-Brown, A. (2010). Adolescent Obesity and Future College Degree Attainment. *Obesity*, 1235-1241.

Fox, M. (2018, May 7). *Restaurant menu label rules go into effect.* Retrieved from NBC News: https://www.nbcnews.com/health/health-news/restaurant-menu-label-rules-go-effect-n872066

Franz, M. (2007). Weight-loss outcomes: a systematic review and meta-analysis of weight-loss clinical trials with a minimum 1-year follow-up. *Journal of the American Dietetic Association*, 1755-1767.

Frazão, E. (1999). *America's Eating Habits: Changes and Consequences.* United States Department of Agriculture.

Fui, M. (2014). Lowered testosterone in male obesity: mechanisms, morbidity and management. *Asian Journal of Andrology*, 223-231.

Fujishiro, K. (2017). Shift work, job strain and changes in the body mass index among women: a prospective study. *Occupational and Environmental Medicine*, 410-416.

Gaesser. (2007). Carbohydrate quantity and quality in relation to body mass index. *Journal of the American Dietetic Association*, 1768-80.

Gallup. (2013, December 19). *In U.S., 40% Get Less Than Recommended Amount of Sleep.* Retrieved from Gallup: https://news.gallup.com/poll/166553/less-recommended-amount-sleep.aspx

Gantz, W. (2007, March). *Food for Thought: Television Food Advertising to Children in the United States.* Retrieved from The Henry J. Kaiser Family Foundation: https://www.kff.org/wp-content/uploads/2013/01/7618.pdf

Garber, J. (2012). Clinical Practice Guidelines for Hypothyroidism In Adults. *Endocrinology Practice.*

Garin, M. (2014). Subclinical Hypothyroidism, Weight Change, and Body Composition in the Elderly: The Cardiovascular Health Study. *The Journal of Clinical Endocrinology and Metabolism*, 1220-1226.

Garvey, W. T. (2012, February). Two-year sustained weight loss and metabolic benefits with controlled-release phentermine/topiramate in obese and overweight adults (SEQUEL): a randomized, placebo-controlled, phase 3 extension study. *Am J Clin Nutr.*, 297-308.

Geliebter, A. (1992). Gastric capacity, gastric emptying, and test-meal intake in normal and bulimic women. *American Journal of Clinical Nutrition*, 656-661.

Gidding, S. S. (2006). Dietary Recommendations for Children and Adolescents: A Guide for Practitioners. *Pediatrics*, Table 3.

Greenway, F. (2018) A Randomized, Double-Blind, Placebo-Controlled Study of Gelesis100: A Novel Nonsystemic oral Hydrogel for Weight Loss. *Obesity*, 205-216.

Glucophage Package Insert. (2018, May). Retrieved from https://packageinserts. bms.com/pi/pi_glucophage.pdf

Goday, A. (2016). Short-term safety, tolerability and efficacy of a very low-calorie-ketogenic diet interventional weight loss program versus hypocaloric diet in patients with type 2 diabetes mellitus. *Nutrition & Diabetes*.

Goldstein, B. (2011). The burden of obesity among adults with bipolar disorder in the United States. *Bipolar Disorders*, 387-395.

Gortmaker, S. (1993). Social and Economic Consequences of Overweight in Adolescence and Young Adulthood. *The New England Journal of Medicine*, 1008-1012.

Greenway, F. (2010). Effect of naltrexone plus bupropion on weight loss in overweight and obese adults (COR-I): a multicentre, randomised, double-blind, placebo-controlled, phase 3 trial. *The Lancet*.

Grynbaum, M. (2014, June 26). *New York's Ban on Big Sodas Is Rejected by Final Court*. Retrieved from NY Times: https://www.nytimes.com/2014/06/27/ nyregion/city-loses-final-appeal-on-limiting-sales-of-large-sodas.html

Guirguis-Blake, J. (2014). Preventing Recurrent Nephrolithiasis in Adults. *American Family Physician*, 461-463.

Guyuron, B. (2009). Factors contributing to the facial aging of identical twins. *Plastic and Reconstructive Surgery*, 1321-31.

Gym Market Research & Industry Stats 2019 . (2019, June 4). Retrieved from Wellness Creative Co.: https://www.wellnesscreatives.com/ gym-market-statistics/

Hajishafiee, M. (2019). Gastrointestinal Sensing of Meal-Related Signals in Humans, and Dysregulations in Eating-Related Disorders. *Nutrients*.

Hall, K. (2016). Energy expenditure and body composition changes after an isocaloric ketogenic diet in overweight and obese men. *The American Journal of Clinical Nutrition*, 324-333.

Hall, K. (2017). Obesity Energetics: Body Weight Regulation and the Effects of Diet Composition. *Gastroenterology*, 1718-1727.

Halls, S. (2019, August 12). *Body Mass Index Versus Body Fat Percentage*. Retrieved from Halls.md: https://halls.md/race-body-fat-percentage/

Hartman, Y. (2017). Insulin-Associated Weight Gain in Type 2 Diabetes Is Associated With Increases in Sedentary Behavior. *Diabetes Care*, e120-e121.

Hartmann-Boyce, J. (2015). Self-Help for Weight Loss in Overweight and Obese Adults: Systematic Review and Meta-Analysis. *American Journal of Public Health*, e43-e57.

HCCIH. (2017, September 24). *Americans Spent $30.2 Billion Out-Of-Pocket On Complementary Health Approaches*. Retrieved from NIH: https://nccih.nih. gov/news/press/cost-spending-06222016

Heindel, J. (2018). Environmental Obesogens: Mechanisms and Controversies. *Annual Review of Pharmacology and Toxicology*, 89-106.

Heldman, D. (2003). In *Encyclopedia of Agricultural, Food, and Biological Engineering* (p. 350). Marcel Dekker, Inc.

Hendricks, E. (2011). Blood Pressure and Heart Rate Effects, Weight Loss and Maintenance During Long-Term Phentermine Pharmacotherapy for Obesity. *Obesity*, 2351-2360.

Henley, S. (2014, January 10). *Lung Cancer Incidence Trends Among Men and Women — United States, 2005–2009*. Retrieved from Centers for Disease Control and Prevention: https://www.cdc.gov/mmwr/preview/mmwrhtml/ mm6301a1.htm

Hill, A. (2007). The psychology of food craving. *Proceedings of the Nutrition Society*, (pp. 277-285).

Hill, J. (1994). *The National Weight Control Registry*. Retrieved from The National Weight Control Registry: http://www.nwcr.ws/default.htm

Hill, J. (2005). The National Weight Control Registry: is it useful in helping deal with our obesity epidemic? *Journal of Nutrition Education and Behavior* , 206-10.

Hirsch, J. (1998). Diet composition and energy balance in humans. *American Journal of Clinical Nutrition*, 551-555.

Hirshkowitz, M. (2015). National Sleep Foundation's sleep time duration recommendations: methodology and results summary. *Sleep Health*, 40-43. Retrieved from National Sleep Foundation: https://www.sleepfoundation. org/excessive-sleepiness/support/how-much-sleep-do-we-really-need

Hitt, H. (2007). Comorbidity of obesity and pain in a general population: results from the Southern Pain Prevalence Study. *Journal of Pain*, 430-436.

Hollingsworth, K. (2012). The Association between Maltreatment in Childhood and Pre-Pregnancy Obesity in Women Attending an Antenatal Clinic in Australia. *Plos One.*

Hollis, J. (2008). Weight Loss During the Intensive Intervention Phase of the Weight-Loss Maintenance Trial. *American Journal of Preventive Medicine,* 118-126.

Holmes, K. (n.d.). *A history of American Snack Foods, From Waffle Cones to Doritos.* Retrieved from www.bonappetit. com: http://www.bonappetit.com/restaurants-travel/ article/a-history-of-american-snack-foods-from-waffle-cones-to-doritos

Holodny, E. (2016, March 10). *The epic collapse of American soda consumption in one chart.* Retrieved from Business Insider: https://www.businessinsider.com/ americans-are-drinking-less-soda-2016-3

Horton, T. (1995). Fat and carbohydrate overfeeding in humans: different effects on energy storage. *American Journal of Clinical Nutrition,* 19-29.

Horvath, T. (2010). Synaptic input organization of the melanocortin system predicts diet-induced hypothalamic reactive gliosis and obesity. *Proceedings of the National Academy of Sciences of the United States of America,* 14875-14880.

Hoyuela, C. (2017). Five-year outcomes of laparoscopic sleeve gastrectomy as a primary procedure for morbid obesity: A prospective study. *World Journal of Gastrointestinal Surgery,* 109-117.

Hu, T. (2012). Effects of Low-Carbohydrate Diets Versus Low-Fat Diets on Metabolic Risk Factors: A Meta-Analysis of Randomized Controlled Clinical Trials. *American Journal of Epidemiology,* S44-S54.

Hurst, Y. (2018). Effects of changes in eating speed on obesity in patients with diabetes: a secondary analysis of longitudinal health check-up data . *BMJ.*

Invokana Package Insert. (2019, 09). Retrieved from Janssen: http://www. janssenlabels.com/package-insert/product-monograph/prescribing- information/INVOKANA-pi.pdf

Jakicic, J. (2008). Effect of exercise on 24-month weight loss maintenance in overweight women. *Archives of Internal Medicine,* 1550-1559.

Janssen, I. (2010). Testosterone and Visceral Fat in Midlife Women: The Study of Women's Health Across the Nation (SWAN) Fat Patterning Study. *Obesity,* 604-610.

Johnson, R. (2007). Potential role of sugar (fructose) in the epidemic of hypertension, obesity and the metabolic syndrome, diabetes, kidney disease, and cardiovascular disease. *The American Journal of Clinical Nutrition*, 899-906.

Kielb, S. (2000). Nephrolithiasis associated with the ketogenic diet. *Journal of Urology*, 464-466.

Kirkova, D. (2013, February 11). *Five Weeks of Willpower*. Retrieved from Daily Mail: https://www.dailymail.co.uk/femail/article-2276930/Five-weeks-willpower-Most-women-diets-weeks-days-43-minutes.html

Klem, L. (1997). A descriptive study of individuals successful at long-term maintenance of substantial weight loss. *The American Journal of Clinical Nutrition*, 239–246.

Kokkinos, A. (2009). Eating Slowly Increases the Postprandial Response of the Anorexigenic Gut Hormones, Peptide YY and Glucagon-Like Peptide-1. *Journal of Clinical Endocrinology & Metabolism*.

Kraschnewski, J. L. (2010). Long-term weight loss maintenance in the United States. *International Journal of Obesity*, 1644–1654.

Kyu, H. (2016). Physical activity and risk of breast cancer, colon cancer, diabetes, ischemic heart disease, and ischemic stroke events: systematic review and dose-response meta-analysis for the Global Burden of Disease Study 2013. *BJM*.

Lampl, M. (1992). Saltation and stasis: a model of human growth. *Science*, 801-803.

Lang, S. (1997, April 1). *Weight relates to dating, marriage and marital satisfaction, Cornell studies find*. Retrieved from Cornell Chronicle: https://news.cornell.edu/stories/1997/04/weight-relates-dating-marriage-and-marital-satisfaction-cornell-studies-find

Lansky, D. (1982). Estimates of food quantity and calories: errors in self-report among obese patients. *American Journal of Clinical Nutrition*, 727-732.

Lavenstein, A. (1962). Effect of cyproheptadine on asthmatic children. Study of appetite, weight gain and linear growth. *Journal of American Medicine*, 912-916.

Layman, D. (2003). A reduced ratio of dietary carbohydrate to protein improves body composition and blood lipid profiles during weight loss in adult women. *Journal of Nutrition*, 411-417.

Lean, M. (2018). Making progress on the global crisis of obesity and weight management. *BJM*, 361:k2538.

Lee, I. (2010). Physical Activity and Weight Gain Prevention. *Journal of the American Medical Association*, 1173-1179.

Lee, I. (2012). Effect of physical inactivity on major non-communicable diseases worldwide: an analysis of burden of disease and life expectancy. *The Lancet*, 219-229.

Lee, J. (2010). *Pounds, The Best Ways to Lose 20*. CBS's Moneywatch.

Lemstra, M. (2016). Weight loss intervention adherence and factors promoting adherence: a meta-analysis. *Patient Preference and Adherence*, 1547-1559.

Leon, A. (1991). Physical activity and 10.5 year mortality in the Multiple Risk Factor Intervention Trial (MRFIT). *International Journal of Epidemiology*, 690-697.

Levitsky, D. (2004). The freshman weight gain: a model for the study of the epidemic of obesity. *International Journal of Obesity*, 1435-1442.

Ley, R. (2006). Human gut microbes associated with obesity. *Nature*, 1022-1023.

Li, J. (2011). Metabolic surgery profoundly influences gut microbial–host metabolic cross-talk. *2011*, 1214-1223.

Lichtman, S. (1992). Discrepancy between self-reported and actual caloric intake and exercise in obese subjects. *New England Journal of Medicine*, 1893-1898.

Liddle, R. (1989). Gallstone Formation During Weight-Reduction Dieting. *Archives of Internal Medicine*, 1750-1753.

Lieverse, R. (1995). Satiety effects of a physiological dose of cholecystokinin in humans. *Gut*, 176-179.

Lifshitz, F. (2008). Obesity in Children. *Journal of Clinical Research in Pediatric Endocrinology*, 53-60.

Lim, J. (2010). The role of fructose in the pathogenesis of NAFLD and the metabolic syndrome. *Nature Reviews Gastroenterology & Hepatology*, 251-264.

Liu, D. (2013). A practical guide to the monitoring and management of the complications of systemic corticosteroid therapy. *Allergy Asthma and Clinical Immunology*, 9-30.

Loevinger, B. (2007). Metabolic syndrome in women with chronic pain. *Metabolism*, 87-93.

men

Loud Commercials. (n.d.). Retrieved from Federal Communications Commission: https://www.fcc.gov/media/policy/loud-commercials

Louis-Sylvestre, J. (1984). Sensory versus dietary factors in cafeteria-induced overweight. *Physiology & Behavior*, 901-905.

Louzada, M. (2015). Consumption of ultra-processed foods and obesity in Brazilian adolescents and adults. *Science Direct*.

Lowery, L. (2004). Dietary Fat and Sports Nutrition: A Primer. *Journal of Sports Science and Medicine*, 106-117.

Ma. (2005). Association between dietary carbohydrates and body weight. *American Journal of Epidemiology*, 359-367.

Maintenance of lost weight and long-term management of obesity. (2018). *Medical Clinics of North America*, 183-197.

Marshall, R. (2015, September 10). *How Many Ads Do You See in One Day?* Retrieved from Red Crow Marketing Inc.: https://www.redcrowmarketing. com/2015/09/10/many-ads-see-one-day/

Martin, C. (2007). Slower eating rate reduces the food intake of men, but not women: implications for behavioral weight control. *Behavior Research and Therapy*, 45(10), 2349-59.

Martin, C. (2010, April). Weight loss and retention in a commercial weight loss program and the effect of corporate partnership. *International Journal of Obesity*, pp. 742-750.

Martínez-González, M. (2019). The Mediterranean Diet and Cardiovascular Health. *Circulation Research*, 779-798.

McCarthy, N. (2018, July 26). *Poll: U.S. Smoking Rate Falls To Historic Low*. Retrieved from Forbes: https:// www.forbes.com/sites/niallmccarthy/2018/07/26/ poll-u-s-smoking-rate-falls-to-historic-low-infographic/#74b03ac13351

McCrory, M. (1999). Overeating in America: association between restaurant food consumption and body fatness in healthy adult men and women ages 19 to 80. *Obesity Research*, 564-571.

McDuffie, J. (2004). Effects of Exogenous Leptin on Satiety and Satiation in Patients with Lipodystrophy and Leptin Insufficiency. *Journal of Clinical Endocrinology & Metabolism*, 4258-4263.

Mechanick, J. (2012). American Association of Clinical Endocrinologists' Position Statement on Obesity and Obesity Medicine. *Endocrine Practice*, 642-648.

Mechanick, J. (3013). Clinical Practice Guidelines for the Perioperative Nutritional, Metabolic, and Nonsurgical Support of the Bariatric Surgery Patient—2013 Update: Cosponsored by American Association of Clinical Endocrinologists, The Obesity Society, and American Society fo. *Surgery for Obesity and Related Diseases*, 159-191.

Mediterranean Diet. (2018, April 18). Retrieved from American Heart Association: https://www.heart.org/en/healthy-living/healthy-eating/ eat-smart/nutrition-basics/mediterranean-diet

Menke, A. (2015). Prevalence of and Trends in Diabetes Among Adults in the United States, 1988-2012. *JAMA*.

Merriam-Webster. (n.d.). Retrieved from Merriam-Webster: https://www.merriam-webster.com/dictionary/dessert

Mikstas, C. (2019, November 21). *WW (Formerly Called Weight Watchers)*. Retrieved from WebMD: https://www.webmd.com/diet/a-z/weight-watchers-diet

Miller, P. (2014). Low-calorie sweeteners and body weight and composition: a meta-analysis of randomized controlled trials and prospective cohort studies. *American Journal of Clinical Nutrition*, 765-777.

Mishori, R. (2011). The dangers of colon cleansing. *Journal of Family Practice*, 454-457.

Mockus, D. (2011). Dietary self-monitoring and its impact on weight loss in overweight children. *International Journal of Pediatric Obesity*, 197-205.

Moellering, D. (2012). Ambient Temperature and Obesity. *Current Obesity Reports*, 26-34.

Monteiro, C. (2016). NOVA. The star shines bright. *World Nutrition*, 28-38.

Moriarty, J. (2012). The effects of incremental costs of smoking and obesity on health care costs among adults: a 7-year longitudinal study. *Journal of Occupational Medicine*, 286-291.

Munro, J. (1968). Comparison of Continuous and Intermittent Anorectic Therapy in Obesity. *British Medical Journal*, 352-254.

Muscogiuri, G. (2019). The management of very low-calorie ketogenic diet in obesity outpatient clinic: a practical guide. *Journal of Translational Medicine*.

Nackers, L. M. (2010). The Association Between Rate of Initial Weight Loss and Long-Term Success in Obesity Treatment: Does Slow and Steady Win the Race? *International Journal of Behavioral Medicine*, 161-167.

Naim, M. (1986). Preference of rats for food flavors and texture in nutritionally controlled semi-purified diets. *Physiology & Behavior*, 15-21.

National Health and Nutrition Examination Survey 2013 to 2016. (n.d.). Retrieved from CDC: https://www.cdc.gov/nchs/nhanes/index.htm

Neumark-Sztainer, D. (2007). Why Does Dieting Predict Weight Gain inAdolescents? Findings from Project EAT-II:A 5-Year Longitudinal Study. *Journal of the American Dietetic Association*, 448-455.

Newmaster, S. (2013). DNA barcoding detects contamination and substitution in North American herbal products. *BMC Medicine*.

Nicklas, T. (2003). Eating patterns and obesity in children: The Bogalusa Heart Study. *American Journal of Preventive Medicine*, 9-16.

Nielsen, S. (2003). Patterns and trends in food portion sizes,. *JAMA*, 450-453.

Nieman, L. (2015). Cushing's Syndrome: Update on signs, symptoms and biochemical screening. *European Journal of Endocrinology*, M33-M38.

Noll, J. (2007). Obesity Risk for Female Victims of Childhood Sexual Abuse: A Prospective Study. *Pediatrics*, e61-e67.

Nursing Your Sweet Tooth. (n.d.). Retrieved from Onlinenursingprograms.com

Nymo, S. (2018). Investigation of the long-term sustainability of changes in appetite after weight loss. *International Journal of Obesity*, 1489-1499.

Ogden, C. (2011). Consumption of sugar drinks in the United Stats, 2005-2008. *NCHS Data Brief*, 1-8.

Ohkawara, K. (2013). Effects of Increased Meal Frequency on Fat Oxidation and Perceived Hunger. *Obestiy*, 336-343.

Ohno, M. (1989). The efficacy and metabolic effects of two different regimens of very low calorie diet. *International Journal of Obesity*, 79-85.

Okifugi, A. (2015). The association between chronic pain and obesity. *Journal of Pain Research*, 399-408.

O'Neil, P. (2018). Efficacy and safety of semaglutide compared with liraglutide and placebo for weight loss in patients with obesity: a randomised, double-blind, placebo and active controlled, dose-ranging, phase 2 trial. *The Lancet*.

Pagoto, S. (2012). Association of post-traumatic stress disorder and obesity in a nationally representative sample. *Obesity*, 200-205.

Painter, S. (2017). What Matters in Weight Loss? An In-Depth Analysis of Self-Monitoring. *Journal of Medical Internet Research*.

Palgi, A. (1985). Multidisciplinary treatment of obesity with a protein-sparing modified fast: results in 668 outpatients. *American Journal of Public Health*, 1190-1194.

Palmisano, G. (2016). Life adverse experiences in relation with obesity and binge eating disorder: A systematic review. *Journal of Behavioral Addictions*, 11-31.

Panossian, L. (2012). Daytime Sleepiness in Obesity: Mechanisms Beyond Obstructive Sleep Apnea—A Review. *Sleep*, 605-615.

Pelchat, M. (1997). Food cravings in young and elderly adults. *Appetite*, 103-113.

Penney, T. (2017). Utilization of Away-From-Home Food Establishments, Dietary Approaches to Stop Hypertension Dietary Pattern. *American Journal of Preventive Medicine*, 155-163.

Pietilainen, K. (2008). Physical Inactivity and Obesity: A Vicious Circle. *Obesity*, 409-414.

Plenity Package Insert (2019), Retrieved from FDA: https://www.gelesis.com/wp-content/uploads/DEN180060_Physician_IFU_FDA_FINAL_4.9.2019Gelesis.pdf

Pomerleau, M. (2004). Effects of exercise intensity on food intake and appetite in women. *The American Journal of Clinical Nutrition*, 1230-1236.

Popkin, B. (2011, June 28). *Energy Density, Portion Size, and Eating Occasions: Conributions to Increased Energy Intake in the United States, 1977 to 2006.* Retrieved from www.plosmedicine.org: http://www.plosmedicine.org/article/Authors/info:doi/10.1371/journal.pmed.1001050

Positive, long-term outcomes in fight against Cushing's syndrome. (2014, June 24). Retrieved from ScienceDaily: https://www.sciencedaily.com/releases/2014/06/140624135805.htm

Poti, J. (2107). Ultra-processed Food Intake and Obesity: What Really Matters for Health – Processing or Nutrient Content? *Current Obesity Reports*, 420-431.

Puhl, R. (2010). Obesity Stigma: Important Considerations for Public Health. *American Journal of Public Health*, 1019-1028.

Purcell, K. (2014). The effect of rate of weight loss on long-term weight management: a randomised controlled trial. *The Lancet*, 954-962.

Qsymia Package Insert. (2012, July). Retrieved from FDA: https://www.accessdata.fda.gov/drugsatfda_docs/label/2012/022580s000lbl.pdf

Qsymia, Full Prescribing Information. (n.d.). Retrieved from https://qsymia.com/pdf/prescribing-information.pdf

Rabot, S. (2016). High fat diet drives obesity regardless the composition of gut microbiota in mice. *Scientific Reports*.

Rader, A. (About 2014). Reference on file with Allen Rader MD FOMA.

Ratliff, J. (2010). Association of prescription H1 antihistamine use with obesity: Results from the National Health and Nutrition Examination Survey. *Obesity*, 2398-2400.

Recalls Background and Definitions. (2014, July 31). Retrieved from U. S. Food and Drug Administration: https://www.fda.gov/safety/industry-guidance-recalls/recalls-background-and-definitions

Reges, O. (2018). Association of Bariatric Surgery Using Laparoscopic Banding, Roux-en-Y Gastric Bypass, or Laparoscopic Sleeve Gastrectomy vs Usual Care Obesity Management With All-Cause Mortality. *JAMA*, 279-290.

Revia Package Insert. (2013, October). Retrieved from FDA: https://www.accessdata.fda.gov/drugsatfda_docs/label/2013/018932s017lbl.pdf

Reynolds, L. (2019). Smoking during pregnancy increases chemerin expression in neonatal tissue. *Experimental Physiology*, 93-99.

Rolls, B. (1991). *Eating slowly may not help you shed pounds.* Retrieved from msnbc.com.

Roque, M. (2006). Gastric Sensorimotor Functions and Hormone Profile in Normal Weight, Overweight, and Obese People. *Gastroeneterology*, 1717-1724.

Rosen, J. C. (1985). Mood and appetite during minimal-carbohydrate and carbohydrate-supplemented hypocaloric diets. *Am J Clin Nutr*, 371-379.

Rosenheck, R. (2008). Fast food consumption and increased caloric intake: a systematic review of a trajectory towards weight gain and obesity risk. *Obesity Reviews*, 535-547.

Rosenstock, J. (2012). Dose-Ranging Effects of Canagliflozin, a Sodium-Glucose Cotransporter 2 Inhibitor, as Add-On to Metformin in Subjects With Type 2 Diabetes. *Diabetes Care*, 1232-1238.

Roux, C. (2017). 3 years of liraglutide versus placebo for type 2 diabetes risk reduction and weight management in individuals with prediabetes: a randomised, double-blind trial. *The Lancet*.

Ruyter, J. d. (2012). A trial of sugar-free or sugar-sweetened beverages and body weight in children. *New England Jounal of Medicine*, 1397-1406.

Ryttig, K. (1997). Long-term effects of a very low calorie diet (Nutrilett) in obesity treatment. A prospective, randomized, comparison between VLCD and a hypocaloric diet+behavior modification and their combination. *International Journal of Obesity Related Metabolic Disorders*, 574-579.

Sacks, F. (2009). Comparison of Weight-Loss Diets with Different compositions of Fat, Protein and Carbohydrates. *New England Journal of Medicine*, 859-873.

Saint-Maurice, P. (2020). Association of Daily Step Count and Step Intensity With Mortality Among US Adults. *JAMA*.

Samuel-Hodge, C. (2009). Randomized Trial of a Behavioral Weight Loss Intervention for Low-income Women: The Weight Wise Program. *Obesity*, 1891-1899.

Sanyal, D. (2016). Hypothyroidism and obesity: An intriguing link. *Indian Journal of Endocrinology and Metabolism*, 554-557.

Saris, W. (2002, September). *Collection of data on products intended for use in very-low-calorie-diets*. Retrieved from http://www.foodedsoc.org/scoop.pdf: http://www.foodedsoc.org/scoop.pdf

Sartorius, K. (2018). Does high-carbohydrate intake lead to increased risk of obesity? A systematic review and meta-analysis. *BMJ Open*.

Savoie, K. (2009, May 18). *http://www.medicalnewstoday.com/articles/150389.php*. Retrieved from www.medicalnewstoday.com.

Saxenda, Full Prescribing Information. (n.d.). Retrieved from http://www.novo-pi.com/saxenda.pdf

Schauer, P. (2003). Open and Laparoscopic Surgical Modalities. *The Society for Surgery of the Alimentary Tract, Inc.*, 468-475.

Schneiderman, E. (2015). *A.G. Schneiderman Asks Major Retailers To Halt Sales Of Certain Herbal Supplements As DNA Tests Fail To Detect Plant Materials Listed On Majority Of Products Tested.* New York State Office of the Attorney General.

Schoeller, D. A. (1997, Sep). How much physical activity is needed to minimize weight gain in previously obese women? *Am J Clin Nutr*, 551-556.

Scirica, B. (2005). Treatment of Elevated Cholesterol. *Circulation*, e360-e363.

Selvin, E. (2014). Trends in Prevalence and Control of Diabetes in the United States, 1988–1994 and 1999–2010. *Annals of Internal Medicine*, 517-525.

Sender, R. (2016). Revised Estimates for the Number of Human and Bacteria Cells in the Body. *PLOS Biology*.

Shah, M. (2014). Effects of GLP-1 on appetite and weight. *Reviews in Endocrine and Metabolic Disorders*, 181-187.

Shai, I. (2008). Weight Loss with a Low-Carbohydrate, Mediterranean, or Low-Fat Diet. *The New England Journal of Medicine*, 229-241.

Shieh, C. (2016). Self-weighing in weight management interventions: A systematic review of literature. *Science Direct*, 493-519.

Shirani, F. (2017). Using rats as a research model to investigate the effect of human adenovirus 36 on weight gain. *ARYA Atherosclerosis*, 167-171.

Sievert, K. (2019). Effect of breakfast on weight and energy intake: systematic review and meta-analysis of randomised controlled trials. *BMJ*, 142.

Signs and Symptoms of Posttraumatic Stress Disorder. (n.d.). Retrieved from Pacific Grove Hospital: https://www.pacificgrovehospital.com/ptsd/symptoms-signs-effects/

Simonds, S. (2019). Determining the Effects of Combined Liraglutide and Phentermine on Metabolic Parameters, Blood Pressure, and Heart Rate in Lean and Obese Male Mice. *Diabetes*, 683-695.

Simpson, K. (2009). Hypothalamic regulation of food intake. *Arquivos Brasileiros de Endocrinologia & Metabologia*, 120-128.

Sjöström, L. (2007). Effects of Bariatric Surgery on Mortality in Swedish Obese Subjects. *The New England Journal of Medicine*, 741-752.

Slattery, M. (1988). Physical fitness and cardiovascular disease mortality. The US Railroad Study. *American Journal of Epidemiology*, 571-580.

Smith, L. (2016). Dulaglutide (Trulicity): The Third Once-Weekly GLP-1 Agonist. *Pharmacy and Therapeutics*, 357-360.

Smuck, M. (2014). Does physical activity influence the relationship between low back pain and obesity? *Spine Journal*, 209-216.

Staiano, A. (2016). Physical Activity, Mental Health, and Weight Gain in a Longitudinal Observational Cohort of Nonobese Young Adults. *Obesity*.

Starr, R. (2015). Too Little, Too Late: Ineffective Regulation of Dietary Supplements in the United States. *American Journal of Public Health*, 478-485.

Statistics About Diabetes. (2018). Retrieved from American Diabetes Association: https://www.diabetes.org/resources/statistics/statistics-about-diabetes

Stavrou, S. (2016). The effectiveness of a stress-management intervention program in the management of overweight and obesity in childhood and adolescence. . *Journal of Molecular Biochemistry*, 63-70.

Steffen, K. (2012). A Review of the Combination of Phentermine and Topiramate Extended-Release for Weight Loss. *Combination Products in Therapy*.

Stevens VL, J. E. (2012). Weight Cycling and Mortality in a Large Prospective US Study. *American journal of epidemiology*, 175 (8), 785-92 PMID: 22287640.

Stockman, M. (2018). Intermittent Fasting: Is the Wait Worth the Weight? *Current Obesity Reports*, 172-185.

Stone, A. (2012). Obesity and pain are associated in the United States. *Obesity*, 1491-1495.

Sturm, R. (2013). A Cash-Back Rebate Program for Healthy Food Purchases in South Africa Results from Scanner Data. *American Journal of Preventitive Medicine*, 567-572.

Sturm, R. (2014). Obesity and economic environments. *CA: A Cancer Journal for Clinicians*, 337-350.

Sugar: The Bitter Truth. (2012). Retrieved from http://kolpinstitute.org/facts-about-sugar/

Sumithran, P. (2011). Long-Term Persistence of Hormonal Adaptations to Weight Loss. *The New England Journal Of Medicine*, 1597-1604.

Sutin, A. (2012). Depressive Symptoms Are Associated with Weight Gain Among Women. *Psychological Medicine*, 2351-2360.

Taheri, S. (2004). Short Sleep Duration Is Associated with Reduced Leptin, Elevated Ghrelin, and Increased Body Mass Index. *PLOS Med*.

Tara, S. (2016, 12 27). *The Mysterious Virus That Could Cause Obesity*. Retrieved from WIRED: https://www.wired.com/2016/12/mysterious-virus-cause-obesity/

Tate, D. (2012). Replacing caloric beverages with water or diet beverages for weight loss in adults: main results of the Choose Healthy Options Consciously Everyday (CHOICE) randomized clinical trial. *American Journal of Clinical Nutrition*, 555-563.

Thalange, N. (1996). Model of normal prepubertal growth. *Archives of Disease in Childhood*, 427-431.

Thaler, J. (2012). Obesity is associated with hypothalamic injury in rodents and humans. *Journal of Clinical Investigation*, 153-162.

The Dangers of Uncontrolled Sleep Apnea. (n.d.). Retrieved from Johns Hopkins Medicine: https://www.hopkinsmedicine.org/health/wellness-and-prevention/the-dangers-of-uncontrolled-sleep-apnea

The impact of food advertising on childhood obesity. (2010, November 17). Retrieved from American Psychological Association: https://www.apa.org/topics/kids-media/food

The Nielsen Total Audience Report: Q1 2018. (2018, July 31). Retrieved from Nielsen: 2018

Thomson, C. (2012). Relationship Between Sleep Quality and Quantity and Weight Loss in Women Participating in a Weight-Loss Intervention Trial. *Obesity*, 1419-1425.

Topamax Package Insert. (2012, October). Retrieved from FDA: https://www.accessdata.fda.gov/drugsatfda_docs/label/2012/020844s041lbl.pdf

Tordoff, M. (2017). Does eating good-tasting food influence body weight? *Physiology & Behavior*, 27-31.

Toubro, S. (1997). Randomised comparison of diets for maintaining obese subjects' weight after major weight loss: ad lib, low fat, high carbohydrate diet v fixed energy intake. *BJM*, 29-34.

Tremblay, A. (1997). Endurance Training With Constant Energy Intake in Identical Twins: Changes Over Time in Energy Expenditure and Related Hormones. *Metabolism*, 499-503.

Trepanowski, J. (2017). Effect of Alternate-Day Fasting on Weight Loss, Weight Maintenance, and Cardioprotection Among Metabolically Healthy Obese Adults: A Randomized Clinical Trial. *JAMA Internal Medicine*, 930-938.

Tronieri, J. S. (2019). Effects of Liraglutide Plus Phentermine in Adults With Obesity Following 1 Year of Treatment by Liraglutide Alone. *Metabolism*.

Tucker, J. (2018). Unapproved Pharmaceutical Ingredients Included in Dietary Supplements Associated With US Food and Drug Administration Warnings. *JAMA*.

Urban, L. (2016). Energy Contents of Frequently Ordered Restaurant Meals and Comparison with Human Energy Requirements and US Department of Agriculture Database Information: A Multisite Randomized Study. *Journal of the Academy of Nutrition and Dietetics*, 590-598.

USDA. (n.d.). *Shifts Needed To Align With Healthy Eating Patterns*. Retrieved from Dietary Guidelines for Americans 2015-2020 Eighth Edition: http://health.gov/dietaryguidelines/2015/guidelines/chapter-2/a-closer-look-at-current-intakes-and-recommended-shifts/#figure-2-13

Vink, R. G. (2016). The effect of rate of weight loss on long-term weight regain in adults with overweight and obesity. *Obesity*, 321-327.

Wang, C. (2011). Low Testosterone Associated With Obesity and the Metabolic Syndrome Contributes to Sexual Dysfunction and Cardiovascular Disease Risk in Men With Type 2 Diabetes. *Diabetes Care*, 1669-1675.

Weintraub, M. (1992). Long-term weight control study. *Clinical Pharmacology and Theraputics*, 581-646.

Weiss, E. C. (2007). Weight regain in U.S. adults who experienced substantial weight loss, 1999-2002. *American Journal of Preventative Medicine*, 34-40.

Wellbutrin SR Package Insert. (2019, November). Retrieved from GSK: https://www.gsksource.com/pharma/content/dam/GlaxoSmithKline/US/en/Prescribing_Information/Wellbutrin_Tablets/pdf/WELLBUTRIN-TABLETS-PI-MG.PDF

Wene, J. (1982). Flavor preferences, food intake, and weight gain in baboons. *Physiology & Behavior*, 569–573.

What is the South Beach Diet. (n.d.). Retrieved from South Beach Diet: https://www.southbeachdiet.com/pdf/sbd/Medical_conditions_letter.pdf

White, W. (2013). Psychotropic-Induced Weight Gain: A Review of Management Strategies. *Consultant 360*, 153-160.

WHO calls on countries to reduce sugars intake among adults and children. (2015, March 4). Retrieved from World Health Organization: http://www.who.int/mediacentre/news/releases/2015/sugar-guideline/en/

Why Electronics May Stimulate You Before Bed. (n.d.). Retrieved from National Sleep Foundation: https://www.sleepfoundation.org/articles/why-electronics-may-stimulate-you-bed

Wien, M. (2003). Long-term maintenance of weight loss: do people who lose weight through various weight loss methods use different behaviors to maintain their weight? *International Journal of Obesity and Related Metabolic Disorders*, 1365-1372.

Wilding, J. (2004). A randomized double-blind placebo-controlled study of the long-term efficacy and safety of topiramate in the treatment of obese subjects. *International Journal of Obesity Related Metabolic Disorders*, 1399-410.

Williams, G. (1996). Motivational Predictors of Weight Loss and Weight-Loss Maintenance . *Journal of Personality and Social Psychology*, 115-126.

Williams, P. (2013). Walking Versus Running for Hypertension, Cholesterol, and Diabetes Mellitus Risk Reduction. *Arteriosclerosis, Thrombosis, and Vascular Biology*, 1085-1091.

Wing, R. (2005). Long-term weight loss maintenance. *American Journal of Clinical Nutrition*, 222-225.

Wing, R. (2006). A self-regulation program for maintenance of weight loss. *New England Journal of Medicine*, 1563-1571.

Wing, R. (2020). *The National Weight Control Registry*. Retrieved 2014, from The National Weight Control Registry: http://www.nwcr.ws/default.htm

Wise, T. (2006). Effects of the Antidepressant Duloxetine on Body Weight: Analyses of 10 Clinical Studies. *The Primary Care Companion to the Journal of Clinical Psychiatry*, 269-278.

Wunsch, N. (2019, September 27). *Soft drink consumption per capita in the European Union (EU) 2010-2017*. Retrieved from Statista: https://www.statista.com/statistics/620186/ soft-drink-consumption-in-the-european-union-per-capita/

Xenaki, N. (2018). Impact of a stress management program on weight loss, mental health and lifestyle in adults with obesity: a randomized controlled trial. *Journal of Molecular Biochemistry*, 78–84.

Xenical Package Insert. (2012, January). Retrieved from FDA: https://www. accessdata.fda.gov/drugsatfda_docs/label/2012/020766s029lbl.pdf

Young, L. (2002). The Contribution of Expanding Portion Sizes to the US Obesity Epidemic. *American Jounal of Public Health*, 246-249.

Yu, Y.-H. (2015). Metabolic vs. hedonic obesity: a conceptual distinction and its clinical implications. *Obesity Reviews*, 234-247.

Zelman, K. M. (2008, August 13). *The Olympic Diet of Michael Phelps*. Retrieved from WebMD: http://www.webmd.com/diet/news/20080813/ the-olympic-diet-of-michael-phelps

Zonegran Package Insert. (2016, April). Retrieved from https://www.accessdata. fda.gov/drugsatfda_docs/label/2016/020789s034lbl.pdf

Zyban Package Insert. (2019, July). Retrieved from GSK: https://www. gsksource.com/pharma/content/dam/GlaxoSmithKline/US/en/Prescribing_ Information/Zyban/pdf/ZYBAN-PI-MG.PDF

TABLE OF FIGURES

ABREVIATIONS AND ACRONYMS

ADA – Americans with Disabilities Act
ADP – Air-Displacement Plethysmography
Adv36 – Adenovirus 36
AHA – American Heart Association
α-MSH – alpha-MSH
AMA – American Medical Association
BIA – Bioelectrical Impedance Analysis
BMI – Body Mass Index
BMR – Basal Metabolic Rate
Carbs – Carbohydrates
CCK – Cholecystokinin
CPAP – Continuous Positive Airway Pressure
CT Scan – Computed Tomography Scan
DSHEA – Dietary Supplement Health and Education Act
DEXA – Dual Energy X-Ray Absorptiometry
ER – Extended Release
FDA – Food and Drug Administration
FOMA – Follow of the Obesity Medicine Association
FTC – Federal Trade Commission
eGFR – Estimated Glomerular Filtration Rate
GI – Gastrointestinal
GLP-1 – Glucagon-Like Peptide 1
HDL – High-Density Lipoprotein
ITT-LOCF – Intent to Treat – Last Observation Carried Forward
LDL – Low-Density Lipoprotein
MRI Scan – Magnetic Resonance Imaging Scan
NEAT – Non-Exercise Activity Thermogenesis

NPY/AgRP neuron – Neural Peptide Y/Agouti-Related Peptide neuron
NWCR – National Weight Control Registry
OMA – Obesity Medicine Association
OSA – Obstructive Sleep Apnea
OXM – Oxyntomodulin
PE – Physical Education
PMS – Pre-Menstrual Syndrome
POMC/CART neuron – Pro-Opiomelanocortin/Cocaine- and Amphetamine-
    Regulated Transcript neuron
PP – Pancreatic polypeptide
PTSD – Post-Traumatic Stress Disorder
PYY – Peptide YY
RDA – Recommend Daily Allowance
RMR – Resting Metabolic Rate
SR – Sustained Release
TSH – Thyroid Stimulating Hormone
US – United States
VLCD – Very Low-Calorie Diet
WHO – World Health Organization
XL – Extended Release
XR – Extended Release

GLOSSARY

Anorexigenic – causing weight loss

Bariatrics – having to do with research on, diagnosis of and treatment of obesity

Completer study results – study results that only include study participants that completed the study

Diet attention span – average length of time a dieter is willing to diet before ending a diet

Fat mass – the weight of the fat of the human body

Ghrelin – hunger hormone released by the stomach and first part of the small intestine

Hangry – excess hunger resulting in increased irritability

ITT-LOCF study results – study results that include results of all study participants, even if they left the study prematurely. If the participants left the study early, the data from the patient's last visit are used as their final study results.

Lean body mass – the weight of the body minus the fat mass

Leptin – satiety hormone produced by fat cells in response to food intake

Lifetime cumulative weight loss – total of all weight lost by any method throughout a patient's life, not including any weight regained and not including any weight lost in the first six months after delivery of a baby

Maximum weight memory – the maladaptive memory by the brain of a new and higher body weight as the weight that the brain will now defend against weight loss

Muse Satiety Type 1 – a person who has the satiety signals of fullness, loss of savor, and nausea with overeating

Muse Satiety Type 2 – a person who has the satiety signals of fullness and nausea with overeating, but not the signal of loss of savor

Muse Satiety Type 3 – a person who has the satiety signal of fullness, but not the signals of loss of savor and nausea with overeating

Muse Satiety Type 4 – a person who has a delayed and weak signal of nausea with overeating, but not the signals of fullness and loss of savor

Muse Satiety Type 5 – a person who does not have the signals of fullness, loss of savor, and nausea with overeating

Muse's Satietopathy – the absence of one or more of the three satiety signals of fullness, loss of savor and nausea with overeating, resulting in progressive weight gain

Orexigenic – causing weight gain

Serial dieting – repeated small 5- to 10-pound diets done during weight maintenance to prevent long-term weight gain

Sympathetic nervous system – the "flight-or-fight" response system of the body that depresses contractility of smooth muscles, decreases appetite, increases heart rate, and prepares the body for activity

Sympathomimetic medications – adrenaline-like medications that are prescribed to assist with compliance on weight-loss diets

Yo-yo dieting – repeated cycles of a dieter losing a large amount of weight and then regaining all the weight they have lost

www.ingramcontent.com/pod-product-compliance
Lightning Source LLC
Chambersburg PA
CBHW052119270326
41930CB00012B/2687